T0226871

Facial Skin: Contemporary Topics for the Surgeon

Editors

DAVID B. HOM
ADAM INGRAFFEA

FACIAL PLASTIC SURGERY CLINICS OF NORTH AMERICA

www.facialplastic.theclinics.com

Consulting Editor
J. REGAN THOMAS

February 2013 • Volume 21 • Number 1

ELSEVIER

1600 John F. Kennedy Boulevard • Suite 1800 • Philadelphia, Pennsylvania, 19103-2899

http://www.theclinics.com

FACIAL PLASTIC SURGERY CLINICS OF NORTH AMERICA Volume 21, Number 1
February 2013 ISSN 1064-7406, ISBN 978-1-4557-7086-1

Editor: Joanne Husovski

Facial Plastic Surgery Clinics of North America (ISSN 1064-7406) is published quarterly by Elsevier Inc., 360 Park Avenue South, New York, NY 10010-1710. Months of issue are February, May, August, and November. Business and Editorial Offices: 1600 John F. Kennedy Blvd., Suite 1800, Philadelphia, PA 19103-2899. Periodicals postage paid at New York, NY, and additional mailing offices. Subscription prices are $373.00 per year (US individuals), $526.00 per year (US institutions), $425.00 per year (Canadian individuals), $628.00 per year (Canadian institutions), $509.00 per year (foreign individuals), $628.00 per year (foreign institutions), $153.00 per year (US students), and $245.00 per year (foreign students). Foreign air speed delivery is included in all *Clinics* subscription prices. All prices are subject to change without notice. POSTMASTER: Send address changes to *Facial Plastic Surgery Clinics*, Elsevier Health Sciences Division, Subscription Customer Service, 3251 Riverport Lane, Maryland Heights, MO 63043. **Customer service: 1-800-654-2452 (US and Canada); 1-314-447-8871 (outside US and Canada); Fax: 314-447-8029; E-mail:journalscustomerservice-usa@elsevier.com (for print support); journalsonline support-usa@elsevier.com (for online support).**

Reprints. For copies of 100 or more of articles in this publication, please contact the Commercial Reprints Department, Elsevier Inc., 360 Park Avenue South, New York, NY 10010-1710. Tel.: 212-633-3812; Fax: 212-462-1935; E-mail: reprints@elsevier.com.

Facial Plastic Surgery Clinics of North America is covered in *MEDLINE/PubMed* (*Index Medicus*).

Printed and bound by CPI Group (UK) Ltd, Croydon, CR0 4YY

Transferred to digital print 2013

Contributors

CONSULTING EDITOR

J. REGAN THOMAS, MD, FACS
Professor and Chairman, Department of Otolaryngology, University of Illinois at Chicago, Chicago, Illinois

EDITORS

DAVID B. HOM, MD, FACS
Professor, Director, Division of Facial Plastic and Reconstructive Surgery, Department of Otolaryngology – Head and Neck Surgery, University of Cincinnati College of Medicine, Cincinnati, Ohio

ADAM INGRAFFEA, MD, FAAD, FACMS
Mohs Surgeon, Clinical Assistant Professor; Assistant Program Director, Department of Dermatology, University of Cincinnati, West Chester, Ohio

AUTHORS

SWATHI BALAJI, PhD
Postdoctoral Research Fellow, Division of Pediatric General, Thoracic and Fetal Surgery, The Center for Molecular Fetal Therapy, Cincinnati Children's Hospital Medical Center, Cincinnati, Ohio

TAPAN K. BHATTACHARYYA, PhD
Research Assistant Professor, Department of Otolaryngology – Head and Neck Surgery, University of Illinois at Chicago, Chicago, Illinois

NITIN CHAUHAN, MD, FRCSC
Division of Facial Plastic and Reconstructive Surgery, Department of Otolaryngology – Head and Neck Surgery, University of Toronto, Toronto, Ontario, Canada

TATIANA K. DIXON, MD
Fellow, Facial Plastic Surgery, Department of Otolaryngology – Head and Neck Surgery, University of Illinois at Chicago, Chicago, Illinois

LAUREN E. DUBAS, MD
Resident Physician, Department of Dermatology, University of Cincinnati College of Medicine, Cincinnati, Ohio

DAVID A.F. ELLIS, MD, FRCSC, FACS
Professor, Division of Facial Plastic and Reconstructive Surgery, Department of Otolaryngology – Head and Neck Surgery, University of Toronto, Toronto, Ontario, Canada

RAVINDHRA G. ELLURU, MD, PhD
Associate Professor, Division of Pediatric Otolaryngology – Head and Neck Surgery, Cincinnati Children's Hospital Medical Center; Department of Otolaryngology – Head and Neck Surgery, University of Cincinnati College of Medicine, Cincinnati, Ohio

FRED G. FEDOK, MD, FACS
Professor and Chief, Facial Plastic and Reconstructive Surgery, Otolaryngology/Head and Neck Surgery, Department of Surgery, Hershey Medical Center, The Pennsylvania State University, Hershey, Pennsylvania

FRANK GARRITANO, MD
Facial Plastic and Reconstructive Surgery, Otolaryngology/Head and Neck Surgery, Department of Surgery, Hershey Medical Center, The Pennsylvania State University, Hershey, Pennsylvania

DAVID B. HOM, MD, FACS
Professor, Director, Division of Facial Plastic and Reconstructive Surgery, Department of Otolaryngology – Head and Neck Surgery, Cincinnati Children's Hospital Medical Center, University of Cincinnati College of Medicine, Cincinnati, Ohio

JEFFREY J. HOULTON, MD
Department of Otolaryngology – Head and Neck Surgery, University of Cincinnati College of Medicine, Cincinnati, Ohio

ADAM INGRAFFEA, MD, FAAD, FACMS
Mohs Surgeon, Clinical Assistant Professor; Assistant Program Director, Department of Dermatology, University of Cincinnati, West Chester, Ohio

SUNDEEP G. KESWANI, MD
Assistant Professor, Division of Pediatric General, Thoracic and Fetal Surgery, The Center for Molecular Fetal Therapy, Cincinnati Children's Hospital Medical Center, Cincinnati, Ohio

ALICE KING, MD
Surgical Research Fellow, Division of Pediatric General, Thoracic and Fetal Surgery, The Center for Molecular Fetal Therapy, Cincinnati Children's Hospital Medical Center, Cincinnati, Ohio

W. JOHN KITZMILLER, MD
Chief, Division of Plastic, Reconstructive and Hand Surgery, Department of Surgery, University of Cincinnati, Cincinnati, Ohio

KRISTEN S. MOE, MD, FACS
Department of Otolaryngology – Head and Neck Surgery, University of Washington, Seattle, Washington

BRIAN S. PAN, MD
Assistant Professor, Division of Plastic, Reconstructive and Hand/Burn Surgery, Department of Surgery, College of Medicine, University of Cincinnati; Division of Plastic Surgery, Cincinnati Children's Hospital Medical Center, Cincinnati, Ohio

ANTONIO PORTELA, MD
Facial Plastic and Reconstructive Surgery, Otolaryngology/Head Neck Surgery, Department of Surgery, Hershey Medical Center, The Pennsylvania State University, Hershey, Pennsylvania

ANTHONY P. SCLAFANI, MD, FACS
Surgeon Director and Director of Facial Plastic Surgery, Division of Facial Plastic Surgery, Department of Otolaryngology, The New York Eye and Ear Infirmary, New York, New York; Professor of Otolaryngology, New York Medical College, Valhalla, New York

GRAHAM MICHAEL STRUB, MD, PhD
Department of Otolaryngology – Head and Neck Surgery, University of Washington, Seattle, Washington

J. REGAN THOMAS, MD
Professor and Head, Department of Otolaryngology – Head and Neck Surgery, University of Illinois at Chicago, Chicago, Illinois

MARTY O. VISSCHER, PhD
Director, Skin Sciences Program, Division of Plastic Surgery, Cincinnati Children's Hospital Medical Center; Associate Professor, Division of Plastic, Reconstructive and Hand/Burn Surgery, Department of Surgery, College of Medicine, University of Cincinnati, Cincinnati, Ohio

Contents

Advisory Board to Facial Plastic Surgery Clinics 2012

J. REGAN THOMAS, MD, CONSULTING EDITOR

Professor and Head
Department of Otolaryngology–Head and Neck Surgery
University of Illinois, Chicago
1855 W. Taylor St. MC 648
Chicago, IL 60612

312.996.6584
thomasrj@uic.edu

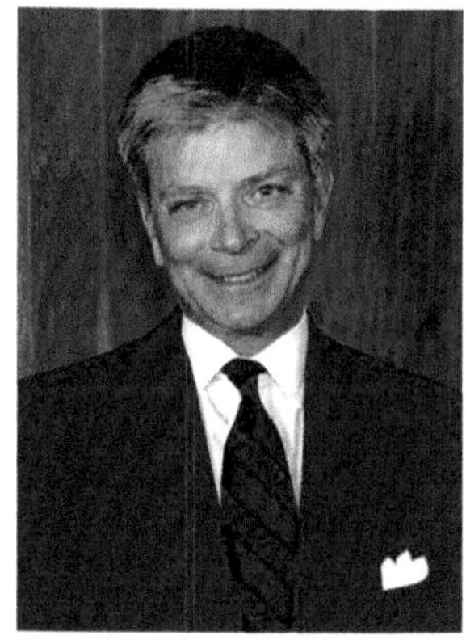

ANTHONY SCLAFANI, MD, BOARD LEADER

Director of Facial Plastic Surgery
The New York Eye & Ear Infirmary
New York, NY

Professor
Department of Otolaryngology
New York Medical College
Valhalla, NY

200 West 57th Street; Suite #1410
New York, NY 10019

212.979.4534
asclafani@nyee.edu
www.nyface.com

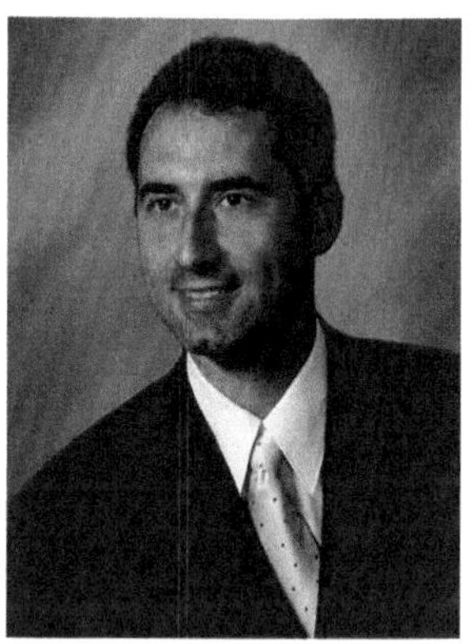

Facial Plastic Surgery Clinics is pleased to introduce the 2012-2013 **Advisory Board**.

Facial Plastic Surgery Clinics is widely available through the media of print, digital e-Reader, online via the Internet, and on iPad and smart phones.

Facial Plastic Surgery Clinics provides professionals access to pertinent point of care answers and current clinical information, along with comprehensive background information for deeper understanding.

Readers are welcome to contact the Clinics Editor or Board with comments.

BOARD MEMBERS 2012

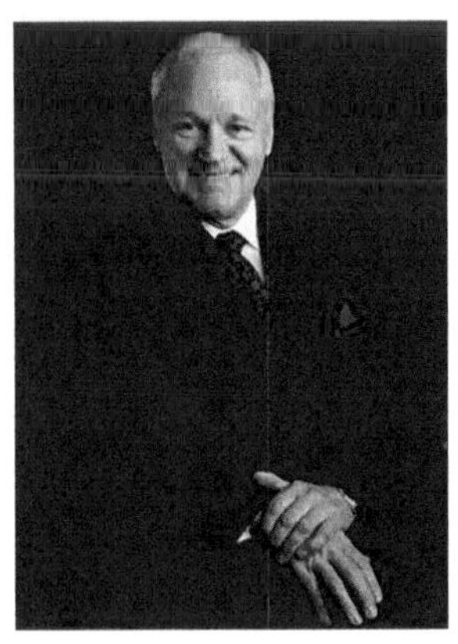

PETER A. ADAMSON, MD

Professor and Head
Division of Facial Plastic and Reconstructive Surgery
Department of Otolaryngology–Head and Neck Surgery
University of Toronto
Toronto, Ontario, Canada

Adamson Cosmetic Facial Surgery
Renaissance Plaza; 150 Bloor Street West; Suite M110
Toronto, Ontario M5S 2X9

416.323.3900
paa@dradamson.com
www.dradamson.com

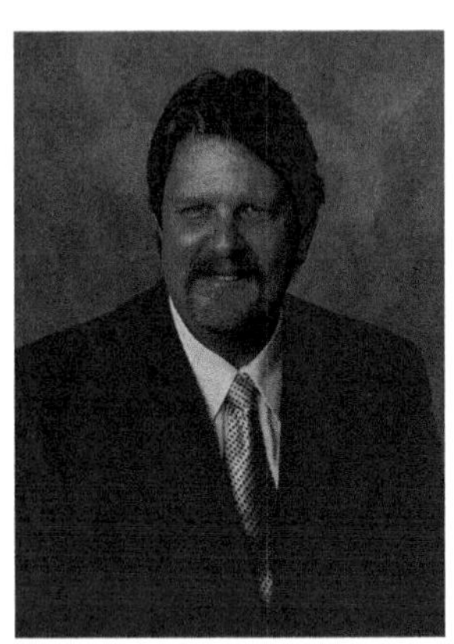

RICK DAVIS, MD

Voluntary Professor
The University of Miami Miller School of Medicine
Miami, Florida

The Center for Facial Restoration
1951 S.W. 172nd Ave; Suite 205
Miramar, Florida 33029

954.442.5191
drd@davisrhinoplasty.com
www.DavisRhinoplasty.com

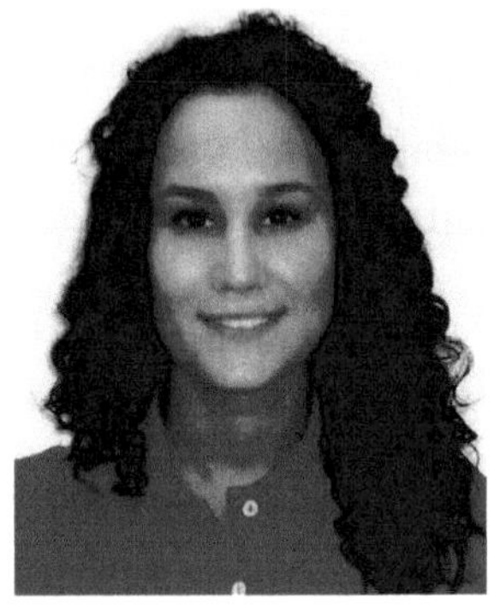

TATIANA DIXON, MD

University of Illinois at Chicago
Resident,
Department of Otolaryngology–Head and Neck Surgery

1855 W. Taylor
Chicago, IL 60612

312.996.6555
TFeuer1@UIC.EDU

STEVEN FAGIEN, MD, FACS

Aesthetic Eyelid Plastic Surgery
660 Glades Road; Suite 210
Boca Raton, Florida 33431

561.393.9898
sfagien@aol.com

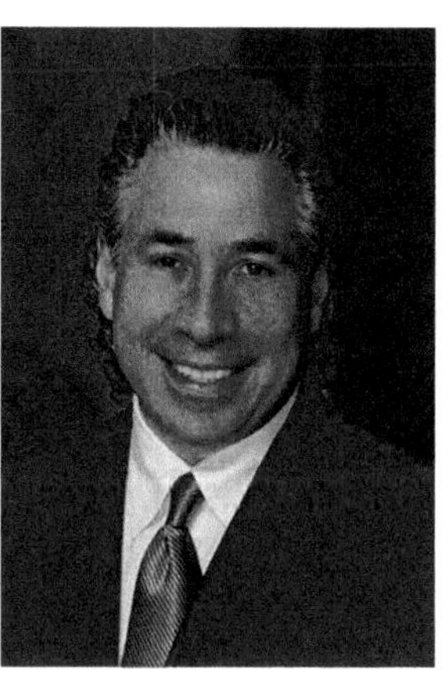

GREG KELLER, MD

Clinical Professor of Surgery, Head and Neck,
David Geffen School of Medicine,
University of California, Los Angeles;

Keller Facial Plastic Surgery
221 W. Pueblo St. Ste A
Santa Barbara, CA 93105

805.687.6408
faclft@aol.com
www.gregorykeller.com

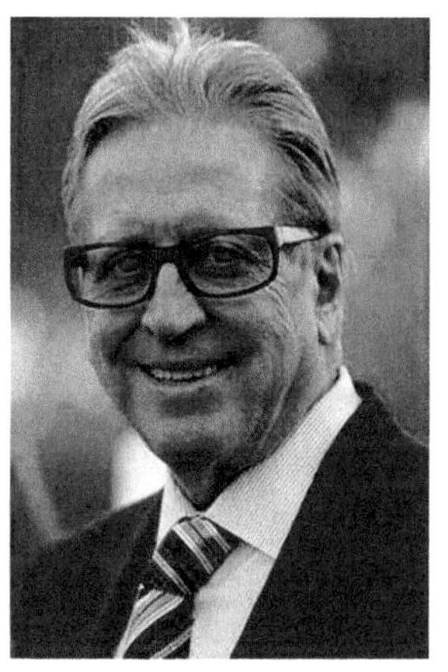

THEDA C. KONTIS, MD

Assistant Professor, Johns Hopkins Hospital
Facial Plastic Surgicenter, Ltd.
1838 Greene Tree Road, Suite 370
Baltimore, MD 21208

410.486.3400
tckontis@aol.com
www.facialplasticsurgerymd.com
www.facial-plasticsurgery.com

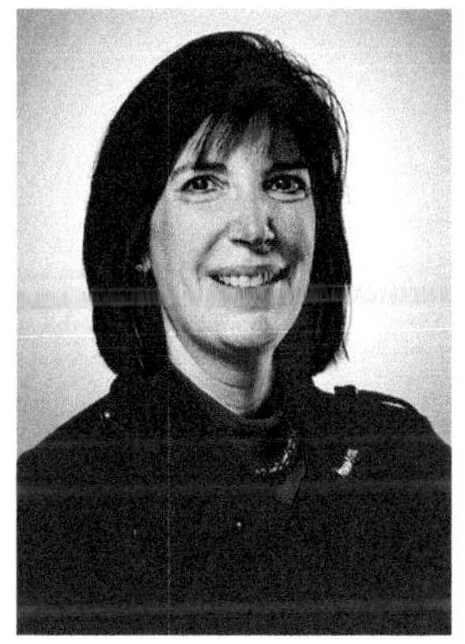

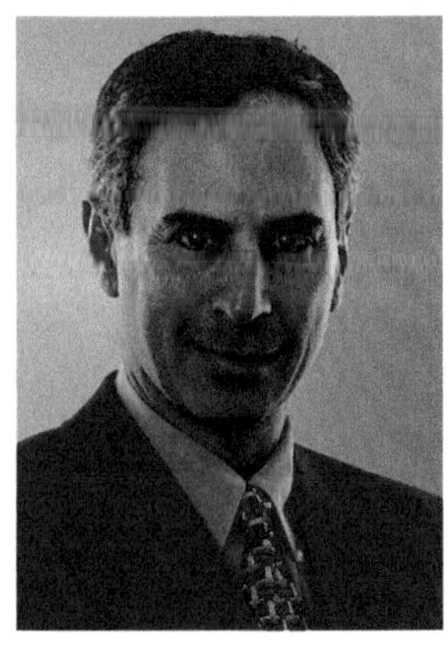

IRA D. PAPEL, MD

Facial Plastic Surgicenter
Associate Professor
The Johns Hopkins University
1838 Greene Tree Road, Suite 370
Baltimore, MD 21208

410.486.3400
idpmd@aol.com
www.facial-plasticsurgery.com

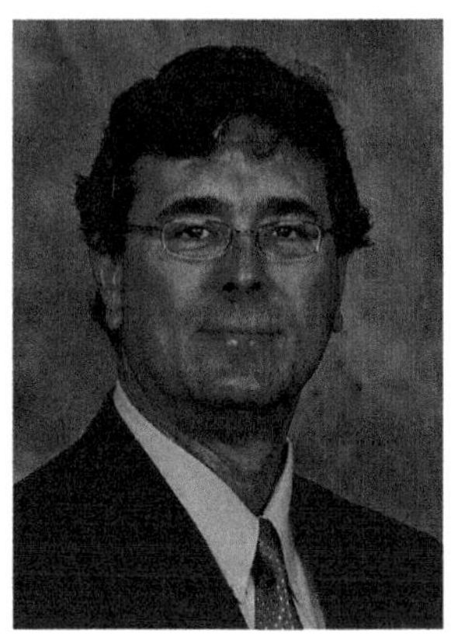

SHERARD A. TATUM, MD

Professor of Otolaryngology and
Pediatrics Cleft and Craniofacial Center
Division of Facial Plastic Surgery
Upstate Medical University
750 E. Adams St.
Syracuse, NY 13210

315.464.4636
TatumS@upstate.edu
www.upstate.edu

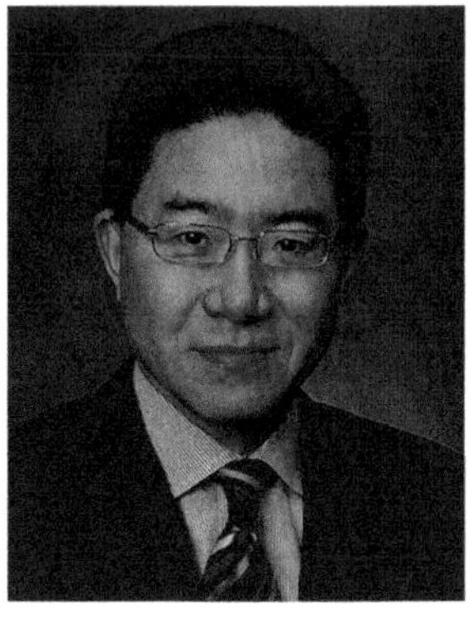

TOM D. WANG, MD

Professor
Facial Plastic and Reconstructive Surgery
Oregon Health & Science University
3181 Southwest Sam Jackson Park Road
Portland, OR 97239

503.494.5678
wangt@ohsu.edu
www.ohsu.edu/drtomwang

FACIAL PLASTIC SURGERY CLINICS OF NORTH AMERICA

FORTHCOMING ISSUES

Minimally Invasive Procedures in Facial Plastic Surgery
Theda Kontis, MD, *Editor*

Hair Restoration
Raymond Konior, MD and Stephen Gabel, MD, *Editors*

Complications in Facial Plastic Surgery
Richard L. Goode, MD and Samuel P. Most, MD, *Editors*

Techniques in Facial Plastic Surgery: Discussion and Debate, Volume 2
Fred Fedok, MD and Robert Kellman, MD, *Editors*

RECENT ISSUES

November 2012
Nonmelanoma Skin Cancer of the Head and Neck
Cemal Cingi, *Editor*

August 2012
Techniques in Facial Plastic Surgery: Discussion and Debate
Fred G. Fedok, MD and Robert M. Kellman, MD, *Editors*

May 2012
Emerging Tools and Trends in Facial Plastic Surgery
Paul J. Carniol, MD, *Editor*

Preface

Facial Skin: Contemporary Topics for the Surgeon

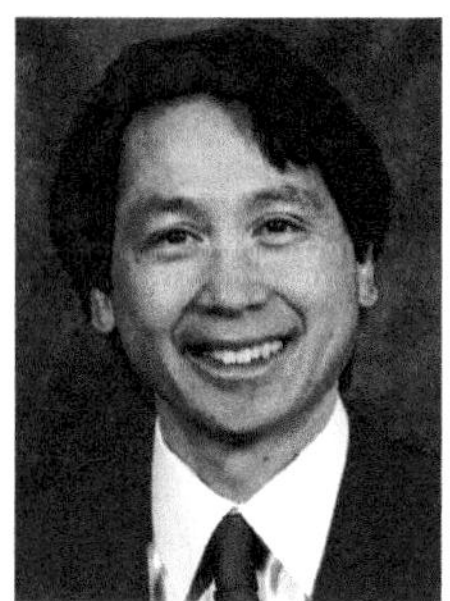
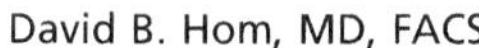
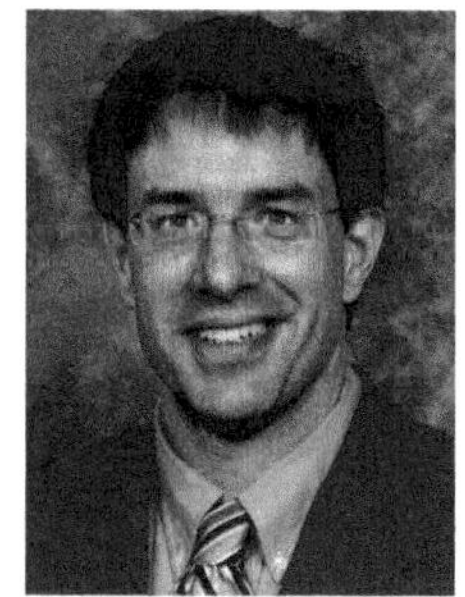

David B. Hom, MD, FACS   Adam Ingraffea, MD, FAAD, FACMS
Editors

The skin is a crucial structure protecting our bodies from the ravages of the external environment. It also serves many other essential purposes throughout our lifetime from fetus to adulthood. This issue on "Facial Skin: Contemporary Topics for the Surgeon" addresses important contemporary topics about the skin relevant to facial plastic surgery.

By increasing our understanding of how skin from the fetus is different from the adult, we may someday manipulate skin wounds to accelerate its healing and to form less of a scar. In addition, recent discoveries have altered the way we now treat certain skin conditions. Such examples described in this issue are the use of propranolol to treat infantile hemangiomas and using negative pressure therapy to help heal difficult cutaneous wounds.

The eclectic subjects covered in this issue range from newer techniques to treat various skin conditions and diseases; innovative ways to measure the skin; and contemporary methods to improve its healing and cosmetic appearance for the facial plastic surgeon.

This issue does not attempt to describe completely all recent clinical skin developments, but instead highlights relevant skin topics for the facial plastic surgeon. We would like to sincerely thank the article authors for sharing their expertise on these diverse topics. As guest editors, we are very pleased to share with you this provocative issue and hope you will find it fascinating.

David B. Hom, MD, FACS
Division of Facial Plastic
and Reconstructive Surgery
Department of Otolaryngology–Head
and Neck Surgery
University of Cincinnati College of Medicine
P.O. Box 670528, 231 Albert Sabin Way
Cincinnati, OH 45267-0528, USA

Adam Ingraffea, MD, FAAD, FACMS
Department of Dermatology
University of Cincinnati
7690 University Court, Suite 3100
West Chester, OH 45069, USA

E-mail addresses:
david.hom@uc.edu (D.B. Hom)
ingrafam@ucmail.uc.edu (A. Ingraffea)

Facial Plast Surg Clin N Am 21 (2013) xv
http://dx.doi.org/10.1016/j.fsc.2012.12.001
1064-7406/13/$ – see front matter

Biology and Function of Fetal and Pediatric Skin

Alice King, MD, Swathi Balaji, PhD,
Sundeep G. Keswani, MD*

KEYWORDS

• Fetal • Pediatric • Skin development • Transepidermal water loss • Skin hydration • Skin acidity

KEY POINTS

- Skin is anatomically mature at birth but continues functional maturity during the first year of life.
- In contrast to adults, infant skin is in a constant state of flux with changes in transepidermal water loss, hydration, lipid content, and skin acidity.
- Mature barrier function is critical for maintenance of thermoregulation, hydration, and protection against infection.
- Impaired barrier function and skin desiccation increases the risk of disease including atopic or contact dermatitis, infection, and even lethal excess water loss.

INTRODUCTION

Fetal and pediatric skin are commonly believed to have advantageous properties for wound repair, with the ability of fetal skin to undergo scarless wound repair and the inherent youthful appearance of pediatric skin.[1] However, infant and pediatric skin are also considered to be more sensitive and prone to injury than adult skin with the cosmetic industry marketing an extensive line of delicate products exclusively for the care and hygiene of infants and children.[2]

SKIN DEVELOPMENT

The development of the dermal/epidermal layers is a continuous process starting early in pregnancy with discrete patterns related to gestational age, developing from the cranial to the caudal pole.[3] At 4 weeks gestation, fetal skin can be visualized as 2 distinct layers: a basal cell layer covered by an outer layer, termed the periderm (**Fig. 1**). The periderm is uniquely found in humans; there is no counterpart in animal models such as mice or rats.[4] Keratinization begincs at 9 weeks gestation, and at 13 weeks gestation, stratification into different layers becomes apparent.[3] Hair follicles begin to form as epidermal buds along the basal layer at 14 weeks gestation. In the subsequent 2 weeks, these epidermal buds are associated with local proliferation of mesenchymal cells associated with the epidermal bud as hair follicles rapidly develop.[3] This is followed by continued elongation of the hair follicles. The development of eccrine sweat glands begins as epidermal buds in the basal layer at 20 weeks gestation and continue to develop over the next 10 weeks, first by elongating and then by coiling.[3] At 24 weeks gestation, fetal skin continues to heal without scar, as keratinization and stratification into mature morphologic layers continues.[4] After 24 weeks gestation, there is a transitional period when skin heals without characteristic scar deposition but fails to reconstitute the dermal appendages. This transitional period has been found in multiple animal models of fetal wound healing. The scarless wound healing

The authors have no disclosures.
Division of Pediatric General, Thoracic and Fetal Surgery, The Center for Molecular Fetal Therapy, Cincinnati Children's Hospital Medical Center, 3333 Burnet Avenue, MLC 11025, Cincinnati, OH 45229-3039, USA
* Corresponding author.
E-mail address: sundeep.keswani@cchmc.org

Facial Plast Surg Clin N Am 21 (2013) 1–6
http://dx.doi.org/10.1016/j.fsc.2012.10.001
1064-7406/13/$ – see front matter

facialplastic.theclinics.com

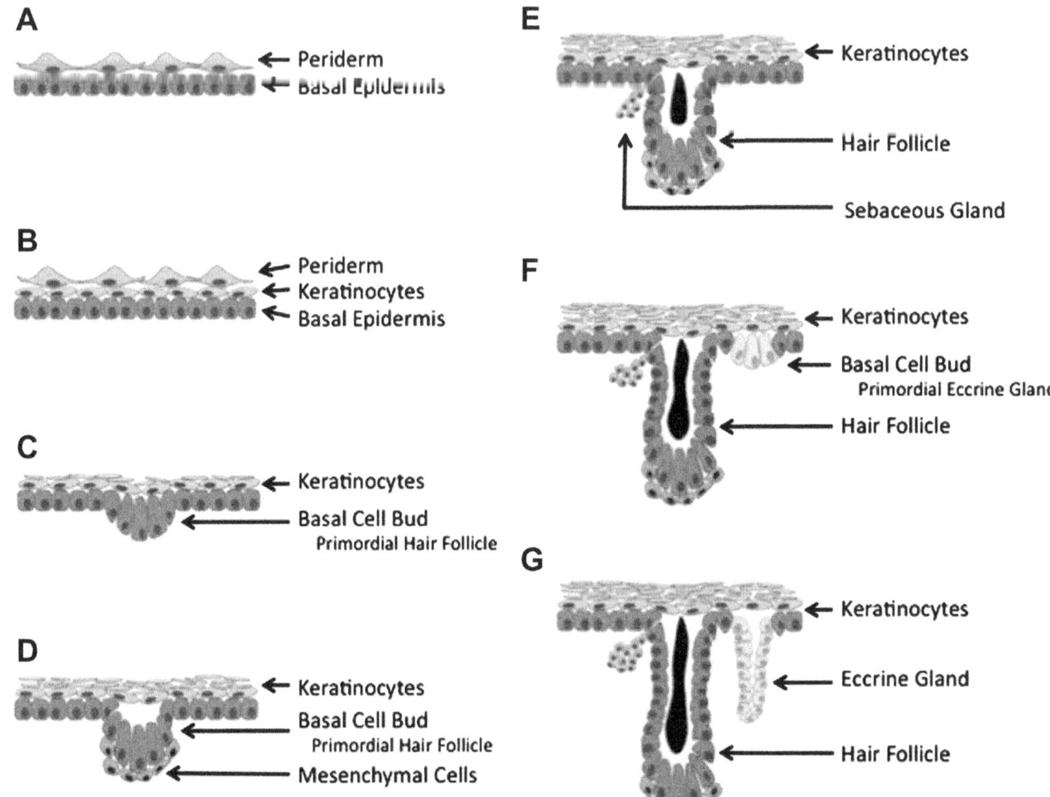

Fig. 1. Fetal development of skin. (*A*) At 4 weeks' gestation, skin is composed of 2 layers, the periderm and basal epidermis. (*B*) At 9 weeks gestation, keratinization becomes apparent. (*C*) At 14 weeks gestation, stratification of the epidermal layer is apparent along with budding of the basal layer as the primordial hair follicle develops. (*D*) At 16 weeks gestation, mesenchymal cells may be seen associated with the epidermal bud. (*E*) At 18 weeks, sebaceous glands become apparent, along with hair follicle elongation. (*F*) At 23 weeks, the hair follicles continue to elongate while the basal layer buds to form primordial eccrine glands. (*G*) At 30 weeks' gestation, the eccrine glands continue to elongate and coil.

phenotype is lost by the third trimester. At 34 weeks gestation, mature keratinocytes characterized by flattened, keratinized morphology are observed in conjunction with adult-type dermoepidermal undulations.[5,6]

In later gestation, the fetal dermis is primarily thickened by an increase in collagen content.[4] This dermis has higher levels of type III collagen, chondroitin sulfate, proteoglycans, and hyaluronan compared with adult dermis.[4] Dermal elastin is also absent in fetal dermis.[7,8]

During the last trimester, the fetus is covered by the vernix caseosa (VC), a protective coat secreted by the sebaceous glands and composed of protein (10%), lipids (10%), and water (80%).[9] The VC is uniquely human, with no counterpart identified in animal models. This coat was initially posited to function as a lubricant in the birthing process. However, as the fetus continues to mature, part of the vernix sloughs from the skin surface into the surrounding amniotic fluid.[10] This physiologic decrease of vernix with advancing gestational age renders this role unlikely. More recent studies of the VC suggest that the layer facilitates the transition from an aqueous in utero environment to the dry extrauterine environment.[11] The vernix helps to protect the fetal epidermis from maceration while immersed in amniotic fluid and permits epidermal cornification and stratum corneum formation.[9] The VC also contains high levels of lysozyme, lactoferrin, linoleic acid, as well as other antiinfective agents.[9,12]

Full-term infants at birth have skin that is anatomically mature when examined histologically with all 5 layers present. These include from deep to superficial: stratum basale, stratum spinosum, stratum granulosum, stratum licidum, and stratum corneum.[13] As epidermal cells mature, their morphology changes from the columnar stratum basale to the tightly overlapping squamous keratinocytes of the stratum corneum.[5,6] The time to fully mature, keratinize, and form this protective horny layer varies depending on body site.[14] This occurs more rapidly in facial skin than in the trunk and limbs.[6] Neonatal skin has a relatively coarse texture compared with older infants and a more homogeneous smooth structure develops during the first 30 days of life.[15] Infants have smaller corneocytes and a significantly thinner stratum corneum until 2 years of age.[13]

During the next developmental period from infancy to puberty, there is little difference in skin between male and female patients. Both genders demonstrate a steady increase in dermal thickness, with boys developing thicker epidermal and dermal layers.[16] At the onset of puberty, there is significant hormonal influence on the skin. After age 12 years, girls accumulate a thick layer of subcutaneous fat, which is absent in boys. On the other hand, boys exhibit a gradual thinning of their thick epidermal and dermal layers. These layers remain a constant thickness in females throughout adolescence and adulthood until menopause.[16] In addition, dermal composition begins to change with advancing age starting at puberty; both sexes show similar rates of linear decrease in skin collagen content with age. Women start with a lower baseline collagen density and they seem to age earlier than men.[4,16]

SKIN FUNCTION

Skin has multiple functions including regulation of body temperature and protection against physical, chemical, and biological insults.[17,18] In full-term neonates at birth, the skin is histologically mature, however it remains functionally immature. Neonatal barrier functions are in a constant state of flux, in contrast to mature adult skin.[5] It has been proposed that this changing infant skin barrier is not a deficit but a benefit because adaptive flexibility allows constant optimization, balancing growth, thermoregulation, water barrier, and protective functions.

BIOPHYSICAL SKIN PARAMETERS

Skin can be defined by a variety of biophysical skin parameters, which permit the study of skin in a noninvasive manner. Multiple parameters, including transepidermal water loss, hydration, and skin acidity, are affected in skin diseases such as atopic dermatitis, psoriasis, and allergic or irritant contact dermatitis.[2]

Transepidermal Water Loss

Transepidermal water loss (TEWL) describes the amount of water loss through the epidermis through evaporation and depends on multiple factors, including skin temperature, skin blood flow, local hemodynamics, degree of corneocyte formation, and stratum corneum lipid content.[19] TEWL is measured by electrical skin impedance; lower impedance indicates higher skin hydration.[20] There is a direct relationship between TEWL and skin development. In full-term infants, there is a significant decrease in TEWL indicating a functional barrier to evaporative water loss. At birth, the sweat glands are anatomically mature, however only a small fraction of these glands are functionally mature with secretory activity.[20] During the first few months of life, impedance values begin to decrease corresponding to the recruitment and maturation of sweat glands. These values stabilize at 4 months in full-term infants.[20]

Premature infants, less than 32 weeks' gestation, have lower impedance and high TEWL at birth. This excess loss is a result of immature barrier function and thinner epidermal layers,[20] relatively increased blood flow to the skin compared with other infants, as well as a high ratio of total body surface area to volume. These factors lead to increased insensible water loss. TEWL in these premature infants can exceed 30% of their total body weight within a 24-hour period. TEWL decreases as skin continues to mature, with improved barrier function. The barrier function regulating evaporative losses varies according to anatomic location. In general, TEWL is higher in the facial region, compared with the body.[19] The highest TEWL is reported in the nasolabial fold and perioral regions, with the lowest TEWL over the cheeks. There are no gender differences noted in the neonatal or pediatric period.[21]

Skin Hydration

At birth, skin is transitioned from continuous immersion in an aqueous solution to exposure to relatively low humidity ambient air. Maintenance of skin hydration is critical for skin function, including plasticity, flexibility, prevention of fissures, and proper desquamation.[22] Neonatal skin responds with a dramatic decrease in hydration at birth.[6] Skin hydration then quickly increases for up to 90 days after birth, as the eccrine glands mature.[23] This increased skin hydration persists for up to the first year of life[5] and subsequently stabilizes to adult levels.[24]

The sebaceous glands also play an important role in maintaining optimal skin hydration, secreting lipid-rich sebum. The highest sebum levels in the face are located in the nasolabial area.[19] These glands are hormonally regulated and are active *in utero*, producing the VC.[9] After birth, there are low levels of sebum protection until puberty, when it markedly increases to adult levels, particularly in boys.[6,24,25]

Skin Acidity

Fully mature skin is characterized by a physiologic acid mantle with the pH maintained between 4.5 and 6.0.[2,26] This acid mantle is an important mechanism in the skin's defense against infection. The enzymes in the upper epidermis are optimized to function at pH 5.6. Neonatal skin is characterized by a higher pH compared with older pediatric and adult patients, regardless of gestational age, sex, mode of delivery, or body weight.[27] This newborn skin has a different chemical composition of skin surface lipids.[2] Maturation and maintenance of the acid mantle depends on lactic acid, free amino acids, and fatty acids found in sebum and sweat. Once established, the acid mantle is more uniformly distributed anatomically in the early pediatric population.[2] At the onset of puberty, the intertriginous areas, such as the axilla and inguinal region, approach a neutral or even alkaline pH, as found in adults.[28]

THERAPEUTIC OPTIONS

As the survival rate of premature infants continues to increase at earlier gestational age, the issue of immature pediatric skin becomes more prevalent. The therapeutic options focus on supporting the barrier function of the infant skin, including thermoregulation, hydration, and attenuating risk of infection. In the neonatal period, thermoregulation can be supported by the use of low-energy infrared radiation, which warms the ambient air.[17] Skin temperature can vary greatly depending on anatomic location; the skin overlying the liver correlates most closely with core temperature.[17]

Table 1
Clinical review of the literature: summary table of various reviews

Author	Groups Compared	Findings
Stamatas et al,[15] 2011	Full-term infants (birth to 3 y) vs Adults	Skin Structure Infants have smaller corneocytes Infants have thinner stratum corneum Skin Function Barrier function: weaker than adults Hydration: decreased at birth, but increased later in infancy TEWL: lower at birth, similar or higher later in infancy (anatomic variance) pH: infant skin is more alkaline Cell proliferation: increased turnover
Fluhr et al,[26] 2012	Newborns (1–15 d) vs Infants (5–6 wk) vs Infants (6 mo) vs Infants (1–2 y) vs Pediatrics (4–5 y) vs Adults (20–35 y)	Skin Function Hydration: newborns have the lowest hydration and water content Skin hydration increases then remains stable through pediatrics and adults TEWL: lowest in the 5–6 wk after birth, highest at 1–2 y pH: skin of newborn infants is more alkaline than all other groups; skin becomes more acidic by 5–6 wk and then remains stable through pediatrics
Giusti et al,[2] 2001	Infants (8–24 mo) vs Adults (25–35 y)	Skin Function Hydration: infants have higher hydration TEWL: no difference between infants and adults pH: infant skin is more alkaline at multiple sites
Firooz et al,[24] 2012	Pediatrics (10–20 y) vs Adults (20–30 y, 30–40 y, 40–50 y)	Skin Function Hydration: no difference between pediatrics and adults TEWL: no difference between pediatrics and adults Sebum: no difference between pediatrics and adults
Man et al,[25] 2009	Prepuberty (0–12 y) vs Young group (13–35 y) vs Middle age (36–50 y) vs Old group (51–70 y)	Skin Function Hydration: higher stratum corneum hydration in young group males compared with females pH: no difference in pH between pediatrics and older groups

Maintenance of a normal core temperature decreases the mortality rate of these premature infants and helps to minimize insensible water loss by optimizing the TEWL. Although barrier function becomes physiologically mature early in the pediatric period, the increased surface area to volume ratio of younger children continues to put them at a higher risk of excess water loss and dehydration due to insensible losses compared with adults and adolescents. Cognizance of this risk and regular oral hydration are necessary to maintain homeostasis.

From birth to puberty, pediatric skin is at risk of desiccation with lower levels of sebum production. Decreased skin hydration is associated with impairment of the skin's barrier function and pathologic conditions such as atopic dermatitis. Desiccation of the skin leads to the early appearance of fine cracks and fissures in pediatric skin.[9] These defects are a route to infection and irritants. Maintenance of hydration can be facilitated by continual use of moisturizers.

CLINICAL OUTCOMES

Skin development continues from birth throughout life. With interim support of skin function in the neonatal period, even the most premature infant progresses to normal skin capable of thermoregulation, maintenance of hydration, and protection against infection (**Table 1**).

COMPLICATIONS AND CONCERNS

Pediatric skin has increased permeability with higher TEWL and increased skin hydration. Increased permeability leads to a tendency to develop xerosis, excessively dry skin that presents as white patches with fine white scales, particularly on the exposed facial skin.[6] Xerosis leads to increased development of irritant or allergic contact dermatitis.[2,6]

Without the support of thermoregulation, hydration, and pathogen barriers in the neonatal and early pediatric period, immature skin can result in lethal consequences secondary to extensive transcutaneous fluid loss or infection.[18]

SUMMARY

Skin development is a continuous process, beginning in utero and continuing throughout life. The skin is anatomically mature at birth, but continues to develop functionally throughout the first year of life. The glandular components of skin are strongly influenced by hormonal changes, with further development seen at the onset of puberty.

REFERENCES

1. Leung A, Crombleholme TM, Keswani SG. Fetal wound healing: implications for minimal scar formation. Curr Opin Pediatr 2012;24:371–8.
2. Giusti F, Martella A, Bertoni L, et al. Skin barrier, hydration, and pH of the skin of infants under 2 years of age. Pediatr Dermatol 2001;18:93–6.
3. Ersch J, Stallmach T. Assessing gestational age from histology of fetal skin: an autopsy study of 379 fetuses. Obstet Gynecol 1999;94:753–7.
4. Satish L, Kathju S. Cellular and molecular characteristics of scarless versus fibrotic wound healing. Dermatol Res Pract 2010;2010:790234.
5. Nikolovski J, Stamatas GN, Kollias N, et al. Barrier function and water-holding and transport properties of infant stratum corneum are different from adult and continue to develop through the first year of life. J Invest Dermatol 2008;128:1728–36.
6. Tagami H. Location-related differences in structure and function of the stratum corneum with special emphasis on those of the facial skin. Int J Cosmet Sci 2008;30:413–34.
7. Coolen NA, Schouten KC, Boekema BK, et al. Wound healing in a fetal, adult, and scar tissue model: a comparative study. Wound Repair Regen 2010;18:291–301.
8. Coolen NA, Schouten KC, Middelkoop E, et al. Comparison between human fetal and adult skin. Arch Dermatol Res 2010;302:47–55.
9. Visscher MO, Utturkar R, Pickens WL, et al. Neonatal skin maturation–vernix caseosa and free amino acids. Pediatr Dermatol 2011;28:122–32.
10. Narendran V, Wickett RR, Pickens WL, et al. Interaction between pulmonary surfactant and vernix: a potential mechanism for induction of amniotic fluid turbidity. Pediatr Res 2000;48:120–4.
11. Hoath SB. Physiologic development of the skin. In: RA P, Fox W, Abman S, editors. Fetal and neonatal physiology. Philadelphia: Elsevier; 2004. p. 679–95.
12. Walker VP, Akinbi HT, Meinzen-Derr J, et al. Host defense proteins on the surface of neonatal skin: implications for innate immunity. J Pediatr 2008;152:777–81.
13. Stamatas GN, Nikolovski J, Luedtke MA, et al. Infant skin microstructure assessed in vivo differs from adult skin in organization and at the cellular level. Pediatr Dermatol 2010;27:125–31.
14. Spearman RI. Vertebrate skin. Nature 1978;276:442.
15. Stamatas GN, Nikolovski J, Mack MC, et al. Infant skin physiology and development during the first years of life: a review of recent findings based on in vivo studies. Int J Cosmet Sci 2011;33:17–24.
16. Tur E. Physiology of the skin–differences between women and men. Clin Dermatol 1997;15:5–16.
17. Friedman F, Adams FH, Emmanouilides G. Regulation of body temperature of premature infants with low-energy radiant heat. J Pediatr 1967;70:270–3.

18. Has C, Bruckner-Tuderman L. Molecular and diagnostic aspects of genetic skin fragility. J Dermatol Sci 2006;44:129–44.
19. Marrakchi S, Maibach HI. Biophysical parameters of skin: map of human face, regional, and age-related differences. Contact Dermatitis 2007;57:28–34.
20. Emery MM, Hebert AA, Aguirre Vila-Coro A, et al. The relationship between skin maturation and electrical skin impedance. J Dermatol Sci 1991; 2:336–40.
21. Ramos-e-Silva M, Boza JC, Cestari TF. Effects of age (neonates and elderly) on skin barrier function. Clin Dermatol 2012;30:274–6.
22. Visscher MO, Chatterjee R, Munson KA, et al. Changes in diapered and nondiapered infant skin over the first month of life. Pediatr Dermatol 2000; 17:45–51.
23. Hoeger PH, Enzmann CC. Skin physiology of the neonate and young infant: a prospective study of functional skin parameters during early infancy. Pediatr Dermatol 2002;19:256–62.
24. Firooz A, Sadr B, Babakoohi S, et al. Variation of biophysical parameters of the skin with age, gender, and body region. ScientificWorldJournal 2012;2012: 386936.
25. Man MQ, Xin SJ, Song SP, et al. Variation of skin surface pH, sebum content and stratum corneum hydration with age and gender in a large Chinese population. Skin Pharmacol Physiol 2009;22:190–9.
26. Fluhr JW, Darlenski R, Lachmann N, et al. Infant epidermal skin physiology: adaptation after birth. Br J Dermatol 2012;166:483–90.
27. Yosipovitch G, Maayan-Metzger A, Merlob P, et al. Skin barrier properties in different body areas in neonates. Pediatrics 2000;106:105–8.
28. Behrendt H, Green M. The relationship of skin pH pattern to sexual maturation in boys. AMA Am J Dis Child 1955;90:164–72.

Update on Techniques for the Quantitation of Facial Skin Characteristics

Marty O. Visscher, PhD[a,b,*], Brian S. Pan, MD[b,c]

KEYWORDS

• Facial skin • Facial skin restoration • Facial skin coloration • Photodamage

KEY POINTS

- Homogeneity of facial skin color strongly influences the perception of age, and increased uniformity can reduce the perceived age by as many as 20 years.
- Visual scales are used to characterize the extent of photoaging, evaluate treatment response, appraise improvement, and determine patient satisfaction; however, none have been established as the universal standard for evaluation.
- The delivery of optimum outcomes and maximum patient satisfaction in the treatment of facial photodamage depends on selection of effective treatment modalities and measurement of changes in perceived age.
- Although it is used routinely in the skin-care industry to demonstrate treatment effects, particularly for cosmetics, color imaging has not been used to evaluate cutaneous conditions in health care.
- Standardized digital imaging techniques can be used successfully to quantify attributes of facial photodamage and treatment response, including dyschromia (solar lentigines, hyperpigmentation), erythema, telangiectasias, elastosis, rhytides, and textural changes. Biomechanical methods quantify elasticity.
- The application of these methods has the potential to assist the plastic surgeon in achieving patient expectations.

INTRODUCTION

Human beings use skin features including color uniformity, color distribution, and texture to infer the physiologic health status of others.[1] For example, visual responses to facial-image sets standardized for shape and surface features were recorded with eye-tracking methods. Those images with more uniform skin coloration drew more attention and were perceived to be younger than those with greater color variability.[2] The distribution of skin color on the face has also been associated with the perception of overall health.[3] These factors can reduce the perceived age by as many as 20 years.[4,5] This homogeneity in skin color is also related to perceived age and health in men.[6] Color itself influences the perception of

Funding Sources: None.
Conflict of Interest: None.

[a] Skin Sciences Program, Division of Plastic Surgery, Cincinnati Children's Hospital Medical Center, 3333 Burnet Avenue, Cincinnati, OH 45229, USA; [b] Division of Plastic, Reconstructive & Hand/Burn Surgery, Department of Surgery, College of Medicine, University of Cincinnati, 231 Albert Sabin Way, Cincinnati, OH 45267, USA; [c] Division of Plastic Surgery, Cincinnati Children's Hospital Medical Center, 3333 Burnet Avenue, Cincinnati, OH 45229, USA

* Corresponding author. Division of Plastic Surgery, Cincinnati Children's Hospital Medical Center, 3333 Burnet Avenue, Cincinnati, OH 45229.
E-mail address: Marty.visscher@cchmc.org

Facial Plast Surg Clin N Am 21 (2013) 7–19
http://dx.doi.org/10.1016/j.fsc.2012.10.002
1064-7406/13/$ – see front matter

health. In one study, observers were asked to adjust the redness of high-resolution facial images to achieve their own perceived "healthy appearance." All of them increased the red coloration, regardless of their inherent pigmentation, but subjects with dark skin increased the red component of dark-skin photos more than for those with lighter skin.[7] The perception of age may vary, however, depending on the person's ethnicity. High-resolution photographs of the cheek region from Japanese women aged 13 to 80 years were viewed by 10 Japanese judges. Using skin lightness (L) and b* color (blue-yellow), those with darker and more yellow skin were perceived to be older.[8,9]

Facial skin texture, such as wrinkling caused by photodamage, also influences the rating of attractiveness and beauty.[10] Periorbital features including the presence of festoons and crow's-feet in addition to perioral features such as the presence of wrinkles and fullness of the lips also influence the perception of age.[11] However, the age of individuals may affect which facial regions are aesthetically important both to themselves and when evaluating others. Sezgin and colleagues[12] grouped female cosmetic-surgery patients by age and asked which facial characteristics they evaluated in themselves or others. The older subjects examined the periorbita and jawline, whereas younger patients concentrated on the nose and skin.

General health questionnaires such as the GHQ 30 have been used to determine the impact of facial skin conditions (eg, acne) as well as the effects of treatment in individuals.[13] Patients undergoing facial rejuvenation procedures reported significant, positive effects on quality-of-life attributes when evaluated with the Derriford Appearance Scale.[14,15] The greatest improvements were in these factors (in descending order): general self-consciousness of appearance, social self-consciousness of appearance, self-consciousness of sexual and bodily appearance, negative self-concept, self-consciousness of facial appearance, and physical distress and dysfunction.

With the population aging in developed countries, attributable in part to improvements in health care and technology, surgical and nonsurgical therapies including cosmeceuticals and cosmetics are highly sought after to reduce one's perceived age.[16] Kosmadaki and Gilchrest[17] found that increased longevity is accompanied by significant interest in the quality of life and appearance. The demand in the United States, driven largely by the baby-boomer generation, has prompted the development of an armamentarium of methods for managing and optimizing facial skin color, texture, and shape. This article and the one that follows address 2 contemporary and relevant topics concerning photodamaged facial skin, because of its increasing prevalence.

This article addresses the strategies and available methods for measuring treatment outcomes, perhaps defined by the consumer/patient as "decrease in perceived age." The second article presents studies on facial rejuvenation that have used these quantitative methods to modify perceived age.

THE NATURE OF PHOTODAMAGED SKIN

Solar exposure at suberythemal levels, or below the exposure required to produce visible skin erythema, is sufficient to cause photodamage.[18] Histologically, photodamaged skin has the following features: increased epidermal thickness, a flattened dermal-epidermal junction, chronic inflammation, thickened walls in the microvascular circulation, lengthened and collapsed fibroblasts, reduced levels of types I and III collagen, increased elastin, and poor organization of the collagen fibrils.[19–23] These changes give rise to observable features including wrinkling, dyschromia, dryness, rough surface texture, rhytides, and keratosis.[24] In general, the extent of photodamage is positively associated with the amount of exposure to ultraviolet (UV) radiation and is observed more commonly in lighter-skinned individuals.[25,26] Skin pigmentation, more specifically melanin content, mitigates the effects of UV exposure in darker-skinned individuals (Fitzpatrick Type VI) having greater inherent photoprotection.

TREATMENT PLANNING AND OUTCOME MEASUREMENT

Plastic surgeons are highly skilled judges of skin damage with significant experience in a variety of techniques and strategies to restore the skin to a "chronologically" younger state. Visual methods are the foundation of clinical care and represent the gold standard for the assessment of skin color; however, assessment of the skin surface relies on clinical judgment.[1] Several visual scales are used to characterize the extent of photoaging, evaluate treatment response, appraise improvement, and determine patient satisfaction. Unfortunately, none have been established as the universal standard for the evaluation of photoaging.[27] Concomitantly, there are no widely accepted descriptions of normal skin. Drawbacks to visual methods of assessment include low reproducibility and variation in interobserver reliability.[28,29] Although the human visual system is uniquely sophisticated and integrative, assessors are limited as to what they can see and palpate at the skin surface. Consequently, the effectiveness of specific interventions is difficult to determine qualitatively and quantitatively. As the health care system emphasizes evidence-based care, prevention, quality, and cost-effectiveness, the requisite for objective measures of the status of cutaneous disease is expected to increase.

LITERATURE REVIEW: GRADING SCALES

Because photodamage affects the entire face, identification of a suitable "normal control" is a limitation of all grading scales. **Table 1** illustrates the visually based methods described in the literature for use by patients and physicians. Visual grading methods commonly use descriptors such as slight, mild, moderate, and severe to indicate the severity of cutaneous damage and area (percentage) of involvement relative to nearby areas of normal skin.[30,31] Scales for degree of cutaneous improvement and satisfaction use similarly vague terminology. The inherent problem with these scales is their subjectivity, in that they are not referenced against standards or quantitative change but rather rely on the evaluator's beliefs. The frame of reference of the judge and the interpretation of these terms is another confounding variable. Logically it follows that analysis of the literature is difficult at best, limiting the applicability of treatment results. The limitations of subjective measurements and the global need for standardized objective measurements have been noted.[32–35]

Alexiades-Armenakas and colleagues[24] have constructed a more objective 8-point grading scale to encompass the attributes of facial photodamage, shown in **Table 2**.[36–38] This schema includes rhytides, elastosis, dyschromia, erythema/telangiectasia, keratoses, texture, and laxity, and can be used as a series of individual scales or as a global composite. Skin color is a feature considered in the assessment of elastosis and erythema. Hyperpigmentation in terms of number and area of spots is graded in the assessment of dyschromia. Textural dimensions include wrinkles, keratoses, and surface roughness. Mechanical properties of tissue are judged based on the presence of folds, jowling, and bands. The attribute scores are based on the extent of involvement and severity. Composite grading scales using high-quality photographic images have also been developed and validated.[39] Specifically, these scales evaluate the effort required for treatment, identify the most problematic region, and estimate the subject's age, thereby providing a framework for the application of objective modalities. The most important individual scales do vary according to sex; however, they do not include other attributes of importance in determining perceived age, namely, color uniformity, hyperpigmentation, red color (erythema), yellow color, or fine surface texture. Together, these grading scales serve as the clinical foundation for selection and application of objective, quantitative methods.

QUANTITATIVE OBJECTIVE MEASUREMENT OF SKIN CHARACTERISTICS

An essential component to delivering optimum outcomes and maximizing patient satisfaction in the treatment of facial photodamage is the capability to identify appropriate treatment modalities and set patient expectations of potential improvement. Arguably, both depend on the capability to measure facial characteristics before and after treatment. The following sections have as a backdrop these questions:

- Are objective, quantitative methods more effective than subjective, experience-based assessment?
- Can clinical judgment adequately predict the treatment effects on the skin at the histologic levels of the dermis, epidermis, and stratum corneum?
- What is the relationship between findings from either the clinical examination or objective assessment and customer/patient perception of improvement?
- Can this be used to predict the outcome of any given procedure for any given patient?
- What is the effect of any particular treatment as a function of initial photoaging severity?

To be effective, objective measurements need to (1) determine whether a real change has occurred as a result of an intervention, (2) accurately show that a condition is different from the normal, (3) be valid as defined by correlating with the gold standard of visual clinical assessment, (4) be reproducible, and (5) be clinically feasible.[40]

TECHNICAL ASPECTS: QUANTITATION OF SKIN COLOR

The human eye perceives color when 3 types of cone cells within the retina receive and mediate light. The peak absorption ranges of these long, medium, and short cones are at 564 to 580 nm, 534 to 545 nm, and 420 to 440 nm, respectively, corresponding roughly to the red, green, and blue

Table 1
Visually based evaluation methods for facial skin[a]

Outcome	Description	Evaluators
Improvement[89] Overall Specific attribute	Five point scale, where 1 = no improvement, 5 = dramatic improvement	Patients, clinicians, nonmedical judges
Satisfaction[90] Overall Specific attribute	Eleven-point scale, where 0 = not satisfied, 10 = most satisfied	Patients
Changes[90] Overall rejuvenation Tone/brightness Pigmented lesions, number Pigmented lesions, lightening Wrinkles Elasticity	Five-point scale, with increments: much worse, slightly worse, no change, slight improvement, improvement[90]	Patients
Improvement[91]	Five-point scale, where 0 = worse, 1 = none, 2 = fair, 3 = good, 4 = excellent	Patients
Satisfaction[92]	Six-point scale, where 0 = none, 1 = mild improvement, 2 = moderate improvement, 3 = good, 4 = very good, 5 = excellent	Patients
Improvement[92] Hyperpigmentation Telangiectasias, skin texture Firmness	Six-point scale for each, where 0 = none, 1 = mild improvement, 2 = moderate improvement, 3 = good, 4 = very good, 5 = excellent	Physicians
Desirability[93] Skin texture, tone, fine lines Age spots, smoothness Softness, pore size Blotchiness Skin moisturization	Ten-point scale for each, where 1 = undesirable, 10 = desirable	Patients
Efficacy[93,94] Fine wrinkling, skin dullness Mottled hyperpigmentation Blotchiness Appearance of milia, acne, large pores	Ten-point scale for each, where 0 = none, 9 = severe	Physicians
Global assessment[93,94] Overall skin texture, tone, appearance	Ten-point scale for each, where 0 = very good, 9 = very poor	Physicians
Glogau Photoaging Classification[95]	Four classifications based on wrinkles, pigmentary changes, keratoses, age, and interaction with makeup Type 1: no wrinkles, early photoaging, mild pigmentary changes, no keratoses, minimal wrinkles Type II: wrinkles in motion, early to moderate photoaging, early senile lentigines visible, keratoses palpable but not visible, parallel smile lines beginning to appear Type III: wrinkles at rest, advanced photoaging, obvious dyschromia, telangiectasia, visible keratoses, wrinkles even when not moving Type IV: only wrinkles, severe photoaging, yellow-gray color, prior skin malignancies, wrinkled throughout, no normal skin	Physicians

(*continued on next page*)

Table 1
(continued)

Outcome	Description	Evaluators
Fitzpatrick Wrinkle Scale[96]	Nine-point scale based on wrinkling and degree of elastosis, where 1–3 is fine wrinkles and mild elastosis (fine textural changes, subtle accentuated skin lines), 4–6 is fine to moderate-depth wrinkles and/or moderate number of lines and moderate elastosis (distinct popular elastosis, individual papules with yellow translucency, dyschromia), 7–9 is fine to deep wrinkles and/or numerous lines with and without redundant skin folds and severe elastosis (multipapular and confluent, thickened yellow and pallid, approaching or consistent with cutis rhomboidalis)	Physicians

[a] References indicate reports in which the method was described and/or used.

regions of the color spectrum.[41,42] The perceived skin color arises when visible light interacts with components within the skin, including the constitutive pigments: melanins (yellow to brown), oxygenated hemoglobin (red), deoxyhemoglobin (blue-purple), bilirubin (yellow), and carotene (yellow).[43] The observed skin color arises from the interplay of light with components of the stratum corneum, epidermis, and dermis, which is determined by diffuse reflection, scattering, and absorption of light within the skin.[43,44] Of the total incident light contacting the skin surface, approximately 5% is reflected back to the eye with the remainder being transmitted, absorbed, or scattered by structural and chemical elements within the aforementioned layers of the skin, as represented in **Fig. 1**.[2] The stratum corneum transmits light while the epidermis and dermis absorb light because of the presence of melanin and hemoglobin. Melanin is synthesized by the melanocytes, a dendritic cell, in the basal layer of the epidermis, and is transferred to keratinocytes throughout the epidermis.[45] Oxygenated blood in the dermal capillaries and vascular plexus, and deoxygenated blood (blue-purple) in the dermal venules also contribute to skin color.[46] The yellow pigmentation is caused by carotene in the epidermis. Bilirubin (yellow) is deposited in the epidermis as a result of precipitation in phospholipid membranes and is leaked into extravascular regions coupled with albumin.[47] Finally, light is scattered within the epidermis, dermis, and subcutaneous fat.[48]

OPTICAL IMAGING METHODS

For more than 50 years plastic surgeons have relied on photography to document patients' characteristics for operative planning and to evaluate surgical outcomes, using standardized lighting, collection, and processing procedures.[49,50] However, though used routinely in the skin-care industry, particularly for cosmetics to demonstrate treatment effects, color imaging has not been widely applied to the evaluation of cutaneous conditions in health care. Recently, imaging techniques have been developed in other dermatologic areas to improve objectivity by quantifying skin features (eg, erythema, depigmentation, abrasion)[48,51,52] as well as wounds, burns, lesions, blanching, skin atrophy, and disease (eg, psoriasis).[29,52–56]

The subject of skin imaging and analysis has been reviewed previously.[50,57,58] This article and the one that follows focus on skin imaging related to photodamage in the context of restoring facial skin.

Skin Color

A standardized procedure for the collection of high-resolution digital images including controlled lighting, white balance, and color correction facilitates the comparison of skin conditions at multiple time points (pretreatment vs posttreatment in real time). To be useful, the detailed color information from photographs must be made available during the live clinical examination. Perception of skin color depends on the illuminating light and skin interactions (see **Fig. 1**) as well as contributions of the observer.[59] The red, green, blue (RGB) tristimulus color space used in digital cameras is an additive model based on the chromaticities (quantity of color specified by dominant wavelength) of red, green, and blue additive primaries.[60] Unfortunately, this system cannot be easily related to the way the human eye perceives color. Consequently, in the process of extracting relevant features, RGB images are first converted to International Commission on Illumination (CIE) 1976 L*b* (CIELAB) space, where colors are in a uniform 3-dimensional space. Specifically, L* is the lightness-darkness (L* of 100 = white and L* of 0 = black), a* is red-green

Table 2
Comprehensive grading scale for photodamage by Alexiades-Armenakas

Grade	Description	Rhytides	Elastosis	Dyschromia	Erythema/ Telangiectasia	Keratoses	Texture	Laxity
0	None	None	None	None	None	None	None	None
1	Mild	In motion, few superficial	Early, minimal, yellow hue	Few (1–3) discrete, small (<5 mm) lentigines	Pink E or few T localized to single site	Few	Subtle irregularity	Localized to NL folds
1.5	Mild	In motion, multiple superficial	Yellow hue or early, localized PO, EB	Several (3–6) discrete small lentigines	Pink E or several T localized to 2 sites	Several	Mild irregularity in few areas	Localized, NL and early ML folds
2	Moderate	At rest, few localized, superficial	Yellow hue, localized PO, EB	Multiple (7–10) small lentigines	Red E or multiple T localized to 2 sites	Multiple, small	Rough in few, localized sites	Localized, NL/ML folds, early jowls, early SM
2.5	Moderate	At rest, multiple localized, superficial	Yellow hue, PO and malar EB	Multiple, small and few large lentigines	Red E or multiple T, localized to 3 sites	Multiple, large	Rough in several localized areas	Localized, prominent NL/ ML folds, jowls and SM
3	Advanced	At rest, multiple forehead, PO and perioral, superficial	Yellow hue, EB involving PO, malar, and other sites	Many (10–20) small and large lentigines	Violaceous E or many T, many sites	Many	Rough in multiple, localized sites	Prominent NL/ML folds, jowls and SM, early neck strands
3.5	Advanced	At rest, few, generalized, superficial, deep	Deep yellow hue, extensive EB, little normal skin	Numerous (>20) or multiple large with little normal skin	Violaceous E, numerous T, little normal skin	Little normal skin	Mostly rough, little normal skin	Deep NL/ML folds, prominent jowls and SM, prominent neck strands
4	Severe	Throughout, numerous, extensively distributed, deep	Deep yellow, EB throughout, comedones	Numerous, extensive, no normal skin	Deep, violaceous E, numerous T throughout	No normal skin	Rough throughout	Marked NL/ML folds, jowls and SM, neck redundancy and strands

Abbreviations: E, erythema; EB, elastotic beads; ML, melolabial; NL, nasolabial; PO, periorbital; SM, submandibular; T, telangiectasia.

Adapted from Alexiades-Armenakas MR, Dover JS, Arndt KA. The spectrum of laser skin resurfacing: nonablative, fractional, and ablative laser resurfacing. J Am Acad Dermatol 2008;58(5):719–37. [quiz: 738–40]; and Alexiades-Armenakas M. A quantitative and comprehensive grading scale for rhytides, laxity, and photoaging. J Drugs Dermatol 2006;5(8):808–9.

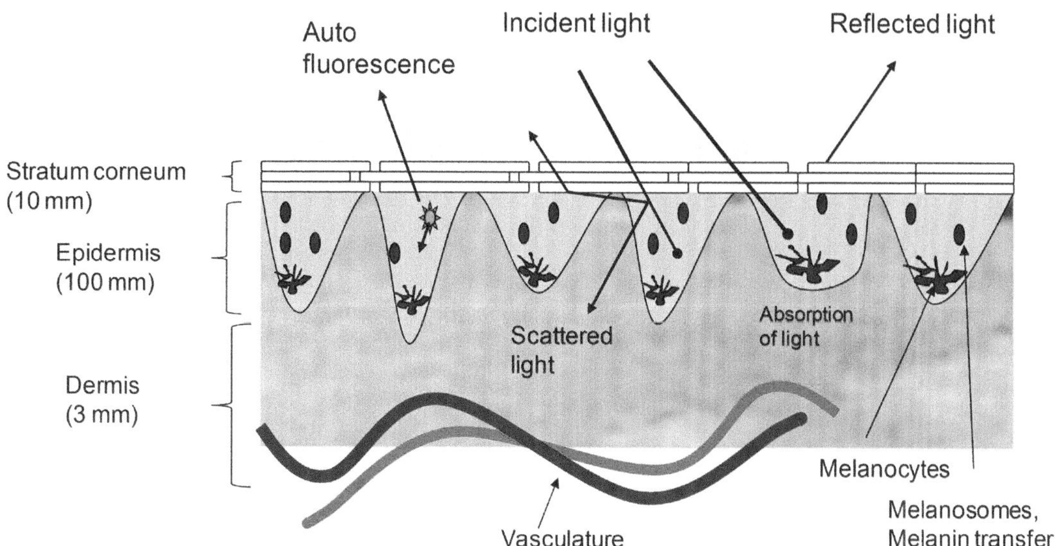

Fig. 1. Energy (light) interactions with the skin.

(positive to negative, respectively) and b* is yellow-blue (positive to negative).[42,61] Images can then be separated into 3 channels, L, a*, and b*, with standard image-processing software (ImagJ freeware; National Institutes of Health) for the analysis of redness (a*, red-green color), blue color (b*, blue-yellow), and lightness (L), without the confounding effects of the full-color digital images. Channel contrasts can be increased further to examine and enhance the areas with more extreme color, for example, areas of greater inflammation. The percentage of red pixels greater than the mean plus 1 or more standard deviations has been calculated to determine excess red color for burn scars, irritant dermatitis, and infantile hemangiomas, and to quantify blue color changes for infantile hemangiomas.[62–65] The use of higher-order statistics has allowed the assessment of glossiness from the L image, red-spot identification from the a* image, and symmetry of yellow color from the b* image.[8] These findings suggest that the area of involvement and severity of elastosis (yellow coloration) and erythema/telangiectasia from the Alexiades-Armenakas grading scale (see **Table 2**) can be quantified with high-resolution color images. Thus, incorporation of these statistical terms may provide an improved model for the evaluation of perceived age and treatment.

Solar Lentigines and Hyperpigmentation

Analysis of hyperpigmented regions such as solar lentigines, caused by UV exposure or injury, is important because these areas are specifically targeted by treatments for facial skin. Controlled digital-image capture and analysis systems have been developed to quantify the total area constituted by multiple hyperpigmented spots on the face (cheek and periorbital regions).[66] Following extraction of the blue channel of the RGB image, the spots have been selected, extracted, and compared with the surrounding skin using CIE L* a* b* values. This method is of sufficient sensitivity to determine the effectiveness of treatment modalities relative to a vehicle control.[67] Miyamoto and colleagues[68] described a facial imaging system with standardized, reproducible positioning of subjects that controlled for facial expression, using black drapes to cover hair and clothing. This precise positioning permitted accurate and unbiased comparison of images. Images were captured using cross-polarization (perpendicular polarizers on the camera and lighting) to eliminate glare from the skin surface caused by variables such as moisture or oil, and to visualize the subepidermal microvasculature.[69] An image-analysis algorithm was then developed to select and measure the hyperpigmented spot size within a region of interest and report them as percent area. The resulting software displayed the affected areas so that the distribution of skin damage could be visualized by the clinician and patient (**Fig. 2**). When this analysis is conducted before and after treatment, the patient can readily observe the changes. This technology can also be used to identify areas of more severe photodamage for targeted resurfacing procedures.

Digital facial images collected with cross-polarization can also be analyzed for specific features of melanin and hemoglobin distribution

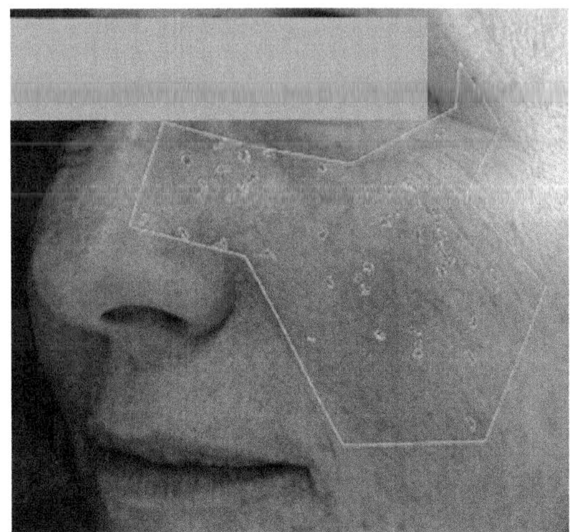

Fig. 2. Facial image showing spots within a region of interest on the cheek.

for further evaluation. By characterizing the type and severity of photodamage, treatment in regard of the selection of resurfacing modality and determination of outcomes may be devised. Two-compartment tissue models and regression methods have been described.[70] A commercially available imaging system (VISIA, VISIA-CR; Canfield Imaging Systems, Fairfield, NJ) has been used for evaluating the effectiveness of facial skin treatments as well as analyzing the skin color and hyperpigmented spot measurements already described.[71] The system also uses proprietary software to quantify melanin (brown spots) and vascular features from the red channel, as shown in **Fig. 3**.[72] Images are analyzed for the total hyperpigmented spot area, texture area, total wrinkle length, and color (erythema, yellow coloration). When images are taken under UV, the melanin pigmentation below the skin surface can be easily visualized and quantified. UV light can also be used to detect the pigment porphyrin that is present in the bacteria *Propionibacterium acnes* found in pores. Porphyrin fluoresces under UV light and can therefore be used to quantify bacteria. **Fig. 4** shows sample images taken with the VISIA system evaluated for percent area of spots, wrinkles, texture, pores, brown spots, red areas, and porphyrins. These imaging methods can be used to measure severity and area of coverage of dyschromia and rhytides as described by Alexiades-Armenakas (see **Table 2**).

The second imaging technique, known as spectrophotometric intracutaneous analysis (SIA), uses

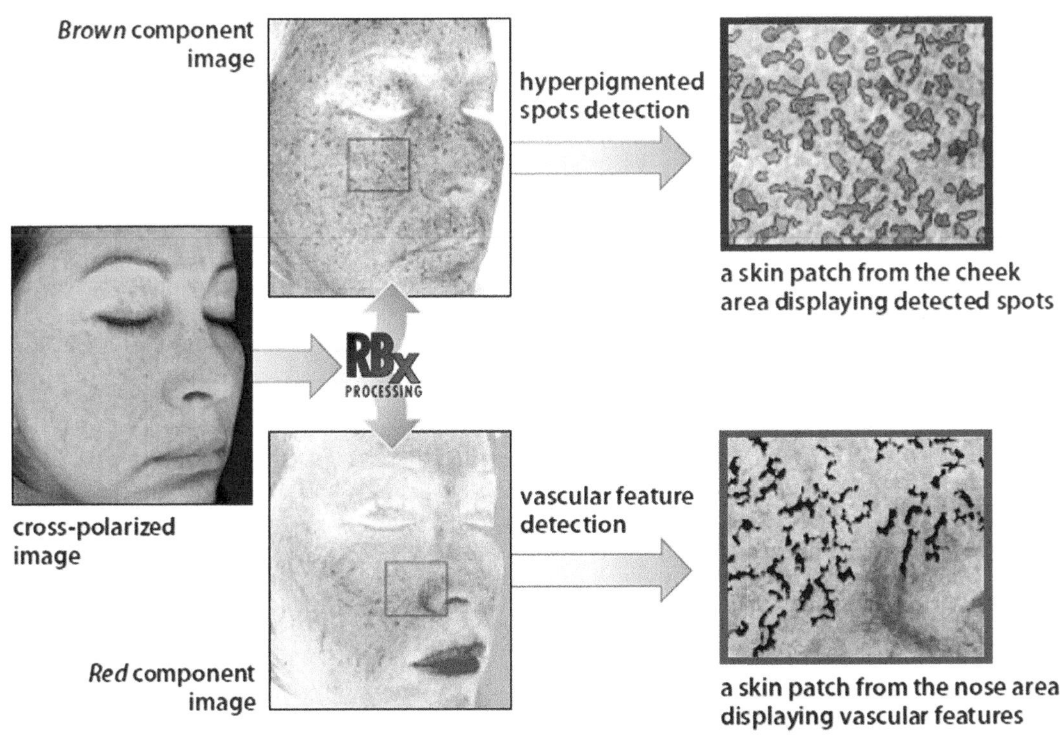

Fig. 3. Image analysis of a facial photograph taken with cross-polarization, showing hyperpigmented spots and redness related to hemoglobin. (*Courtesy of* Canfield Imaging Systems, Fairfield, NJ. Available at http://www.canfieldsci.com/FileLibrary/RBX%20tech%20overview-LoRz1.pdf).

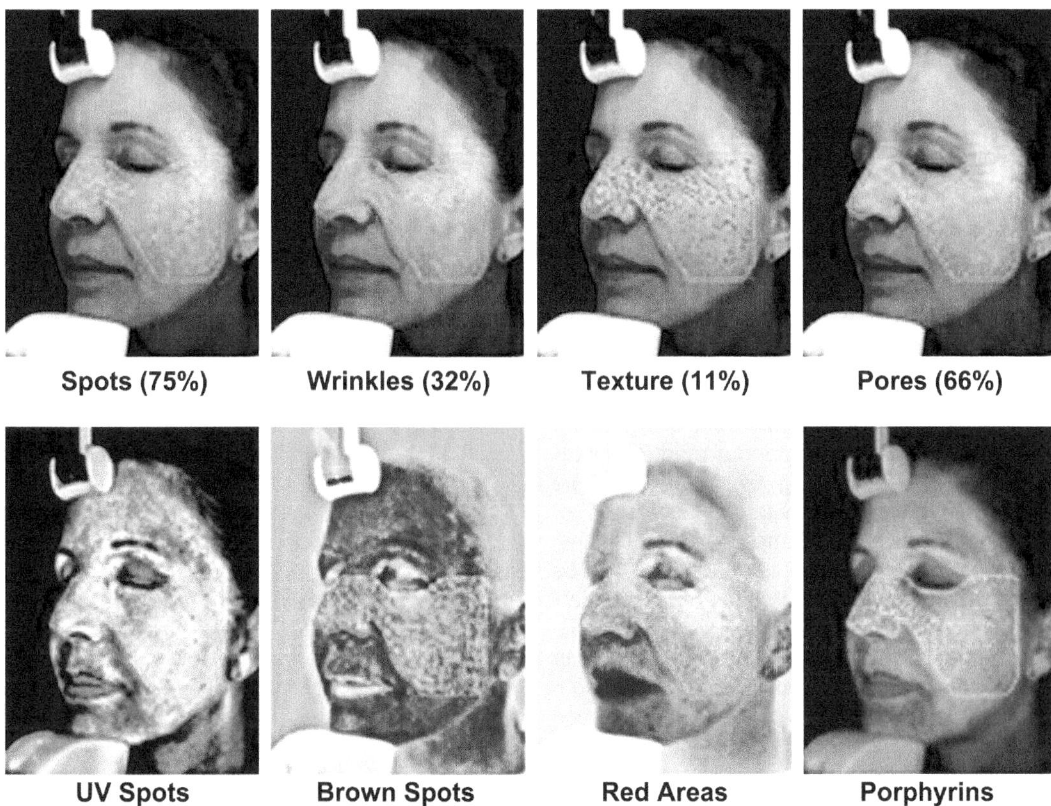

Fig. 4. Sample images collected and processed using the VISIA complexion analysis system. (*Courtesy of* Canfield Imaging Systems, Fairfield, NJ. Available at http://www.canfieldsci.com/FileLibrary/RBX%20tech%20overview-LoRz1.pdf).

diffuse reflectance spectroscopy over 400 to 1000 nm. SIA has the capability of extracting features of skin-lesion morphology, including papillary dermal collagen, total melanin, oxyhemoglobin, and deoxyhemoglobin, for a region of 12 to 24 mm diameter[73] or for the entire area of involvement.[74,75] Because of the presence of melanin, SIA has also been applied to quantify the effects of long-term UV exposure leading to hyperpigmented spots, and to evaluate the perception of age, health status, and common skin conditions.[73,76,77]

Skin Elasticity and Laxity

Exposure to UV radiation also results in dermal changes, as evidenced by reduced levels of types I and III collagen, increased elastin, and poor organization of the collagen fibrils. These effects are manifested in the loss of tissue elasticity and slower recovery from applied mechanical stress.

Skin restoration methods, including dermabrasion, ablative CO_2 laser resurfacing, and fractional CO_2 laser treatment, have been shown to increase the elasticity of facial skin as measured with biomechanical methods[78,79] Quantitative assessment of the mechanical properties of tissue has been used to understand the factors that influence scar formation[80–83] and to evaluate treatments.[84] Biomechanical skin properties have been quantified with various suction devices,[85,86] including the Cutometer 575 (Courage and Khazaka GmbH, Cologne, Germany) and the BTC-2000 (Surgical Research Laboratory Inc, Nashville, TN).[87] The changes in skin elasticity may be inferred from visual or photographic methods, but the dynamic interaction of tissue deformation and assessment of skin recovery are likely to be related to functional tissue changes. Biomechanical measurements measure the changes in laxity (see **Table 2**).

FUTURE PERSPECTIVE

Imaging methods used for assessing outcomes are always related to, and usually correlated with, clinical judgment.[58] The relationship between the clinician's assessment of outcomes and customer/patient perception of treatment success is important, particularly because of the elective and discretionary nature of skin-restoration procedures. Differences between clinicians and patients in perceived outcomes, whereby "technical" or clinician perceived improvements are inconsistent with the patient's self-analysis, have been reported and may occur frequently.[78,88,89] For instance, patients and physicians may be measuring different attributes, particularly those of neurosensory origin that cannot be observed or palpated.

The finding that optimization of skin coloration can reduce perceived age by up to 20 years is particularly intriguing and potentially serves as a benchmark for the measurement of treatment effectiveness. The use of standardized, quantitative energy-based imaging techniques has the potential to generate substantial databases of treatment effectiveness. Patients of similar ages, skin types, and degrees of photodamage can be compared and the findings used to optimize treatment. The VISIA system has a feature whereby the patient's facial images can be compared with a large dataset of similar skin types and/or age. Therefore, this system can be used to determine "perceived age" to assess how the treatment outcome corresponds to the appearance of younger subjects. To date, however, the data suggest that the quantitation of facial skin characteristics will need to be multimodal, as one method will be unable to provide sufficient measures to predict outcome or patient satisfaction.

The early detection of photodamage or tissue injury depends on objective, quantitative skin-imaging methods. In this era of globalization, assessment tools and models demand that skin imaging is done successfully and completely across an extraordinarily diverse population of humans. The need for clinical tools and techniques that can be rapidly learned and used to direct patient care is driven by an increased understanding of the complex processes in the skin as well as a desire to deliver cost-effective care that meets patient/consumer expectations of good quality of life. In conclusion, the generation of a coherent framework with quantitative end points may be facilitated by the reapplication of validated, published methods from one condition to another.

REFERENCES

1. Galdino GM, Vogel JE, Vander Kolk CA. Standardizing digital photography: it's not all in the eye of the beholder. Plast Reconstr Surg 2001;108(5):1334–44.
2. Anderson RR, Parrish JA. The optics of human skin. J Invest Dermatol 1981;77(1):13–9.
3. Taylor S, Westerhof W, Im S, et al. Noninvasive techniques for the evaluation of skin color. J Am Acad Dermatol 2006;54(5 Suppl 2):S282–90.
4. Fink B, Grammer K, Matts PJ. Visual skin color distribution plays a role in the perception of age, attractiveness, and health of female faces. Evol Hum Behav 2006;27(6):433–42.
5. Matts PJ, Fink B. Chronic sun damage and the perception of age, health and attractiveness. Photochem Photobiol Sci 2010;9(4):421–31.
6. Fink B, Bunse L, Matts PJ, et al. Visible skin colouration predicts perception of male facial age, health and attractiveness. Int J Cosmet Sci 2012;34(4):307–10.
7. Caspers PJ, Lucassen GW, Carter EA, et al. In vivo confocal Raman microspectroscopy of the skin: noninvasive determination of molecular concentration profiles. J Invest Dermatol 2001;116(3):434–42.
8. Arce-Lopera C, Igarashi T, Nakao K, et al. Image statistics on the age perception of human skin. Skin Res Technol 2012. http://dx.doi.org/10.1111/j.1600-0846.2012.00638.x. [Epub ahead of print].
9. Dobke M, Chung C, Takabe K. Facial aesthetic preferences among Asian women: are all oriental Asians the same? Aesthetic Plast Surg 2006;30(3):342–7.
10. Fink B, Grammer K, Thornhill R. Human (*Homo sapiens*) facial attractiveness in relation to skin texture and color. J Comp Psychol 2001;115(1):92–9.
11. Nkengne A, Bertin C, Stamatas GN, et al. Influence of facial skin attributes on the perceived age of Caucasian women. J Eur Acad Dermatol Venereol 2008;22(8):982–91.
12. Sezgin B, Findikcioglu K, Kaya B, et al. Mirror on the wall: a study of women's perception of facial features as they age. Aesthet Surg J 2012;32(4):421–5.
13. Samson N, Fink B, Matts PJ. Visible skin condition and perception of human facial appearance. Int J Cosmet Sci 2010;32(3):167–84.
14. Litner JA, Rotenberg BW, Dennis M, et al. Impact of cosmetic facial surgery on satisfaction with appearance and quality of life. Arch Facial Plast Surg 2008;10(2):79–83.
15. Gunn DA, Rexbye H, Griffiths CE, et al. Why some women look young for their age. PLoS One 2009;4(12):e8021.
16. Mayes AE, Murray PG, Gunn DA, et al. Ageing appearance in China: biophysical profile of facial skin and its relationship to perceived age. J Eur Acad Dermatol Venereol 2009;24(3):341–8.
17. Kosmadaki MG, Gilchrest BA. The demographics of aging in the United States: implications for dermatology. Arch Dermatol 2002;138(11):1427–8.
18. Seite S, Fourtanier A, Moyal D, et al. Photodamage to human skin by suberythemal exposure to solar ultraviolet radiation can be attenuated by sunscreens: a review. Br J Dermatol 2010;163(5):903–14.

19. El-Domyati M, Attia S, Saleh F, et al. Intrinsic aging vs. photoaging: a comparative histopathological, immunohistochemical, and ultrastructural study of skin. Exp Dermatol 2002;11(5):398–405.
20. Lavker RM. Cutaneous aging: chronic versus photoaging. In: Gilchrest BA, editor. Photodamage. Cambridge (England): Blackwell Science; 1995. p. 123–35.
21. Lavker RM, Kligman AM. Chronic heliodermatitis: a morphologic evaluation of chronic actinic dermal damage with emphasis on the role of mast cells. J Invest Dermatol 1988;90(3):325–30.
22. Lewis KG, Bercovitch L, Dill SW, et al. Acquired disorders of elastic tissue: part I. Increased elastic tissue and solar elastotic syndromes. J Am Acad Dermatol 2004;51(1):1–21 [quiz: 22–4].
23. Varani J, Schuger L, Dame MK, et al. Reduced fibroblast interaction with intact collagen as a mechanism for depressed collagen synthesis in photodamaged skin. J Invest Dermatol 2004;122(6):1471–9.
24. Alexiades-Armenakas MR, Dover JS, Arndt KA. The spectrum of laser skin resurfacing: nonablative, fractional, and ablative laser resurfacing. J Am Acad Dermatol 2008;58(5):719–37 [quiz: 738–40].
25. Kligman A, Kligman L. Photoaging. In: Freedberg IM, Eisen AZ, Wolff K, et al, editors. Fitzpatrick's dermatology in general medicine. New York: McGraw-Hill; 1999. p. 1717–23.
26. Timilshina S, Bhuvan KC, Khanal M, et al. The influence of ethnic origin on the skin photoageing: nepalese study. Int J Cosmet Sci 2011;33(6):553–9.
27. Elsner P, Fluhr JW, Gehring W, et al. Anti-aging data and support claims–consensus statement. J Dtsch Dermatol Ges 2011;9(Suppl 3):S1–32.
28. Kawai K, Kawai J, Nakagawa M, et al. Effects of detergents. In: Wilhelm K, Elsner P, Berardesca E, et al, editors. Bioengineering of the skin: skin surface imaging and analysis. Boca Raton (FL): CRC Press; 1997. p. 303–14.
29. Mattsson U, Jonsson A, Jontell M, et al. Digital image analysis (DIA) of colour changes in human skin exposed to standardized thermal injury and comparison with laser Doppler measurements. Comput Methods Programs Biomed 1996;50(1):31–42.
30. Wagner JK, Jovel C, Norton HL, et al. Comparing quantitative measures of erythema, pigmentation and skin response using reflectometry. Pigment Cell Res 2002;15(5):379–84.
31. Jordan WE, Lawson KD, Berg RW, et al. Diaper dermatitis: frequency and severity among a general infant population. Pediatr Dermatol 1986;3(3):198–207.
32. Kim SC, Kim DW, Hong JP, et al. A quantitative evaluation of pigmented skin lesions using the L*a*b* color coordinates. Yonsei Med J 2000;41(3):333–9.
33. O'Doherty J, McNamara P, Clancy NT, et al. Comparison of instruments for investigation of microcirculatory blood flow and red blood cell concentration. J Biomed Opt 2009;14(3):034025.
34. Pickering J, Mordon S, Brunetaud J. The objective reporting of laser treatment of port wine stains. Lasers Med Sci 1992;7(1):415–21.
35. Haedersdal M, Efsen J, Gniadecka M, et al. Changes in skin redness, pigmentation, echostructure, thickness, and surface contour after 1 pulsed dye laser treatment of port-wine stains in children. Arch Dermatol 1998;134(2):175–81.
36. Alexiades-Armenakas M. A quantitative and comprehensive grading scale for rhytides, laxity, and photoaging. J Drugs Dermatol 2006;5(8):808–9.
37. McCollough EG. The McCollough Facial Rejuvenation System: a condition-specific classification algorithm. Facial Plast Surg 2011;27(1):112–23.
38. McCollough EG, Ha CD. The McCollough Facial Rejuvenation System: expanding the scope of a condition-specific algorithm. Facial Plast Surg 2012;28(1):102–15.
39. Rzany B, Carruthers A, Carruthers J, et al. Validated composite assessment scales for the global face. Dermatol Surg 2012;38(2 Spec No):294–308.
40. Bendeck SE, Jacobe HT. Ultrasound as an outcome measure to assess disease activity in disorders of skin thickening: an example of the use of radiologic techniques to assess skin disease. Dermatol Ther 2007;20(2):86–92.
41. Hunt RW. The reproduction of color. 6th edition. Chichester (England): Wiley; 2004.
42. Wyszecki G, Stiles WS. Color science: concepts and methods, quantitative data and formulae. 2nd edition. New York: Wiley; 1982.
43. Chardon A, Cretois I, Hourseau C. Skin colour typology and suntanning pathways. Int J Cosmet Sci 1991;13(4):191–208.
44. Stamatas GN, Zmudzka BZ, Kollias N, et al. Non-invasive measurements of skin pigmentation in situ. Pigment Cell Res 2004;17(6):618–26.
45. Nordlund JJ, Boissy RE. The biology of melanocytes. In: Freinkel RK, Woodley DT, editors. The biology of the skin. New York: Parthenon Publishing Group; 2001. p. 113–31.
46. Morgan JE, Gilchrest B, Goldwyn RM. Skin pigmentation. Current concepts and relevance to plastic surgery. Plast Reconstr Surg 1975;56(6):617–28.
47. Knudsen A, Brodersen R. Skin colour and bilirubin in neonates. Arch Dis Child 1989;64(4):605–9.
48. Takiwaki H. Measurement of skin color: practical application and theoretical considerations. J Med Invest 1998;44(3–4):121–6.
49. Imaging. In: The American heritage science dictionary. Orlando (FL): Houghton Mifflin Company; 2005.
50. Perednia DA. What dermatologists should know about digital imaging. J Am Acad Dermatol 1991;25(1 Pt 1):89–108.
51. Coelho SG, Miller SA, Zmudzka BZ, et al. Quantification of UV-induced erythema and pigmentation

using computer-assisted digital image evaluation. Photochem Photobiol 2006;82(3):651–5.

52. Setaro M, Sparavigna A. Quantification of erythema using digital camera and computer-based colour image analysis: a multicentre study. Skin Res Technol 2002;8(2):84–8.
53. Aspres N, Egerton IB, Lim AC, et al. Imaging the skin. Australas J Dermatol 2003;44(1):19–27.
54. Fogelberg A, Ioffreda M, Helm KF. The utility of digital clinical photographs in dermatopathology. J Cutan Med Surg 2004;8(2):116–21.
55. Nystrom J, Geladi P, Lindholm-Sethson B, et al. Objective measurements of radiotherapy-induced erythema. Skin Res Technol 2004;10(4):242–50.
56. Oduncu H, Hoppe A, Clark M, et al. Analysis of skin wound images using digital color image processing: a preliminary communication. Int J Low Extrem Wounds 2004;3(3):151–6.
57. Rallan D, Harland CC. Skin imaging: is it clinically useful? Clin Exp Dermatol 2004;29(5):453–9.
58. Visscher MO. Imaging skin: past, present and future perspectives. G Ital Dermatol Venereol 2010;145(1): 11–27.
59. Weatherall IL, Coombs BD. Skin color measurements in terms of CIELAB color space values. J Invest Dermatol 1992;99(4):468–73.
60. Susstrunk S, Buckley R, Swen S. Standard RBG color spaces. In: IS&T/SID 7th Color Imaging Conference. Scottsdale, November 16–19, 1999. p. 127–34.
61. CIE publications No. 15.2. Colorimetry. 2nd edition. Vienna (Austria): Central Bureau of the CIE; 1986.
62. Canning J, Barford B, Sullivan D, et al. Use of digital photography and image analysis techniques to quantify erythema in health care workers. Skin Res Technol 2009;15(1):24–34.
63. Bailey JK, Burkes SA, Visscher MO, et al. Multimodal quantitative analysis of early pulsed-dye laser treatment of scars at a pediatric burn hospital. Dermatol Surg 2012;38(9):1490–6.
64. Visscher M, Burkes S, Wickett R, et al. Use of multimodal quantitative imaging to determine stage and treatment response of infantile hemangiomas. In: International Society for the Study of Vascular Anomalies. Malmo (Sweden); June 16–19, 2012.
65. Whitmer K, Barford B, Turner M, et al. Digital image analysis of facial erythema over time in persons with varied skin pigmentation. Skin Res Technol 2011. http://dx.doi.org/10.1111/j.1600-0846.2011.00505.x. [Epub ahead of print].
66. Serup J. Skin irritation: objective characterization in a clinical perspective. In: Wilhelm KP, Elsner P, Berardesca E, et al, editors. Bioengineering of the skin: skin surface imaging and analysis. Boca Raton (FL): CRC Press; 1997. p. 261–73.
67. Stephen ID, Coetzee V, Law Smith M, et al. Skin blood perfusion and oxygenation colour affect perceived human health. PLoS One 2009;4(4): e5083.
68. Miyamoto K, Takiwaki H, Hillebrand GG, et al. Development of a digital imaging system for objective measurement of hyperpigmented spots on the face. Skin Res Technol 2002;8(4):227–35.
69. O'Doherty J, Henricson J, Anderson C, et al. Sub-epidermal imaging using polarized light spectroscopy for assessment of skin microcirculation. Skin Res Technol 2007;13(4):472–84.
70. Nishidate I, Aizu Y, Mishina H. Estimation of melanin and hemoglobin in skin tissue using multiple regression analysis aided by Monte Carlo simulation. J Biomed Opt 2004;9(4):700–10.
71. Bissett DL, Oblong JE, Berge CA. Niacinamide: A B vitamin that improves aging facial skin appearance. Dermatol Surg 2005;31(7 Pt 2):860–5 [discussion: 865].
72. Demirli R, Otto P, Viswanathan R, et al. RBX^{TM} technology overview. Fairfield (CA): Canfield Imaging Systems; 2007.
73. Moncrieff M, Cotton S, Claridge E, et al. Spectrophotometric intracutaneous analysis: a new technique for imaging pigmented skin lesions. Br J Dermatol 2002;146(3):448–57.
74. Matts PJ, Dykes PJ, Marks R. The distribution of melanin in skin determined in vivo. Br J Dermatol 2007;156(4):620–8.
75. Preece S, Cotton SD, Claridge E. Imaging the pigments of skin with a technique which is invariant to changes in surface geometry and intensity of illuminating light. In: Barber D, editor. Proceedings of Medical Image Understanding and Analysis. Malvern (PA): British Machine Vision Association; 2003. p. 145–8.
76. Kollias N, Seo I, Bargo PR. Interpreting diffuse reflectance for in vivo skin reactions in terms of chromophores. J Biophotonics 2010;3(1–2):15–24.
77. Jerajani HR, Mizoguchi H, Li J, et al. The effects of a daily facial lotion containing vitamins B3 and E and provitamin B5 on the facial skin of Indian women: a randomized, double-blind trial. Indian J Dermatol Venereol Leprol 2010;76(1):20–6.
78. Kitzmiller WJ, Visscher M, Page DA, et al. A controlled evaluation of dermabrasion versus CO_2 laser resurfacing for the treatment of perioral wrinkles. Plast Reconstr Surg 2000;106(6):1366–72 [discussion: 1373–4].
79. Naouri M, Atlan M, Perrodeau E, et al. Skin tightening induced by fractional CO(2) laser treatment: quantified assessment of variations in mechanical properties of the skin. J Cosmet Dermatol 2012; 11(3):201–6.
80. Corr DT, Gallant-Behm CL, Shrive NG, et al. Biomechanical behavior of scar tissue and uninjured skin in a porcine model. Wound Repair Regen 2009;17(2):250–9.

81. Gordon A, Kozin ED, Keswani SG, et al. Permissive environment in postnatal wounds induced by adenoviral-mediated overexpression of the anti-inflammatory cytokine interleukin-10 prevents scar formation. Wound Repair Regen 2008;16(1):70–9.
82. McHugh AA, Fowlkes BJ, Maevsky EI, et al. Biomechanical alterations in normal skin and hypertrophic scar after thermal injury. J Burn Care Rehabil 1997; 18(2):104–8.
83. Hollander DA, Erli HJ, Theisen A, et al. Standardized qualitative evaluation of scar tissue properties in an animal wound healing model. Wound Repair Regen 2003;11(2):150–7.
84. Burkes S, Bailey J, Visscher M, et al. Multimodal quantitative analysis of pediatric burn scars treated with the pulse dye laser. Chicago: American Burn Association; 2011.
85. Balbir-Gurman A, Denton CP, Nichols B, et al. Non-invasive measurement of biomechanical skin properties in systemic sclerosis. Ann Rheum Dis 2002; 61(3):237–41.
86. Cua AB, Wilhelm KP, Maibach HI. Elastic properties of human skin: relation to age, sex, and anatomical region. Arch Dermatol Res 1990;282(5):283–8.
87. Smalls LK, Randall Wickett R, Visscher MO. Effect of dermal thickness, tissue composition, and body site on skin biomechanical properties. Skin Res Technol 2006;12(1):43–9.
88. Coimbra M, Rohrich RJ, Chao J, et al. A prospective controlled assessment of microdermabrasion for damaged skin and fine rhytides. Plast Reconstr Surg 2004;113(5):1438–43 [discussion: 1444].
89. Kitzmiller WJ, Visscher MO, Maclennan S, et al. Comparison of a series of superficial chemical peels with a single midlevel chemical peel for the correction of facial actinic damage. Aesthet Surg J 2003; 23(5):339–44.
90. Shin JW, Lee DH, Choi SY, et al. Objective and non-invasive evaluation of photorejuvenation effect with intense pulsed light treatment in Asian skin. J Eur Acad Dermatol Venereol 2011;25(5):516–22.
91. Kunzi-Rapp K, Dierickx CC, Cambier B, et al. Minimally invasive skin rejuvenation with erbium: YAG laser used in thermal mode. Lasers Surg Med 2006;38(10):899–907.
92. Mezzana P. "Multi Light and Drugs": a new technique to treat face photoaging. Comparative study with photorejuvenation. Lasers Med Sci 2008;23(2): 149–54.
93. Spencer JM, Kurtz ES. Approaches to document the efficacy and safety of microdermabrasion procedure. Dermatol Surg 2006;32(11):1353–7.
94. Pagnoni A. Photoaging and photodocumentation. Cosmetics & Toiletries 2002;39–44.
95. Glogau RG. Aesthetic and anatomic analysis of the aging skin. Semin Cutan Med Surg 1996;15(3): 134–8.
96. Fitzpatrick RE, Goldman MP, Satur NM, et al. Pulsed carbon dioxide laser resurfacing of photo-aged facial skin. Arch Dermatol 1996;132(4):395–402.

Benign Skin Neoplasms

Adam Ingraffea, MD*

KEYWORDS

• Benign neoplasms • Nevi • Vascular malformations • Hemangiomas • Cysts • Lipoma • Syringoma • Angiofibroma

KEY POINT

• It is essentially to rule out malignant melanoma before trying to remove nevi Propanolol is a safe and effective treatment for infantile hemangiomas Benign cysts and lipomas are generally best treated with surgical exsion.

DISORDERS OF MELANOCYTES

Key Points

1. It is vital, especially in patients with multiple nevi, to rule out malignant melanoma, especially before removal with CO_2, Er:YAG, and Nd:YAG lasers.
2. Blue nevi can be misdiagnosed as melanoma, but dermatoscopic results of homogeneous pigmentation support the diagnosis of blue nevi.
3. In patients with multiple halo nevi, screening for vitiligo is essential, especially in patients with family history of autoimmune disorders.

Acquired Nevi (Moles)

Acquired nevi are one of the most frequently acquired new growths in white patients, with average adults accumulating, on average, 20 nevi. They tend to appear in early childhood and reach a maximum in young adulthood. One recent study noted that 83% of newborns examined within 48 hours of birth presented with nevi. They undergo gradual fibrosis, with most disappearing by age 60. African Americans and Asians tend to less frequently present with nevi; however, when they do, the nevi are more likely to occur on palms, soles, and nail beds. Sun exposure and ultraviolet radiation have been identified throughout literature as the major factors that induce nevi on exposed surfaces.[1]

Benign nevi are common, small (<1 cm diameter), circumscribed, pigmented macules, papules, or nodules. They tend to be asymptomatic with uniform shape and color, ranging from pink to black.[1] Nevi are composed of nests of nevus cells located in the epidermis, dermis, and/or (rarely) subcutaneous tissue, with the following progression.

Junctional melanocytic nevi

Defined as nevus cell nests on the epidermal side of the basement membrane, making them intraepidermal structures (**Fig. 1**), these tend to be flat dark nevi because the melanocytes have the greatest capacity to form melanin in this layer.[2]

Compound melanocytic nevi

Defined as nevus cell nests invading the papillary dermis, making these lesions intraepidermal and dermal (**Fig. 2**), these present as raised lesions of variable color.[2]

Dermal melanocytic nevi

Defined as nevus cells located exclusively in the dermis, due to melanocytes losing their capacity to make melanin as they penetrate into the dermis,[2] these present as elevated, pink to light brown lesions (**Fig. 3**).

The author has nothing to disclose.
University of Cincinnati College of Medicine, Cincinnati, OH 45202, USA
* 7690 Discovery Drive, Suite 3100, West Chester, OH 45069.
E-mail address: ingrafam@ucmail.uc.edu

Facial Plast Surg Clin N Am 21 (2013) 21–32
http://dx.doi.org/10.1016/j.fsc.2012.11.002
1064-7406/13/$ – see front matter

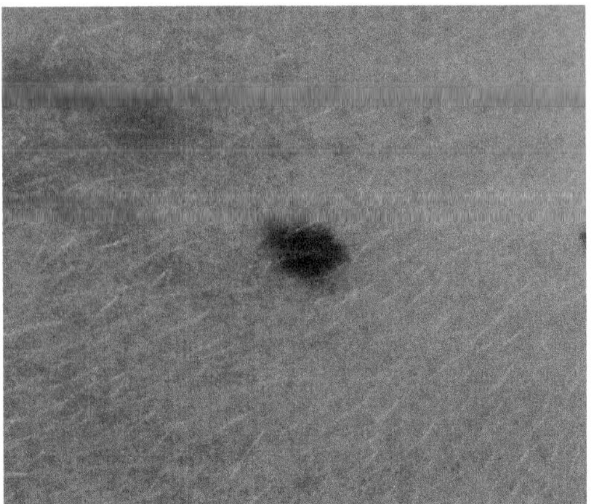

Fig. 1. Junctional melanocytic nevi.

Although nevi are benign findings individually, the risk of melanoma is related to the number and size of the nevi. Physicians must be aware of the dysplastic nevus syndrome in which dysplastic nevi are precursors to malignant melanoma.[3] Treatment, although not necessary, usually involves surgical excision. Recently, it has been reported that, although traditionally CO_2 or Er:YAG lasers have been used to remove melanocytic nevi, 1064 nm Q-switched Nd:YAG lasers also provide a safe and effective treatment modality.[4]

Blue Nevi

Blue nevi appear as small, sharply defined, round, dark blue, or grayish-blue lesions that most commonly develop during childhood (**Fig. 4**). These tend to be slow growing nodules covered by smooth, intact epidermis. These lesions are composed of melanocytes limited to the dermis, with an intimate association with the fibroblasts of the dermis. Blue nevi may occur anywhere on the body, but most commonly on the face, neck, hands, and arms.[5] Unfortunately, because they can be acquired lesions, they can frequently be misdiagnosed as melanoma or cutaneous metastasis of melanoma. Therefore, when melanoma is suspected, surgical excision is mandatory.[6,7]

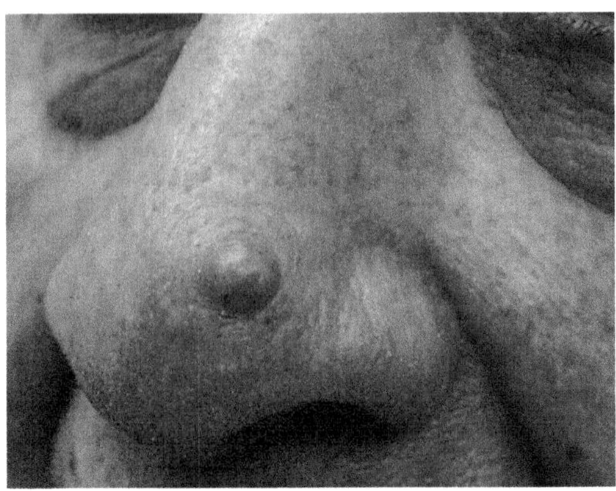

Fig. 2. Compound melanocytic nevi.

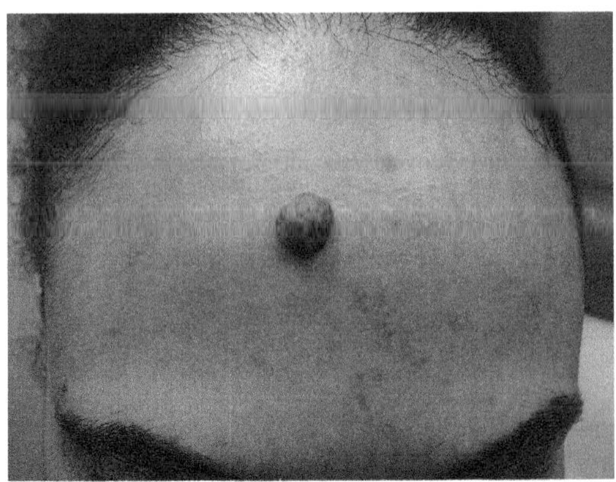

Fig. 3. Dermal melanocytic nevi.

Halo Nevus

Halo nevi appear as nevi encircled by an oval to round halo of sharply demarcated leukoderma or depigmentation. The leukoderma is based on the decrease of melanin in melanocytes and/or disappearance of melanocytes at the dermal-epidermal junction.[8] These halo nevi can occur around blue nevi, congenital nevomelanocytic nevi, Spitz nevi, primary melanoma, melanoma metastases, dermatofibroma, or neurofibroma. Overall prevalence is 1%, seen with spontaneous onset within the first three decades of life, generally with multiple lesions on the back.[9]

Many recent studies have identified that those patients with multiple halo nevi may be more likely to develop vitiligo, especially in those with family

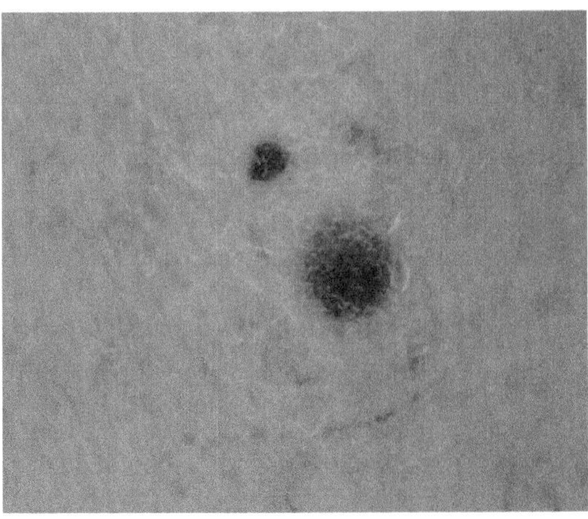

Fig. 4. Blue nevi.

history of autoimmune disorders.[10,11] This lesion is considered an autoimmune response, mediated by T lymphocytes and, therefore, has been associated with other autoimmune conditions, including vitiligo, celiac disease, atopic dermatitis, alopecia areata, and Hashimoto thyroiditis.[12]

Spitz Nevus

Spitz Nevi can occur across all ages, though typically they occur in patients less than 10 years old (**Fig. 5**). The lesions arise rapidly, usually over several months, and are distributed most frequently on the head and neck (37%) and lower extremities (28%), with less than 6% located on the back.[13]

The lesions are solitary, well-defined, dome-shaped, hairless, firm, small (<1 cm) papules or nodules. They are typically pink to red due to the limited melanin content and increased vascularity within these nevi. About 10% may be pigmented, however, ranging in color from tan to brown to black. Nevi that are greater than 1 cm diameter, present with asymmetry, and/or irregular borders, shape, and color, should be examined more closely for potential malignancy.[13]

Spitz tumors have long been histologically challenging diagnoses; however, histologic examination must be done to confirm the clinical diagnosis of Spitz nevi. Evidence of neat organizational attributes, such as symmetry, maturation with descent, distinct margins, and small size are typical. Epidermal hyperplasia is common with melanocytic nests weaving neatly between keratinocytes (unlike melanoma, which tends to be more disordered). Furthermore, Kamino bodies (eosinophilic aggregates) may be present intraepidermally and at the dermoepidermal junction. Histopathologic features that suggest more aggressive behavior are increased mitotic activity, mitoses near the base of the lesion, ulceration, deeper extension, and inflammation.[14]

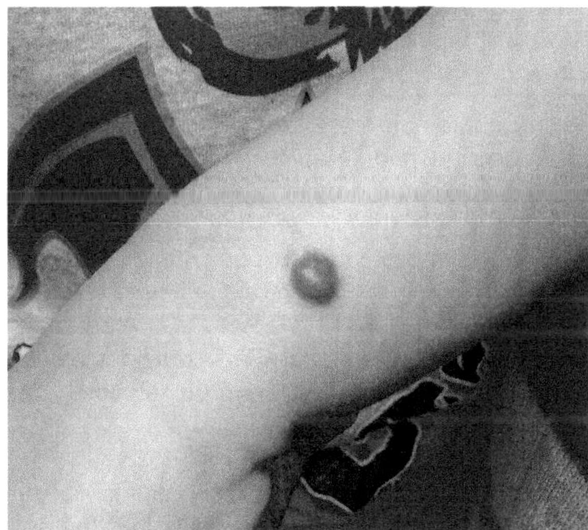

Fig. 5. Spitz nevus.

Rare instances of metastasis have been observed with Spitz tumors. Atypical Spitz tumors greater than 1 cm diameter and ulcerated, with subcutaneous involvement and mitotic figures, are more likely to show micrometastasis. Adult Spitz nevi are usually excised, whereas pediatric cases are sometimes managed nonsurgically due to the lower probability of true melanoma. When these nevi are removed, it is advised that the lesion be completely excised due to a high frequency of recurrence. Due to this risk, it is advisable also to re-excise a Spitz nevus if the margins are involved. Sentinel node biopsy has been suggested as a possible diagnostic technique, but it has not been met with favor as a global screening tool. Up to 40% of Spitz nevi cases were associated with regional metastasis, which was associated with an extremely low rate of mortality.[15]

Nevus Sebaceous

Nevus sebaceous presents at birth or within the first few months of life, with equal incidence in males and females. This hamartoma most commonly presents as a solitary papillomatous yellow-orange linear or oval plaque on the scalp or face. Lesions on the scalp are associated with alopecia. This lesion has been seen in association with the SCALP syndrome, which describes a constellation of sebaceous nevus with associated central nervous system malformations, aplasia cutis congenita, limbal dermoid, and pigmented nevi.[16]

These lesions, similar to other types of nevi, progress through several stages. During the first few months after birth there are an increased number of sebaceous glands with diminution in hair follicles due to hormonal influences. During the next phase, there is a slight papillomatous epithelial hyperplasia and increased number of underdeveloped sebaceous glands, eccrine glands, and miniature hairs. Then rapid growth occurs at puberty with enlarged sebaceous glands, apocrine gland maturation, verrucous hyperplasia of the epidermis, and decreased number of normal hair follicles.[17]

Benign tumors, including syringocystadenoma papilliferum, trichoblastoma, and trichilemmoma, have been reported developing secondarily within nevus sebaceous at an incidence of 16%. Malignant tumors such as basal cell carcinoma were reported at an incidence of 8%. There has been recent controversy about the utility of prophylactic excision of these nevi to avoid development of such malignancies and, therefore, further studies must be performed before a recommendation is made. Definitive treatment would involve surgical excision with narrow margins. In many cases, patients also desire removal secondary to cosmetic concerns because these nevi tend to occur on the face or cause alopecia when on the scalp.[18]

VASCULAR TUMORS OR MALFORMATIONS

Key Points

1. Propranolol has been shown to be safe and efficacious in the treatment of hemangiomas.
2. Pulsed dye laser (PDL) is the gold standard for port-wine stain treatment. Combining this with imiquimod is superior to laser alone.
3. Laser therapy, including Potassium titanyl phosphate (KTP), PDL, and Nd:YAG, has been effective in cherry angioma treatment.
4. Clinicians should maintain a high index of suspicion when diffuse angiokeratomas are identified.

CONGENITAL

Hemangiomas

Hemangiomas are the most common tumor of infancy with an incidence of 1% to 2.5% of all newborns. White children reach an incidence of 10% by 1 year of age with a three to one predilection for females.[19]

These lesions progress through an initial proliferative phase of 3 to 9 months during which they enlarge rapidly, after which they regress over 2 to 6 years, usually completely by age 10. Typically there are no residual skin changes at the site of the lesion. They present as soft, bright red to deep purple, 1 to 8 cm, compressible nodules or plaques that do not blanch completely with pressure. The lesions tend to be solitary and localized, with 50% on the head and neck and 25% on the trunk. The final 25% are on the legs or oral mucous membrane.

The clinical course generally consists of waiting for spontaneous resolution of the lesion, with treatment indicated if lesions ulcerate or obstruct vital structures, including eyes, ears, or the larynx. Surgical and medical interventions include continuous wave or PDL, cryosurgery, intralesional and systemic high-dose glucocorticoids, and interferon (IFN-alpha). There have been numerous recent studies demonstrating the superior safety profile and efficacy of propranolol in the treatment of hemangiomas.[20–22]

Nevus Flammeus (Port-wine Stains)

Port-wine stains are a relatively common occurrence, affecting 0.3% of all newborns.[19] They may be associated with vascular malformations in the eye and leptomeninges in Sturge-Weber syndrome, resulting in neurologic and orbital abnormalities.[23] Acquired port-wine stains have also been reported, usually secondary to trauma. It is morphologically identical to congenital port-wine stains but is usually unilateral and affects the face.[24]

These lesions tend to be irregularly shaped, generally unilateral, red or violaceous, macular capillary malformations. They most commonly involve the face in the distribution of the trigeminal nerve, but can involve the conjunctiva and mouth. With increasing age, the color deepens and macules progress to papules, causing disfigurement.

These lesions never disappear spontaneously and, therefore, laser treatment is recommended for aesthetic concerns. Pulsed dye laser (PDL) is the gold standard for treatment of port-wine stain birthmarks given the minimal risk of scarring but multiple sessions are required. Posttreatment vessel recurrence limits the efficacy of laser treatment.[25,26] Recent literature has indicated that a combination of PDL and imiquimod is superior to PDL alone. One study indicated that treatment intervals of 2 weeks were superior to the standard 6 week intervals currently used. Acquired PWS tends to have a quicker and better response to the laser than congenital.[27]

ACQUIRED

Cherry Angioma, De Morgan Spots

Cherry angiomas are extremely common lesions that occur in middle-aged and elderly patients, tending to appear first at age 30 and increasing in number over the years. They usually occur as multiple asymptomatic lesions, most commonly on the upper trunk and arms. They present as dome-shaped, small (0.1–0.5 cm diameter), bright red to violaceous, soft, compressible papules with a smooth surface. They always blanch with pressure and bleed profusely with any traumatic rupture.

Treatment is only necessary for patients who are bothered by these lesions. Even after therapy, however, new lesions are likely to develop. Several treatment modalities are available, including electrocautery or laser coagulation for small lesions and shave excision for larger lesions. KTP, PDL, and Nd:YAG lasers have been found to be effective treatments.[28]

Angiokeratoma

Angiokeratoma is a vascular tumor with keratotic elements presenting as solitary dark violaceous to black, keratotic papules or plaques (**Fig. 6**). These lesions tend to be hard on palpation and cannot be compressed. They are found predominantly on the thighs, umbilicus, buttocks, lower abdomen, and groin. These lesions can generally be followed clinically, although if desired, excision, laser therapy, cryotherapy, or electrocautery may be used for cosmetic reasons.

Diffuse angiokeratomas have been associated with Fabry syndrome, which is a rare X-linked recessive genetic disorder caused by a deficiency of the lysosomal enzyme α-galactosidase. This allows for accumulation of glycosphingolipids in the dermis, heart, and kidneys, resulting in a wide range of effects, including renal failure, cardiomyopathy, anhidrosis, gastrointestinal distress, and neuropathy. Given that the syndrome generally has a delay of more than 10 years from the onset of symptoms to diagnosis and that there is a window of opportunity for successful treatment if caught early, clinicians should maintain a high index of suspicion when diffuse angiokeratomas are identified.[29]

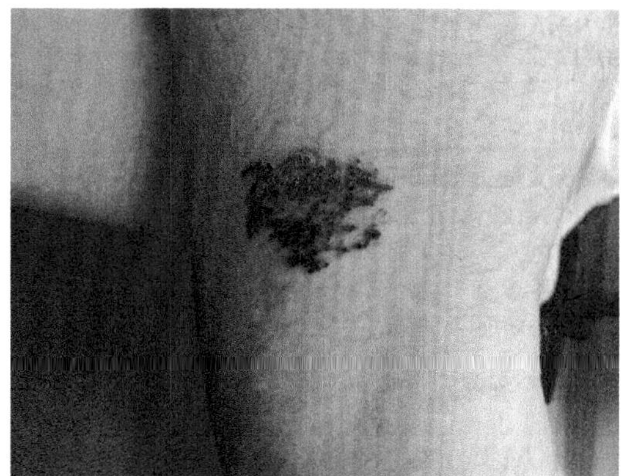

Fig. 6. Angiokeratoma.

CYSTS

Key Points

1. Cysts are generally treated by surgical excision.
2. Wait 4 to 6 weeks to remove epidermal cysts if acutely inflamed. Intralesional injection of triamcinolone into the dermis can hasten resolution of the inflammation.
3. Pilar cysts resemble epidermal inclusion cysts but lack the central punctum.
4. Thyroglossal duct cysts are treated by the Sistrunk procedure, which involves removing the midsection of the hyoid bone to prevent recurrence.

Epidermal Inclusion Cyst

Epidermal inclusion cysts are the most common type of cutaneous cysts. They typically present in the head and neck followed by the trunk (**Fig. 7**). They reach their maximum incidence in the third to fourth decade of life.[30] They result from a proliferation of epidermal cells within the dermis. These cysts have been found to be associated with Gardner syndrome, a rare autosomal dominant condition of multiple epidermal inclusion cysts, often in atypical locations, such as the fingers and toes, associated with colonic polyps and skull osteomas. Importantly, the skin cysts often occur before the intestinal polyps are detectable and, therefore, the presence of the epidermoid cysts in children should be an indication for sigmoidoscopy.[31]

Treatment is not necessary unless desired by the patient because inflamed, uninfected epidermoid cysts often resolve spontaneously without therapy, although they tend to recur. Intralesional injection of triamcinolone into the surrounding inflamed dermis can hasten resolution of the inflammation and may prevent infection and the need for incision and drainage. Excision is best accomplished when the lesion is not inflamed; when acutely inflamed, the cyst wall is friable, making recurrence more likely. Instead, waiting

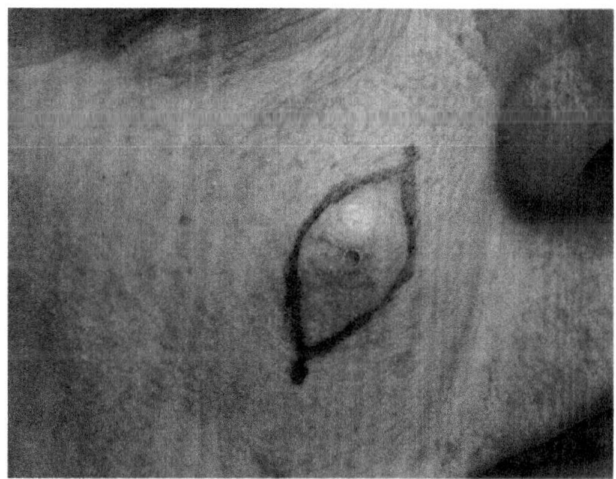

Fig. 7. Epidermal inclusion cyst.

4 to 6 weeks after the inflammation has resolved is suggested before excision.[32]

Dermoid Cyst

Dermoid cysts occur when skin becomes sequestered during fetal development. This relatively uncommon cyst is usually present at birth and, otherwise, presents in adolescents and young adults. Dermoid cysts occur mostly on the face, neck, or scalp with a predilection for the forehead, primarily around the eyes and nose. In addition to the skin, dermoid cysts can be also be intracranial, intraspinal, or perispinal, as well as intra-abdominal.

Dermoid cysts appear as painless solitary, occasionally multiple, 1 to 4 cm hamartomatous tumors. They are not attached to skin and are frequently attached to or extend through underlying bony structures. They may extend to meningeal structures as well, necessitating imaging to determine their full extent. Those presenting on the forehead and brow are known to cause pressure-related erosion of the underlying bony tissue. These lesions may enlarge over time due to accumulation of sebaceous contents, which could potentially lead to cyst rupture and granulomatous inflammation of the surrounding skin and soft tissues.

Treatment is by complete surgical excision while avoiding rupture of the cyst. Recurrence is predicted by incomplete excision of all the epithelial elements and by intraoperative rupture of the cyst.

Trichilemmal or Pilar Cyst

Trichilemmal cysts are the second most common type of cutaneous cysts after epidermoid cysts, affecting 5% to 10% of the population. They tend to present after puberty, peaking in the third decade, with a female predilection. Seventy percent of patients have a familial component.

Pilar cysts resemble epidermal inclusion cysts but lack the central punctum. They present as smooth, firm, slow growing, dome-shaped, subcutaneous nodules. They are most commonly located on the scalp (90%) and are generally multiple (70%). The cysts can slowly enlarge up to 5 cm. Similarly to epidermoid cysts, rupture causes them to become inflamed and painful. The cyst itself contains dense keratin and homogenous, often calcified material. Trichilemmal cysts are derived from the outer root sheath of the hair follicle and are surrounded by an epithelial lined wall.

Two percent of pilar cysts can develop into tumors known as proliferating trichilemmal cysts, which grow rapidly and can progress to squamous cell carcinoma. They rarely metastasize but may, become large and ulcerated.

Definitive treatment, if desired, is complete excision of the cyst. Several methods, including a small linear incision, an elliptical excision, and a circular dermal punch incision, may be used to remove these cysts. Removal tends to be easier than excising epidermoid cysts because the pilar cyst wall is firm and thick and tends not to rupture as easily.

Branchial Cleft Cyst

Branchial cleft cysts most commonly present in the second to third decade of life. There are two proposed theories regarding their origin: either they arise from the failure of obliteration of the second branchial cleft in embryonic development or they represent cystic alteration of embryologic or tonsillar epithelium within cervical lymph nodes.[33]

These cysts occur in the lateral part of the neck, preauricular area, mandibular region, or along the anterior border of sternocleidomastoid muscle. Most cysts are asymptomatic, presenting as solitary, smooth, painless masses but, commonly, becoming tender, enlarged, or inflamed. They can also get infected and develop abscesses, particularly during periods of upper respiratory tract infections due to lymphoid tissue underneath the epithelium. Spontaneous rupture of the abscess may result in a purulent draining sinus to the skin or pharynx. Depending on the size, local symptoms, such as dysphagia, dysphonia, dyspnea, and stridor, may occur. Fine-needle aspiration may be performed to help distinguish branchial cleft cysts from malignant neck masses.

Treatment consists of excising the cyst and its tortuous tract. Surgery is best delayed until the patient is at least 3 months of age.

Thyroglossal Duct Cyst

Thyroglossal duct cysts typically present in children and young patients, with an average age of 6 years. Fifty percent of patients present before 20 years of age, but a significant percentage (15%) present after 50 years of age.[34]

Between the fourth and eighth weeks of development, the thyroid gland descends from the foramen cecum of the tongue to the anterior neck; this tract is called the thyroglossal duct. Failure of the duct to obliterate results in its persistence during development and after birth. There is generally a tract connecting these cysts to the hyoid bone (65% of cases).[34]

Unlike the branchial cleft cysts, thyroglossal duct cysts present as painless midline (vs lateral) cystic nodules on the anterior neck in the region of the hyoid bone in children and young adults. There is movement of the cyst with swallowing and tongue protrusion. It is usually diagnosed clinically, but ultrasonography is the preferred imaging technique in children. Most cysts appear as unilocular lesions with thin walls and posterior acoustic enhancement. CT scan or MRI can be performed to determine the full extent of the lesion and its relationship to surrounding structures. The two most common complications of these cysts are infection and malignancy, the former occurring in about one-third of patients, the latter in 1% to 4% of cases. Because the thyroglossal duct remnants can contain functional thyroid tissue, every type of thyroid carcinoma has been identified within the cyst, with 80% of papillary cell origin.[33]

DERMAL AND SUBCUTANEOUS NEOPLASMS

Key Points

1. Injections of phosphatidylcholine solubilized with deoxycholate are safe and effective in lipoma treatment.
2. Dermatofibromas exhibit a dimple sign and can be treated with PDL therapy.
3. CO_2 lasers have indicated promising results in keloid treatment.

Lipoma

Lipomas are single or multiple soft, flesh-colored nodules that are movable against the overlying skin. They are frequently found on the neck, trunk, and extremities. Though these lesions are generally diagnosed clinically, one study recently found that, whereas the sensitivity for the diagnosis of lipoma with palpation was 54.8%, the sensitivity with ultrasound was 88.1%, suggesting the use of this noninvasive procedure could be helpful clinically.[35]

Several options are available for lipoma removal if chosen for aesthetic concerns by the patient. Surgery and liposuction are methods that have been used traditionally, though the later can only be performed if the lipomas are soft. Recently, injections of phosphatidylcholine solubilized with deoxycholate have come to favor due to their noninvasiveness, with a 75% reduction in size of lipomas after three treatments.[36–38]

Familial multiple lipomatosis is a rare benign hereditary syndrome with a proposed autosomal-dominant inheritance and an incidence of 0.002%.[39] This syndrome is characterized by multiple lipomas found on the trunk and extremities with relative sparing of the head and shoulders. These lesions tend to appear in the third decade of life, with men affected twice more commonly than women. These lipomas tend to be painless and can be treated in the same manner as solitary lipomas, including surgical excision or injection with phosphatidylcholine.[40]

Dermatofibroma, Fibrous Histiocytoma

Dermatofibromas are most commonly located on the lower extremities of adults and, less commonly, on the upper extremities or trunk (**Fig. 8**). Eighty percent of the cases occur between the ages of 20 to 49, with a female predominance. These lesions can occur as a result of trauma or insect bites, but often are idiopathic.[41]

Dermatofibromas are oval, hyperpigmented, typically solitary, firm papules, 0.3 to 1.0 cm in diameter. They have variable color, ranging from skin colored to pink and brown and tend to be darker at the center and fade to normal skin color at the margin. They exhibit a dimple sign (a depression on lateral compression of the lesion with thumb and index finger) due to the fibrous nature of the lesion because dermatofibromas represent a proliferation of fibroblasts. These papules are typically asymptomatic and not tender but can be pruritic. They tend to appear gradually over months and may persist for years or decades.[41]

Usually, no treatment is required unless a lesion is symptomatic, has recently changed in size or color, or is bleeding. If the lesion protrudes above the skin surface and is irritated from repeated trauma, it can be partially removed with cryosurgery or shave excision. The lesion may recur, however, and the scar can look worse than the

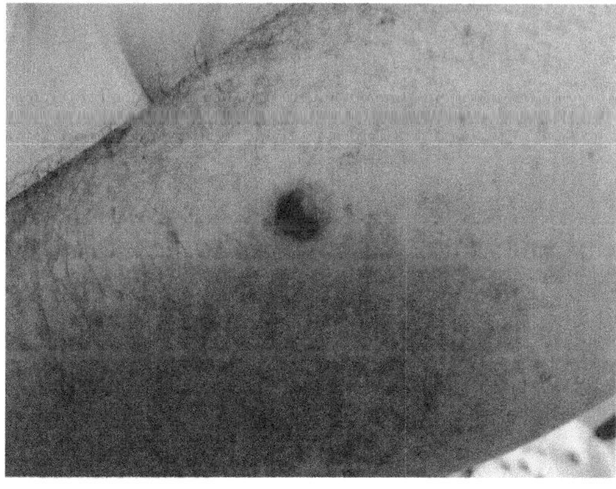

Fig. 8. Dermatofibroma.

initial lesion. Recently, a study examined 22 dermatofibromas treated with PDL therapy at a 595 nm wavelength, using a spot size of 7 mm, a pulse duration of 2 ms, and a fluence of 11 J/cm^2 with 2 or 3 stacked pulses. Global clinical improvement was higher than 50% in all 12 lesions. Patient satisfaction assessment showed 73% of patients as satisfied or very satisfied with this treatment.[42,43]

Hypertrophic Scars or Keloids

Hypertrophic scars and keloids occur in all ages with equal gender distribution but tend to occur more commonly in African Americans, Hispanics, and Asians (**Fig. 9**). These occur because of exuberant fibrous repair with excessive accumulation of type I collagen in the dermis of tissues after a cutaneous injury. They can range from firm, hard papules to nodules to large tuberous lesions. Hypertrophic scars remain confined to the site of original injury, whereas keloids extend beyond the original site. Whereas hypertrophic scars tend to regress and become flatter and softer with time, keloids tend to require treatment because they can cause pain, itching, functional limitation, and disfigurement, leading to significant psychological distress.

No treatment has been proven to be fully effective for keloids. Several methods can be used, including intralesional glucocorticoids,[44] surgical excision with postoperative radiation, silicon cream, and laser treatments. The most effective method for those patients with keloid predilection, however, is prevention.

Radiotherapy following surgical excision has been an additional modality for treating recalcitrant recurrent keloids. However, a major disadvantage in using radiation is an increased risk for developing other types of cancer (including primary cutaneous melanoma, parotid tumors, and thyroid cancers).[45] Thus, if radiation therapy is considered, the surrounding tissues must be shielded.

Compared with radiotherapy, the use of CO_2 laser after surgical excision of keloids has shown promising results with few recurrences and without the risk of carcinogenesis.[46] Ablative fractional CO_2 laser seems to be an encouraging approach in the treatment of keloids and hypertrophic scars, not only for its efficacy, but also for its low side-effect profile.[46] For those still desiring to use radiation, a study of 81 patients found intralesional excision of keloids with postoperative radiotherapy with 15 to 20 Gy within 6 hours for 5 days was effective at preventing keloid recurrence.[47]

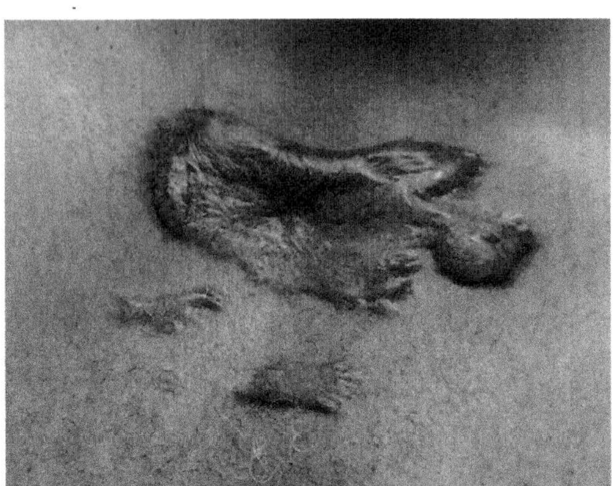

Fig. 9. Hypertrophic scars and keloids.

EPIDERMAL PROLIFERATIONS AND TUMORS

> **Key Points**
>
> 1. The Leser-Trélat sign is an abrupt eruption of multiple seborrheic keratosis appearing in association with an underlying malignancy (often adenocarcinoma), most commonly of solid organ tumors.
> 2. Syringomas have been effectively treated by intralesional insulated needles.
> 3. Verrucae should first by treated by salicylic acid, followed by cryotherapy, and finally physical destruction if the former treatments fail.
> 4. Sebaceous adenomas are found in the Muir-Torre syndrome (MTS), in which patients present with at least one sebaceous gland neoplasm and at least one internal malignancy.
> 5. When multiple neurofibromas are present, neurofibromatosis or von Recklinghausen disease must be suspected.

Seborrheic Keratosis

Seborrheic keratoses are the most common benign epithelial tumor (**Fig. 10**). They tend to be hereditary lesions that do not appear until age 30 and continue to occur throughout life.[48] They present as multiple, well-circumscribed, yellow to brown, raised lesions that feel slightly greasy, velvety, or warty. They are described as having a "stuck-on" appearance and are symmetrically distributed on the trunks of older people.[49]

The Leser-Trélat sign is the abrupt eruption of multiple seborrheic keratosis appearing in association with an underlying malignancy (often adenocarcinoma), most commonly of solid organ

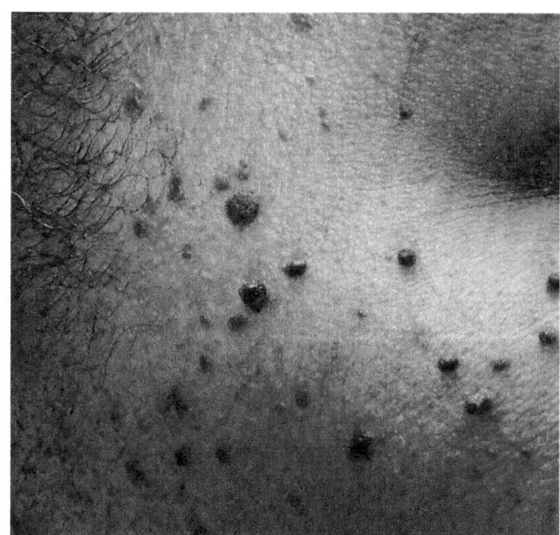

Fig. 10. Seborrheic keratoses.

tumors. Though this generally signals poor prognosis, the seborrheic keratoses may resolve with treatment of the underlying malignancy and reappear with its recurrence.

Seborrheic keratoses generally do not require treatment unless they become irritated or traumatized with pain and bleeding. At that point, they may be treated with light electrocautery, shave excision (preferred if biopsy is required to rule out malignancy), ablative laser therapy (YAG or CO_2), curettage, or, most commonly, cryotherapy. Cryotherapy generally involves spray cooling for 5 to 10 seconds with longer duration or second treatment of thicker tumors.

Syringoma

Syringomas are benign adnexal tumors of intradermal eccrine ducts. They predominately occur in women, beginning at puberty. They present as 1 to 2 mm, skin-colored or yellow, firm papules. They are most often multiple and occur most frequently on the lower periorbital area. They also occur on face, axilla, umbilicus, upper chest, and vulva. Syringomas are generally treated by surgical excision, electrodessication, cryosurgery, chemical peeling, and laser ablation, but complete removal is often unsuccessful and recurrence is frequent. Furthermore, because these treatments lead to hyperpigmentation or scarring, they are not ideal treatments.

Pilomatricoma

Pilomatricomas are uncommon neoplasms, arising from hair matrix cells, which occur most commonly in childhood and adolescence with a female predominance, mostly on the head or upper trunk.[50] These lesions present as asymptomatic, slow growing, solitary, skin-colored to faint blue nodules or cysts, typically being firm and adherent to the skin though not to the underlying tissues. Calcification accompanies these lesions and it can elicit fibrosis and inflammation.[51]

Because spontaneous regression is never observed and malignant transformation can occur, the standard treatment of pilomatricoma is complete surgical excision. Recurrence after surgery is rare, with an incidence of 0% to 3%. Malignant transformation to a pilomatrix carcinoma should be suspected in cases with repeated local recurrences.

These lesions are treated by simple excisional biopsy and rarely recur. If there are multiple recurrences, complete excision with negative margins should be performed to exclude the possibility of pilomatrical carcinoma.[52]

Sebaceous Adenoma

Sebaceous adenomas present as benign sebaceous neoplasms with glandular differentiation (**Fig. 11**). Clinically, they appear as small, circumscribed, yellowish papules or nodules, usually less than a centimeter in diameter and are distributed on the head, neck, and, occasionally, upper trunk. Generally, no treatment is obligatory for these lesions, but conservative complete excision of such lesions is appropriate to exclude the possibility of carcinoma. Photodynamic therapy has been reported to be successful in the treatment of these lesions.[53]

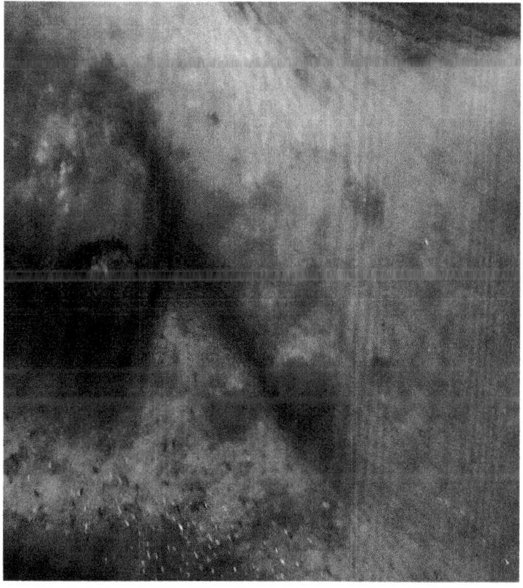

Fig. 11. Sebaceous adenoma.

Sebaceous adenomas are found in the Muir-Torre syndrome in which patients present with at least one sebaceous gland neoplasm and at least one internal malignancy. Sebaceous adenomas are highly specific for Muir-Torre syndrome. The median age of onset for this syndrome is 55 years, with a male to female ratio of three to two. This syndrome has an autosomal dominant inheritance of a mutation in DNA mismatch repair genes, but with variable penetrance and expression. Sixty one percent of the visceral malignancies occur in the gastrointestinal tract (colorectal carcinoma), with 22% occurring in the urogenital tract. These malignancies tend to be less aggressive carcinomas than sporadic cases, so most patients have good long-term survival even with metastatic disease.[54]

Angiofibroma

Angiofibromas present as fibrous papules, located on the face of adults, most commonly on the nose. They have two distinct presentations, including a solitary, skin-colored, shiny, dome-shaped papule that can be treated by shave excision or electrodessication. The other is pearly penile papules, which are white, dome-shaped, closely aggregated, small papules located on the glans penis. This is a relatively common condition, affecting 30% of young postpubertal men, more commonly in those who are uncircumcised. Angiofibromas are generally treated by shave excision, dermabrasion, electrodessication and curettage, or laser therapy. Once the lesions are treated, they seldom recur, though new lesions may form.

Multiple facial angiofibromas has been linked with tuberous sclerosis, at an incidence of 75%. They tend to be distributed bilaterally on the cheeks, nasolabial folds, chin, and nose. Patients can also have multiple periungual fibromas and significant epidermal hyperplasia and orthokeratosis.

Neurofibroma

Neurofibromas present as solitary, sporadic, soft papules or nodules that range from skin to tan in color. They slowly grow to 0.2 to 2 cm but may become pedunculated. Neurofibromas exhibit a "buttonhole sign," with the tumor easily invaginating on palpation. Neurofibromas are caused by a proliferation of neuromesenchymal tissue including Schwann cells, perineural cells, fibroblasts, and mast cells. These lesions are treated by simple surgical excision.

When multiple lesions are present, neurofibromatosis or von Recklinghausen disease must be suspected. These lesions tend to be large, pigmented, bag-like masses that favor the trunk and proximal extremities.

SUMMARY

Benign neoplasms are very common pathological conditions encountered in general practice and surgical clinics. Patients desire removal due to cosmetic and/or symptomatic reasons, as well as fear of malignant potential. Many treatment options have been studied regarding these lesions, including excision, cryotherapy, laser therapy, curettage, and pharmacotherapy. Regardless of the treatment choice, however, it is pivotal to rule out malignant lesions before removal.

ACKNOWLEDGMENTS

The author would like to gratefully acknowledge the contributions of Sphoorthi Jinna, MSIV, University of Cincinnati College of Medicine.

REFERENCES

1. Rhodes AR. Common acquired nevomelanocytic nevi and the fourth dimension. Arch Dermatol 2000;136(3):400–5.
2. Kim JK, Nelson KC. Dermoscopic features of common nevi: a review. G Ital Dermatol Venereol 2012;147(2):141–8.
3. Skender-Kalnenas TM, English DR, Heenan PJ. Benign melanocytic lesions: risk markers or precursors of cutaneous melanoma? J Am Acad Dermatol 1995;33(6):1000–7.
4. Kim YJ, Whang KU, Choi WB, et al. Efficacy and safety of 1,064 nm Q-switched Nd:YAG laser treatment for removing melanocytic nevi. Ann Dermatol 2012;24(2):162–7.
5. Phadke PA, Zembowicz A. Blue nevi and related tumors. Clin Lab Med 2011;31(2):345–58.
6. Di Cesare A, Sera F, Gulia A, et al. The spectrum of dermatoscopic patterns in blue nevi. J Am Acad Dermatol 2012;67(2):199–205.
7. Lee HY, Na SY, Son YM. A malignant melanoma associated with a blue nevus of the lip. Ann Dermatol 2010;22(1):119.
8. Pearl H, Jaber R, Mehregan D. Acquired leukoderma in a regressing congenital nevomelanocytic nevus. Int J Dermatol 2009;48(8):870.
9. Wayte DM, Helwig EB. Halo nevi. Cancer 1968; 22(1):69–90.
10. Hofmann UB, Bröcker EB, Hamm H. Simultaneous onset of segmental vitiligo and a halo surrounding a congenital melanocytic naevus. Acta Derm Venereol 2009;89:402–6.
11. Stierman SC, Tierney EP, Shwayder TA. Halo congenital nevocellular nevi associated with extralesional vitiligo: a case series with review of the literature. Pediatr Dermatol 2009;26(4):414–24.

12. Kim HS, Goh BK. Vitiligo occurring after halo formation around congenital melanocytic nevi. Pediatr Dermatol 2009;26(6):755–6.
13. Luo S, Sepehr A, Tsao H. Spitz nevi and other spitzoid lesions: part I. Background and diagnoses. J Am Acad Dermatol 2011;65(6):1073–84.
14. Miteva M, Lazova R. Spitz nevus and atypical spitzoid neoplasm. Semin Cutan Med Surg 2010;29(3):165–73.
15. Luo S, Sepehr A, Tsao H. Spitz nevi and other Spitzoid lesions: part II. Natural history and management. J Am Acad Dermatol 2011;65(6):1087–92.
16. Hsieh CW, Wu YH, Lin SP, et al. Sebaceous nevus syndrome, central nervous system malformations, aplasia cutis congenita, limbal dermoid, and pigmented nevus syndrome. Pediatr Dermatol 2012;29(3):365–7.
17. Moody MN, Landau JM, Goldberg LH. Nevus sebaceous revisited. Pediatr Dermatol 2012;29(1):15–23.
18. Kim JH, Park HY, Ahn SK. Nevus sebaceous accompanying secondary neoplasms and unique histopathologic findings. Ann Dermatol 2011;23(0):S231–4.
19. Kanada KN, Merin MR, Munden A, et al. A prospective study of cutaneous findings in newborns in the United States: correlation with race, ethnicity, and gestational status using updated classification and nomenclature. J Pediatr 2012;161(2):240–5.
20. Bertrand J, Sammour R, McCuaig C, et al. Propranolol in the treatment of problematic infantile hemangioma: review of 35 consecutive patients from a vascular anomalies clinic. J Cutan Med Surg 2012;16(2):115–21.
21. Talaat AA, Elbasiouny MS, Elgendy DS, et al. Propranolol treatment of infantile hemangioma: clinical and radiologic evaluations. J Pediatr Surg 2012;47(4):707–14.
22. Chung SH, Park DH, Jung HL, et al. Successful and safe treatment of hemangioma with oral propranolol in a single institution. Korean J Pediatr 2012;55(5):164–70.
23. Piram M, Lorette G, Sirinelli D, et al. Sturge-Weber syndrome in patients with facial port-wine stain. Pediatr Dermatol 2012;29(1):32–7.
24. Kirkland CR, Mutasim DF. Acquired port-wine stain following repetitive trauma. J Am Acad Dermatol 2011;65(2):462–3.
25. Faurschou A, Olesen AB, Leonardi-Bee J, et al. Lasers or light sources for treating port-wine stains. Cochrane Database Syst Rev 2011;(11):CD007152.
26. Nelson JS, Jia W, Phung TL, et al. Observations on enhanced port wine stain blanching induced by combined pulsed dye laser and rapamycin administration. Lasers Surg Med 2011;43(10):939–42.
27. Tremaine AM, Armstrong J, Huang YC, et al. Enhanced port-wine stain lightening achieved with combined treatment of selective photothermolysis and imiquimod. J Am Acad Dermatol 2012;66(4):634–41.
28. Pancar GS, Aydin F, Senturk N, et al. Comparison of the 532-nm KTP and 1064-nm nd:YAG lasers for the treatment of cherry angiomas. J Cosmet Laser Ther 2011;13(4):138–41.
29. Zampetti A, Orteu CH, Antuzzi D, et al. Angiokeratoma: decision-making aid for the diagnosis of Fabry disease. Br J Dermatol 2012;166(4):712–20.
30. Handa U, Chhabra S, Mohan H. Epidermal inclusion cyst: cytomorphological features and differential diagnosis. Diagn Cytopathol 2008;36(12):861–3.
31. Leppard B, Bussey HJ. Epidermoid cysts, polyposis coli and Gardner's syndrome. Br J Surg 1975;62(5):387–93.
32. Zuber TJ. Minimal excision technique for epidermoid (sebaceous) cysts. Am Fam Physician 2002;65(7):1409–12.
33. Al-Khateeb TH, Al-Masri NM, Al-Zoubi F. Cutaneous cysts of the head and neck. J Oral Maxillofac Surg 2009;67(1):52–7.
34. Foley DS, Fallat ME. Thyroglossal duct and other congenital midline cervical anomalies. Semin Pediatr Surg 2006;15(2):70–5.
35. Kuwano Y, Ishizaki K, Watanabe R, et al. Efficacy of diagnostic ultrasonography of lipomas, epidermal cysts, and ganglions. Arch Dermatol 2009;145(7):761–4.
36. Bechara FG, Mannherz HG, Jacob M, et al. Induction of fat cell necrosis in human fat tissue after treatment with phosphatidylcholine and deoxycholate. J Eur Acad Dermatol Venereol 2012;26(2):180–5.
37. Nanda S. Treatment of lipoma by injection lipolysis. J Cutan Aesthet Surg 2011;4(2):135–7.
38. Rotunda AM, Ablon G, Kolodney MS. Lipomas treated with subcutaneous deoxycholate injections. J Am Acad Dermatol 2005;53(6):973–8.
39. Rosmaninho A, Pinto-Almeida T, Fernandes IC, et al. Do you know this syndrome? An Bras Dermatol 2012;87(2):324–5.
40. Veger HT, Ravensbergen NJ, Ottenhof A, et al. Familial multiple lipomatosis: a case report. Acta Chir Belg 2010;110(1):98–100.
41. Han TY, Chang HS, Lee JH, et al. A clinical and histopathological study of 122 cases of dermatofibroma (benign fibrous histiocytoma). Ann Dermatol 2011;23(2):185–92.
42. Alonso-Castro L, Boixeda P, Segura-Palacios J, et al. Dermatofibromas treated with pulsed dye laser: clinical and dermoscopic outcomes. J Cosmet Laser Ther 2012;14(2):98–101.
43. Wang SQ, Lee PK. Treatment of dermatofibroma with a 600 nm pulsed dye laser. Dermatol Surg 2006;32(4):532–5.
44. Hayashi T, Furukawa H, Oyama A, et al. A new uniform protocol of combined corticosteroid injections and ointment application reduces recurrence

rates after surgical keloid/Hypertrophic scar excision. Dermatol Surg 2012;38(6):893–7.

45. Fish LM, Duncan L, Gray KD, et al. Primary cutaneous melanoma arising in a long-standing irradiated keloid. Case Rep Surg 2012;2012:165310.
46. Scrimali L, Lomeo G, Tamburino S, et al. Laser CO2 versus radiotherapy in treatment of keloid scars. J Cosmet Laser Ther 2012;14(2):94–7.
47. Li PC, Jia CY, Li YM, et al. Clinical efficacy of keloids treated by surgical ablation and immediate postoperative adjuvant radiotherapy. Zhonghua Yi Xue Za Zhi 2011;91(45):3223–4.
48. Kyriakis KP, Alexoudi I, Askoxylaki K, et al. Epidemiologic aspects of seborrheic keratoses. Int J Dermatol 2012;51(2):233–4.
49. Hafner C, Vogt T. Seborrheic keratosis. J Dtsch Dermatol Ges 2008;6(8):664–77 [in English, German].
50. Guinot-Moya R, Valmaseda-Castellon E, Berini-Aytes L, et al. Pilomatrixoma. Review of 205 cases. Med Oral Patol Oral Cir Bucal 2011;16(4):552–5.
51. Simi CM, Correa M, Rajalakshmi T. Pilomatricoma: a tumor with hidden depths. Indian J Dermatol Venereol Leprol 2010;76(5):543–6.
52. Pant I, Joshi SC, Kaur G, et al. Pilomatricoma as a diagnostic pitfall in clinical practice: report of two cases and review of literature. Indian J Dermatol 2010;55(4):390–2.
53. Kim SK, Lee JY, Kim YC. Treatment of sebaceous adenoma with topical photodynamic therapy. Arch Dermatol 2010;146(10):1186–8.
54. Eisen DB, Michael DJ. Sebaceous lesions and their associated syndromes: part I. J Am Acad Dermatol 2009;61(4):549–60.

Melanoma

Adam Ingraffea, MD*

KEYWORDS

• Melanoma • Skin cancer • BRAF • Immunotherapy • Noninvasive imaging

KEY POINTS

- In the United States, the incidence of melanoma is increasing with an estimated 76,250 cases in 2012.
- New 2009 AJCC staging criteria allows for increased accuracy of diagnosis and treatment.
- The new adjuvant therapies, ipilimumab and vemurafenib, offer promising options for therapy.
- Melafind, a new innovation computer-based visual technology, may improve the accuracy in diagnosis of cutaneous melanoma.

INTRODUCTION

In simple terms, melanoma is described as malignancy of the melanocyte, a melanin-producing cell located in the stratum basale of the epidermis. Normal-functioning melanocytes remain responsible for the basic pigmentation of the skin, in addition to protection versus harmful UV light. Practitioners commonly refer to this malignancy as either cutaneous or malignant melanoma.

EPIDEMIOLOGY

Worldwide, the incidence of cutaneous melanoma is increasing continuously, especially among whites.[1] Estimated cases in the United States in 2012 were 76,250 new diagnoses with concurrent 9180 deaths expected because of melanoma alone.[2] Surveillance Epidemiology and End Results data collected from the National Cancer Institute also conclude that this cancer is steadily increasing among whites with a 60% increase observed within the last 30 years. These data quote melanoma as the fifth and seventh most common new diagnosis of malignancy among men and women, respectively.[3]

Incidence rates of melanoma per year vary between women and men from 3% to 4.1% per year and 5.1% to 6.1% per year, respectively.[3,4] These rates have been reported as high as 21.6, 1, and 4.5 per 100,000 among non-Hispanics, African Americans, and Hispanics, respectively.[3,5] Overall incidence seems to be higher among females; the elderly; and non-Hispanic whites versus Hispanic whites, African Americans, American Indians, Alaskans, Asians, and Pacific Islanders.[6] However, minority groups demonstrate increased metastasis, advanced stages, thicker lesions, earlier age at diagnosis, and poorer outcomes overall.[7]

Anatomic location of these lesions also helps study the evolution of melanoma throughout the last several decades. During the 1970s, cutaneous melanoma was mainly observed on the trunk of males and extremities of females. However, most likely because of changes in lifestyle habits and clothing, current reports state lesions are most common on the chests of females and lower extremities of males.[8] Different patterns of sun exposure help predict location of such lesions. Head, neck, and extremity lesions are associated with chronic sun exposure versus truncal lesions associated with intermittent UV radiation.[1,9]

Many suggest that there is currently no decline in the mortality rate of this disease.[10] Median survival rates after metastasis occurs have been reported

Funding Sources: None.
Conflict of Interest Disclosure: None declared.

Department of Dermatology, University of Cincinnati College of Medicine, 7690 Discovery Dr Suite 3100. West Chester, OH 45069, USA
* Department of Dermatology, University of Cincinnati College of Medicine, 7690 Discovery Drive, Suite 3100, West Chester, OH 45069.
E-mail address: ingrafam@ucmail.uc.edu

Facial Plast Surg Clin N Am 21 (2013) 33–42
http://dx.doi.org/10.1016/j.fsc.2012.11.007
1064-7406/13/$ – see front matter

facialplastic.theclinics.com

as a mere average of 6 to 9 months, with records of a 5-year survival rate less than 5% to 10%.[1,11,12]

RISK FACTORS

Several risk factors are linked to the development of cutaneous melanoma. Genetic predisposition plays a large role and several susceptibility genes have been identified. An important gene, CDKN2A, codes for a tumor-suppressor protein, p16INK4A. This is a CDK4 inhibitor causing the phosphorylation of Rb, which regularly restricts the G1-S interface during cell division in mitosis. This mutation, witnessed in a third of the cases of hereditary melanoma, thus disrupts the normal cell division pathway.[13–15]

Another significant gene, BRAF (V600E), is thought to be crucial to the pathogenesis of melanoma. Several studies implicate that a single mutation in this gene is observed in 50% to 60% of cutaneous melanomas.[15] These mutations are often associated with younger patients (86% between 20 and 30 years old); a predilection for the trunk and extremities; high nevus counts; few freckles; individuals that tan easily; and the superficial spreading subtype.[16] Other susceptibility genes include NRAS (15%–20%); CKIT (2%, 10%–20% acral or mucosal melanomas); GNAQ/GNA11 (50% uveal cases); BRCA2; MCR1; OCA1; and those with an inherited defect causing xeroderma pigmentosum.[16–19]

Studies report that 1% to 11% of patients with prior history of melanoma develop additional primary melanomas.[20–22] Additionally, family history cannot be ignored, especially with the implication of genetic susceptibility. As many as 8% to 12% of patients with melanoma showed familial propensity in certain studies, with an individual with one first-degree showing a 1.7-fold increased risk, whereas a ninefold increase was appreciated in those patients with two affected first-degree relatives.[17,20,23,24]

Age plays a large role in melanoma with the median age of diagnosis at 62 and 54 for men and women, respectively.[25] In addition to standard screening used for skin cancer, men older than age 50 should be specifically targeted because of this increased propensity.[20] Other risk factors include moles that are new, changing, or symptomatic, and patients with prior removal of suspicious moles.[20] Chronic immunosuppression also seems to play a large role, especially in those patients with prior cancer (chronic lymphocytic leukemia and non-Hodgkin's lymphoma especially), AIDS, or posttransplant.[26,27] Melanoma was observed in 6% to 15% of posttransplant cases of skin cancers.[27]

In summary, the strongest causes of melanoma can be linked to a personal or family history of melanoma, male gender, older age, presence of dysplastic or atypical nevi, history of intense intermittent sun exposure, and increased sunburns during childhood.[20,28] Researchers have found that the HARMM acronym can help identify the five most important independent factors for increased likelihood of melanoma. A score of five represents high-risk patients, whereas 0 to 1 confers lower risk.[29] This simplifies the importance of history of prior melanoma (H), age greater than 50 years (A), the absence of a regular dermatologist (R), a changing mole (M), and the male gender (M).

Furthermore, environmental exposures play an important role in melanoma. Researchers have concluded that consistent residence in medium or high UVR locations is associated with an incremental risk of two Non-Melanoma Skin Cancer or greater later in life.[30] Concomitantly, sun exposure is the most important environmental risk and the only one that remains potentially modifiable.[20] Sun exposure and its' association with melanoma seems to increasingly affect those individuals who experience a pattern of intense intermittent exposure versus chronic exposure, thus concluding that vacationing and recreational activities are modifiable risk factors.[23]

Artificial UV exposure by tanning is an additional modifiable risk factor. This source of intermittent radiation became popular in the 1980s and emits UVA and UVB radiation. UVB rays are the putative factor in the carcinogenesis of skin cancer; however, individuals must remember that UVA can also be absorbed by melanocytes and is much higher in artificial sources than in natural exposure.[1,31] A study in Minnesota observed that a strong dose response relationship between the risks of malignant melanoma existed between the total hours, sessions, or total years that individuals spent with indoor tanning. Cutaneous malignant melanoma was observed higher among indoor tanners versus those who never used it (odds ratio, 1.74).[32] An additional analysis of artificial sources concluded that an increased risk (relative risk, 1.15) existed for any individual that had ever used a sunbed, and even higher was observed (relative risk, 1.75) if this occurred before the age of 35.[31] These studies concluded that no artificial device is safe, regardless of the UVA/UBV emission ratio.

A clear link exists between atypical or dysplastic nevi and malignant melanoma. Typical features of dysplastic nevi include lesions that are greater than 6 mm in diameter, are flat, possess irregular borders, and contain a variability in color.[13] However, dysplastic nevi individually rarely evolve into melanoma. Although a single dysplastic nevus does not hold much malignant potential, multiple nevi are markers for malignancy.[33] Congenital nevi, melanocytic nevi that are present at birth, also confer risk for future melanocytic lesions. These are sometimes evident in 1% to 6% of neonates and risk is dependent on size. A small (<1.5 cm) or medium lesion has a low (<1%) lifetime and nonexistent risk before puberty. However, a larger lesion (>20 cm) contains a 5% risk of evolving into either a cutaneous or extracutaneous melanoma.[34]

DIAGNOSIS

For a clinician to properly identify and manage cutaneous melanoma, it is imperative to be aware of the array of lesions encompassing the differential diagnosis for melanoma. These lesions include seborrheic keratosis, pigmented actinic keratosis, pigmented basal cell carcinoma, blue nevi, and benign nevi.

After proper identification of a lesion that is suspected to be melanoma, the clinician must do a proper clinical examination to determine if it is consistent with melanoma. This must include a total skin examination from head to toe with emphasis placed on sun-exposed areas including the scalp, face, extremities, and back. Caution must be taken to include intertriginous regions, palms, soles, and the nail beds because in situ lesions may show up here. Afterward, the five critical fundamentals of determination can be explored: (1) asymmetry, (2) border, (3) color, (4) diameter, and (5) elevation.

Important parameters to consider include examining the pattern and the shape of the lesion. Irregular borders of melanoma are often attributed to the propensity of the lesion for uneven growth within it. The most important determination of color includes irregularity and specific colors. Cutaneous melanomas are often blue-black; however, numerous colors, such as brown, tan, red, gray, or white, can be demonstrated within these lesions. A specific shade of gray or white often represents an area of regression within the lesion, one where melanin production has concurrently stopped and left behind a lesion resembling a pale scar. Color can also help determine subtypes of melanoma. Uniformly black lesions are often small and nodular in type.[13]

An important method to aid in the diagnosis of melanotic lesions includes dermoscopy. A dermatoscope allows for the magnification of lesions while simultaneously providing a polarized light source rendering the stratum cornea translucent. Two key objectives of dermoscopy are decreasing the number of biopsies of benign skin lesions in addition to providing increased diagnostic accuracy of melanoma.[35] Several dermatoscopic structures associated with an atypical proliferation include an atypical pigment network, pigment pseudonetwork, irregular dots and globules, streaks, and even a blue-white veil overlying the suspected lesion. An atypical lesion has grid lines of varying thickness and color, whereas a benign lesion demonstrates a regular meshlike appearance.[35]

CLASSIFICATION

Melanoma is classified as superficial spreading, nodular, lentigo maligna, acral lentiginous, and desmoplastic melanoma.[16] Further subtyping in the future could result in a more refined classification system possibly personalizing specific treatments.

Superficial spreading melanoma is often seen in younger patients with a median age in the fifth decade (**Fig. 1**). Lesions present as flat, slow-growing, irregularly bordered lesions with variegated pigment. These lesions enlarge radially and are present on areas of intermittent sun exposure including the trunk, back, and extremities.[16] Histology demonstrates large pleomorphic epitheloid melanocytes in nested and single cells, upward migration demonstrating pagetoid epidermal invasion (**Fig. 2**). Nodular melanomas can present on any location as rapidly expanding nodules, which may ulcerate and hemorrhage (**Fig. 3**). Epidemiologically, this is often seen in older patients near the seventh decade of life.[16] Histology demonstrates no epidermal portion of the lesion extending beyond the dermal component (**Fig. 4**).

An additional subtype found in the elderly includes lentigo maligna, mainly observed near the eight decade (**Fig. 5**). These lesions are typically found on chronically sun-exposed areas including the head, neck, and forearms. Lesions demonstrate large variegated pigmented macules with irregular

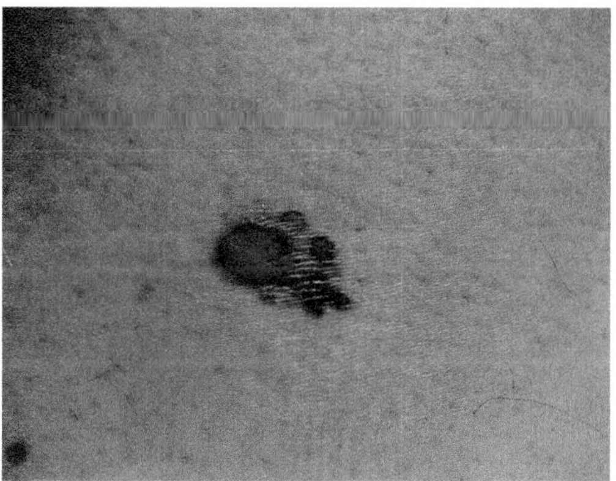

Fig. 1. Superficial spreading melanoma.

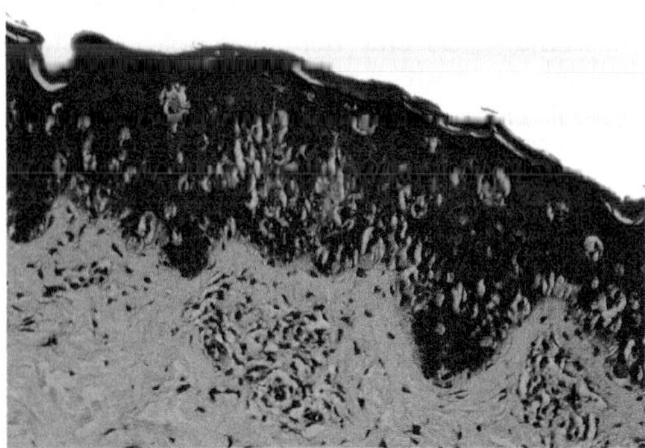

Fig. 2. Superficial spreading melanoma histopathology (H&E, original magnification 20×).

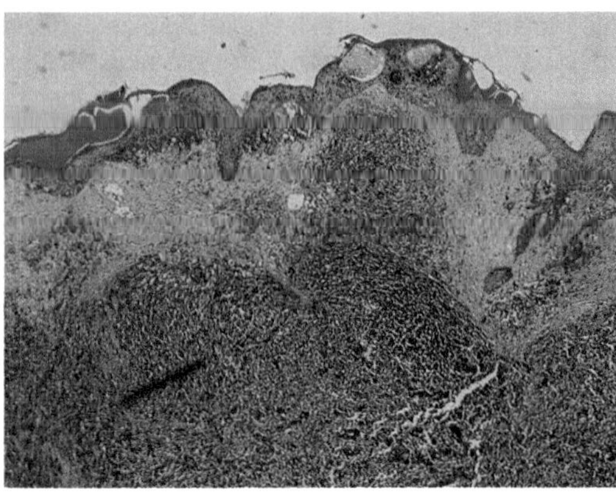

Fig. 4. Nodular melanoma histopathology (H&E, original magnification 4×).

edges, which can further become raised if dermal invasion occurs.[16] Histologically, severe dermal solar elastosis and epidermal thinning with confluent melanocytes, and pagetoid epidermal invasion in the epidermis are characteristic (**Fig. 6**). Acral lentiginous melanoma is found specifically on the palm, soles, or subungal locations (**Fig. 7**). These are very slow growing and demonstrate variegated pigmented macules.[16] Desmoplastic melanoma demonstrates more sarcoma-like tendencies with increased hematogenous spread when compared with other subtypes.[16,36] Postoperative radiotherapy must be offered to these patients because of the increased local recurrence rates even with adequate excision margins.[37]

STAGING

New staging criteria by the American Joint Committee on Cancer published in 2009 allow for increased accuracy and precision for clinicians managing malignant melanoma compared with the 2002 guidelines (**Tables 1** and **2**). The American Joint Committee on Cancer 2009 guidelines reiterated the importance of several prognostic factors including tumor thickness and mitotic rate, and significantly the mitotic rate now replaces previous Clark's level of invasion for criteria in defining stage T1b melanomas. Any patient with microscopic nodal metastases is now officially classified as stage III.[38]

Staging within the N category now includes the number of metastatic nodes, tumor burden, and ulceration of the primary lesions. The M category is now defined by any distant metastases, visceral metastases, in addition to an elevated serum lactate dehydrogenase level.[38]

PREVENTION

Because many risk factors for melanoma are modifiable factors, the importance of prevention and education must be stressed. Early detection remains one of the most important features ofdisease burden reduction. Although no major prevention task force recommends formal screening for

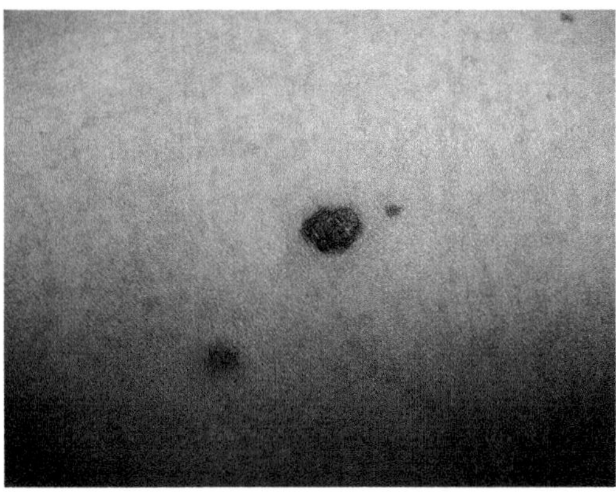

Fig. 3. Nodular melanoma.

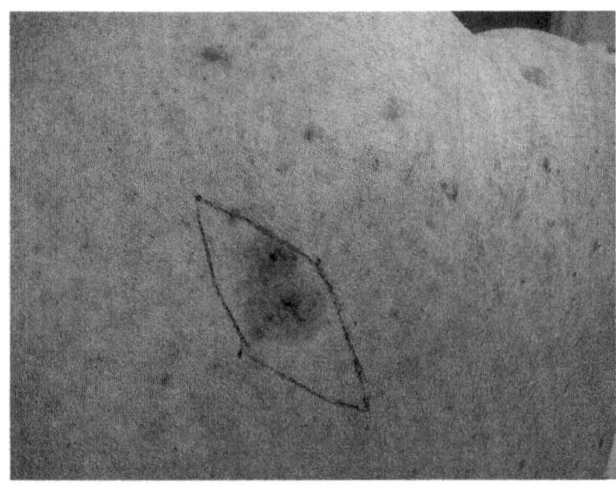

Fig. 5. Lentigo maligna melanoma.

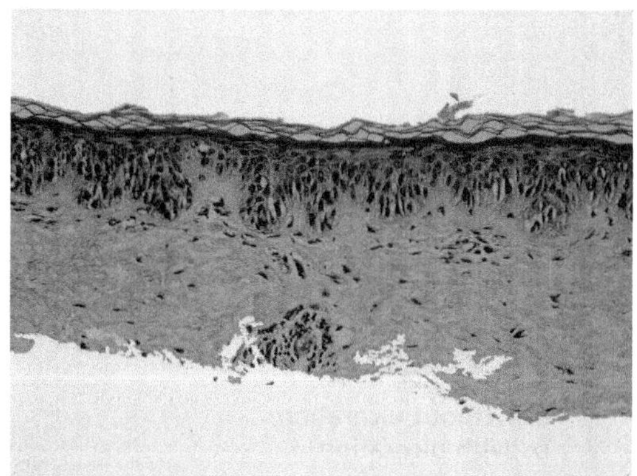

Fig. 6. Lentigo maligna melanoma histopathology (H&E, original magnification 10×).

melanoma, skin examinations by an experienced dermatologist should be performed in any patient with risk factors.[20] Preferred biopsy technique for any suspicious lesion is a narrow excision encompassing the entire breath with sufficient depth to ensure the lesion is not transected. Clinicians may also approach these lesions with an elliptical excision, punch, or shave biopsy. A partial sampling by incisional biopsy is acceptable in lesions of the facial or acral location where complete biopsy is unattainable or if the clinician has low suspicion.[39]

Education plays a large factor in the prevention and diagnosis of melanoma. Middle to older aged men and those within lower socioeconomic class should be targeted for increased screening.[40] In addition, education of other medical profession is of crucial importance for the recognition and proper referral to dermatologists. Most Americans do not have a dermatologist and only 25% of white Americans have screenings for skin cancer.[40] In addition, middle-aged and older white men visit their primary care physician frequently, providing opportune times for diagnosis or further referral. Even partial skin examinations by physicians were found to be a practical approach for early

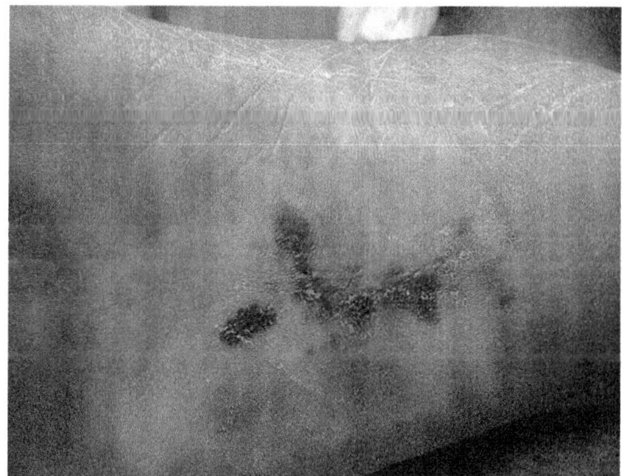

Fig. 7. Acral lentiginous melanoma.

detection within this subgroup of men older than 60 years and were associated with thinner tumors.[41]

TREATMENT

Approach to treatment of malignant melanoma depends on several important prognostic factors, including histologic classification and extent of disease, demonstrated by staging criteria. To date, surgical management through wide local excision continues to be the standard of care.[39] Several expert studies demonstrate that excision for invasive melanoma should include a minimum of 1-cm margins and no more than 2 cm around the primary tumor. Excision with 0.5- to 1-cm margins is appropriate for in situ tumors.[39,42] Lesions less than 2 mm in thickness can be excised with 1-cm margins and any tumor more than 2-mm thickness probably warrants excision with 2-cm margins.[39,42]

Additionally, management of the draining lymph nodes is of utmost importance. Because of the spread of melanomas to lymph nodes, excision of draining lymph nodes has been previously studied. Currently, sentinel lymph node biopsy (SLNB) remains the most sensitive and specific test for detection of micrometastatic melanoma in regional lymph nodes, allowing for proper staging. SLNB status seems to be the most important prognostic indicator for disease-specific survival in patients with primary cutaneous melanoma. However, no improvement in overall survival has been demonstrated in patients undergoing SLNB versus observation. Currently, clinicians can recommend SLNB in all patients with T2, T3, and T4 staged melanomas.[38] All patients with stage T1b melanoma can be considered selectively and specific importance should be focused on lesions with greater than 1-mm thickness, positive ulceration, increased mitotic rate, positive deep margins, or those associated with younger age.[38,39]

The efficacy of SLNB has decreased the need for elective lymph node dissection. Current data from several trials demonstrate no significant difference in overall survival exists for elective node dissection when compared with CLND.[43] Elective dissection can often lead to unnecessary complications and procedures for patients in which metastasis may not have occurred. Currently, a multicenter selective trial is underway to demonstrate whether or not completion dissection is necessary for patients with a positive SLNB, which could further guide treatment strategies.[39]

Of note, specifically focusing on head and neck lesions, radiotherapy for malignant melanoma has demonstrated efficacy in preventing recurrence.[1] Clinicians can consider radiotherapy for unresectable

Table 1
TNM staging categories for cutaneous melanoma

Classification	Thickness (mm)	Ulceration Status/Mitoses
T		
Tis	NA	NA
T1	≤1.00	a: Without ulceration and mitosis <1/mm^2 b: With ulceration or mitoses ≥1/mm^2
T2	1.01–2.00	a: Without ulceration b: With ulceration
T3	2.01–4.00	a: Without ulceration b: With ulceration
T4	>4.00	a: Without ulceration b: With ulceration
N	**No. of Metastatic Nodes**	**Nodal Metastatic Burden**
N0	0	NA
N1	1	a: Micrometastasis[a] b: Macrometastasis[b]
N2	2–3	a: Micrometastasis[a] b: Macrometastasis[b] c: In transit metastases/satellites without metastatic nodes
N3	4+ metastatic nodes, or matted nodes, or in transit metastases/satellites with metastatic nodes	
M	**Site**	**Serum LDH**
M0	No distant metastases	NA
M1a	Distant skin, subcutaneous, or nodal metastases	Normal
M1b	Lung metastases	Normal
M1c	All other visceral metastases Any distant metastasis	Normal Elevated

Abbreviations: LDH, lactate dehydrogenase; NA, not applicable.

[a] Micrometastases are diagnosed after sentinel lymph node biopsy.

[b] Macrometastases are defined as clinically detectable nodal metastases confirmed pathologically.

From Balch CM, Gershenwald JE, Soong SJ, et al. Final version of 2009 AJCC melanoma staging and classification. J Clin Oncol 2009;27(36):6199–206; with permission.

cutaneous malignant melanoma and sinonasal, nasopharyngeal, and oral lesions in which excision may not be appropriate.[1,44]

ADJUVANT THERAPY

Malignant melanoma provides an important model for the development of treatment strategies for human cancer.[13] Immunotherapy for malignant melanoma strives to provide stimulation for an individual's immune response to battle the cancer.

One approach includes targeting cytokines, several of which have demonstrated a role in melanoma treatment including interleukin (IL)-2, IL-5, IL-7, IL-21, interferon (IFN)-a, and granulocyte-macrophage colony–stimulating factor (GM-CSF). Treatment with IL-2, the first Food and Drug Administration approved immunotherapy option for unresectable melanoma, has demonstrated some efficacy in treatment.[11] Response rates range from 6% to 10% in treatment trials, which also demonstrate that response is increased with combination therapy with IFN and chemotherapy.[45,46]

Additionally, IL-21 also has antitumor effects and in several trials demonstrated partial response in 9 of 37 patients, stable response in 16 of 37 patients, and progressive disease in 12 of 37 patients.[11,47] Side effects include mild to minor fatigue, muscle pain, flulike symptoms, and the possibility of a transient lymphopenia or unclassified rash.[11,47] This treatment also demonstrated synergistic effects with GM-CSF.[11,48] Treatment with INF-a to date

Table 2
Anatomic stage groupings for cutaneous melanoma

	Clinical Staging[a]				Pathologic Staging[b]		
	T	N	M		T	N	M
0	Tis	N0	M0	0	Tis	N0	M0
IA	T1a	N0	M0	IA	T1a	N0	M0
IB	T1b	N0	M0	IB	T1b	N0	M0
	T2a	N0	M0		T2a	N0	M0
IIA	T2b	N0	M0	IIA	T2b	N0	M0
	T3a	N0	M0		T3a	N0	M0
IIB	T3b	N0	M0	IIB	T3b	N0	M0
	T4a	N0	M0		T4a	N0	M0
IIC	T4b	N0	M0	IIC	T4b	N0	M0
III	Any T	N > N0	M0	IIIA	T1-4a	N1a	M0
					T1-4a	N2a	M0
				IIIB	T1-4b	N1a	M0
					T1-4b	N2a	M0
					T1-4a	N1b	M0
					T1-4a	N2b	M0
					T1-4a	N2c	M0
				IIIC	T1-4b	N1b	M0
					T1-4b	N2b	M0
					T1-4b	N2c	M0
					Any T	N3	M0
IV	Any T	Any N	M1	IV	Any T	Any N	M1

[a] Clinical staging includes microstaging of the primary melanoma and clinical/radiologic evaluation for metastases. By convention, it should be used after complete excision of the primary melanoma with clinical assessment for regional and distant metastases.
[b] Pathologic staging includes microstaging of the primary melanoma and pathologic information about the regional lymph nodes after partial (ie, sentinel node biopsy) or complete lymphadenectomy. Pathologic stage 0 or stage IA patients are the exception; they do not require pathologic evaluation of their lymph nodes.
From Balch CM, Gershenwald JE, Soong SJ, et al. Final version of 2009 AJCC melanoma staging and classification. J Clin Oncol 2009;27(36):6199–206; with permission.

has not demonstrated significant improvement in survival either as a single agent or combination therapy and also holds an increased side effect profile.[11,46] GM-CSF is another cytokine , which activates macrophages and dendritic cells responsible in the T-cell immune response.[49] One trial demonstrated efficacy of treatment showing improvement of survival of 72.1 months in patients versus a placebo at 59.8 months.[50] Furthermore, the use of temozolomide, an alkylating agent, along with subcutaneous GM-CSF, INF-a, and recombinant IL-2 demonstrated complete response in 13% of patients and partial response in 13% patients.[51]

Other treatment options include the use of antibodies targeting immune molecules. Ipilimumab (Yervoy) is the first Food and Drug Administration approved treatment of unresectable melanoma targeting the cytotoxic T-lymphocyte antigen-4 demonstrating increased overall survival in Phase III studies.[7] The antibody is dosed at 3 mg/kg in unresectable or metastatic melanoma. Randomized, double-blinded studies have demonstrated an overall survival of 10.1 months (95% confidence interval [CI], 8–13.8) for Ipilimumab; 6.4 months for vaccination with gp100 (95% CI, 5.5–8.7); compared with 10 months for a combination of therapy (95% CI, 8.5–11.5).[7,52] One percent of patients demonstrated complete response, whereas 5% to 10% had partial responses.[52] Ipilimumab demonstrated 1- and 2-year survivals at 46% and 24%, respectively, compared with gp100, demonstrating 25% and 14.2% survival rates.[7] Side effects include diarrhea, nausea, constipation, abdominal pain, vomiting, vitiligo, and dermatitis.[52] Severe effects included enterocolitis, hepatitis, dermatitis, toxic epidermal necrolysis, neuropathy, and endocrinopathy.[7,11]

Vemurafenib (Zelboraf) is a new BRAF inhibitor approved for use in metastatic or unresectable melanomas expressing BRAFV600E. Several studies have demonstrated that the 6-month survival versus chemotherapy with dacarbazine is 84% and 64%, respectively, and a 52% rate of shrinkage.[7] Additional studies demonstrated a near 50% response rate in metastatic melanoma.[53] Side effects include arthralgias, unspecified rash, fatigue, alopecia, photosensitivity, nausea, diarrhea, and reports of keratoacanthoma and squamous cell carcinoma.[7] Tremelimumab, an antibody against cytotoxic T-lymphocyte antigen 040, may be useful for the treatment of melanoma. Investigation has demonstrated that although this drug is well tolerated, no additional benefits exist versus standard chemotherapy with either temozolomide or dacarbazine.[11,54] Administration of this drug with High Dose Interferon demonstrates promising antitumor effects with tolerable toxicities for malignant melanoma and further testing through randomized controlled trials is warranted.[55]

NEW TECHNOLOGIES

An innovative computer-vision system, Melafind, MELA Sciences, Irvington, New York has recently been designed to aid dermatologists in the detection of early pigmented cutaneous melanoma. It is indicated to aid in the diagnosis of atypical pigmented lesions with a minimum of one characteristic for melanoma. In addition, guidelines state it should be used on lesions that are between 2 and 22 mm; with significant pigment; void of trauma, scars, fibrosis, ulceration, or bleeding; and be located greater than 1 cm area away from the eye.[56] Testing with Melafind has demonstrated high sensitivities of 98% versus dermoscopists of 39% and dermatologists 72%.[56–58] This new computer vision technique will aid dermatologists in early detection of malignant melanoma and may limit the number of unnecessary biopsies.

Vaccinations to induce effector mechanisms against cancer cells are also a new hot topic in melanoma. A study has demonstrated that a triple peptide vaccine that targets against gp100, tyrosinase, and MART-1 has shown some promising results in increasing T-cell activity against malignant melanoma.[59] Augmented immunologic responses in patients with malignant melanoma were also demonstrated to be successful in those with vaccinations with adjuvant Toll-Like receptors agonists.[60,61] Immunotherapy and vaccinations against malignant melanoma open a new door for treatment of melanoma and demonstrate promising results.

FOLLOW-UP

Although official guidelines for follow-up for patients with malignant melanoma do not exist, several important principles must be kept in mind. Physicians can teach patients to perform monthly skin examinations and encourage the examination of important and inaccessible areas. High-risk patients with a positive family history of melanoma should have examinations starting in the adolescent years to monitor congenital nevi. Baseline photography or dermoscopy during these visits can serve as an excellent tool for further follow-up for changing lesions. A patient with more than five atypical moles is at moderate risk for developing malignant melanoma, and therefore should follow-up every 6 to 12 months depending on the heterogeneity of their nevi.[20,62] All patients with a history of malignant melanoma or other NMSC must receive annual skin examinations.

ACKNOWLEDGMENTS

The author gratefully acknowledges Mona Mislankar BS, Medical Student IV at University of Cincinnati College of Medicine for her valued assistance in preparing this manuscript.

REFERENCES

1. Erdei E, Torres SM. A new understanding in the epidemiology of melanoma. Expert Rev Anticancer Ther 2010;10(11):1811–23.
2. Melanoma. National Cancer Institute. Available at: http://www.cancer.gov/cancertopics/types/melanoma. Accessed September 17, 2012.
3. Melanoma. Available at: http://nci.nih.gov/aboutnci/servingpeople/snapshots/melanoma.pdf. Accessed August 24, 2012.
4. Jemal A, Devesa SS, Hartge P, et al. Recent trends in melanoma incidence among whites in the United States. J Natl Cancer Inst 2001;93:678–83.
5. Eide MJ, Weinstock MA. Association of UV index, latitude, and melanoma incidence in nonwhite populations: US Surveillance, Epidemiology, and End Results (SEER) Program, 1992-2001. Arch Dermatol 2005;141(4):477–81.
6. Melanoma. Available at: http://www.cdc.gov/cancer/dcpc/research/articles/melanoma_supplement.htm. Accessed March 19, 2012.
7. Hu S, Parmet Y, Allen G, et al. Disparity in melanoma: a trend analysis of melanoma incidence and stage at diagnosis among whites, Hispanics, and blacks in Florida. Arch Dermatol 2009;145(12):1369–74.
8. Clark LN, Shin DB, Troxel AB, et al. Association between the anatomic distribution of melanoma and sex. J Am Acad Dermatol 2007;56:768–73.
9. Chang YM, Barrett JH, Bishop DT, et al. Sun exposure and melanoma risk at different latitudes: a pooled analysis of 5700 cases and 7216 controls. Int J Epidemiol 2009;38:814–30.

10. Jemal A, Siegel R, Ward E, et al. Cancer statistics, 2008. CA Cancer J Clin 2008;58(2):71–96.
11. Zito CR, Kluger HM. Immunotherapy for metastatic melanoma. J Cell Biochem 2012;113(3):725–34.
12. Houghton AN, Polsky D. Focus on melanoma. Cancer Cell 2002;2(4):275–8.
13. Thompson JF, Morton DL, Kroon BB. Textbook of melanoma. London: Martin Dunitz; 2004.
14. Goldstein AM, Struewing JP, Chidambaram A, et al. Genotype-phenotype relationships in U.S. melanoma-prone families with CDKN2A and CDK4 mutations. J Natl Cancer Inst 2000;92:1006–10.
15. Jemal A, Siegel R, Xu J, et al. Cancer statistics, 2010. CA Cancer J Clin 2010;60(5):277–300.
16. Scolyer RA, Long GV, Thompson JF. Evolving concepts in melanoma classification and their relevance to multidisciplinary melanoma patient care. Mol Oncol 2011;5(2):124–36.
17. High WA, Robinson WA. Genetic mutations involved in melanoma: a summary of our current understanding. Adv Dermatol 2007;23:61–79.
18. Kraemer KH, et al. The role of sunlight and DNA repair in melanoma and nonmelanoma skin cancer. The xeroderma pigmentosum paradigm. Arch Dermatol 1994;130:1018–21.
19. Easton D. Cancer risks in BRCA2 mutation carriers. The Breast Cancer Linkage Consortium. J Natl Cancer Inst 1999;91:1310–6.
20. Psaty EL, Scope A, Halpern AC, et al. Defining the patient at high risk for melanoma. Int J Dermatol 2010;49(4):362–76.
21. Ferrone CR, et al. Clinicopathological features of and risk factors for multiple primary melanomas. JAMA 2005;294:1647–54.
22. Stam-Postguna JJ, et al. Multiple primary melanomas. J Am Acad Dermatol 2001;44:22–7.
23. Gandini S, et al. Meta-analysis of risk factors for cutaneous melanoma: III. Family history, actinic damage and phenotypic factors. Eur J Cancer 2005;41:2040–59.
24. Hemminki K, Zhang H, Czene K. Familial and attributable risks in cutaneous melanoma: effects of proband and age. J Invest Dermatol 2003;120:217–23.
25. Jemal A, Thun MJ, Ries LA, et al. Annual report to the nation on the status of cancer, 1975-2005, featuring trends in lung cancer, tobacco use, and tobacco control. J Natl Cancer Inst 2008;100(23).1672–94.
26. Levi F, et al. Non-Hodgkin's lymphomas, chronic lymphocytic leukaemias and skin cancers. Br J Cancer 1996;74:1847–50.
27. Euvrard S, Kanitakis J, Claudy A. Skin cancers after organ transplantation. N Engl J Med 2003;348: 1681–91.
28. Wei-Passanese EX, Han J, Lin W, et al. Geographical variation in residence and risk of multiple nonmelanoma skin cancers in US women and men. Photochem Photobiol 2012;88:483–9.
29. Goldberg MS, et al. Risk factors for presumptive melanoma in skin cancer screening: American Academy of Dermatology National Melanoma/Skin Cancer Screening program experience 2001-2005. J Am Acad Dermatol 2007;57:60–6.
30. Goodson AG, Grossman D. Strategies for early melanoma detection: approaches to the patient with nevi. J Am Acad Dermatol 2009;60:719–35.
31. The International Agency for Research on Cancer Working Group on Artificial Ultraviolet (UV) Light, Skin Cancer. The association of use of sunbeds with cutaneous malignant melanoma and other skin cancers: a systematic review. Int J Cancer 2007;120:1116–22.
32. Olsen CM, Zens MS, Stukel TA, et al. Nevus density and melanoma risk in women: a pooled analysis to test the divergent pathway hypothesis. Int J Cancer 2009;124(4):937–44.
33. Albert LS, Sober AJ. The dysplastic nevus as precursor and marker of increased risk for melanoma. In: Balch CM, Houghton AN, Milton GW, et al, editors. Cutaneous melanoma. 2nd edition. Philadelphia: Lippincott; 1992. p. 60–9.
34. Price HN, Schaffer JV. Congenital melanocytic nevi: when to worry and how to treat. Facts and controversies. Clin Dermatol 2010;28(3):293–302.
35. Hirokawa D, Lee JB. Dermatoscopy: an overview of subsurface morphology. Clin Dermatol 2011;29(5): 557–65.
36. Murali R, Shaw HM, Lai K, et al. Prognostic factors in cutaneous desmoplatic melanoma: a study of 252 patient. Cancer 2010;116:4130–8.
37. Chen JY, Hruby G, Scolyer RA, et al. Desmoplastic neurotropic melanoma: a clinicopathologic analysis of 128 cases. Cancer 2008;113:2770–8.
38. Balch CM, Gershenwald JE, Soong SJ, et al. Final version of 2009 AJCC melanoma staging and classification. J Clin Oncol 2009;27(36):6199–206.
39. Bichakjian CK, Halpern AC, Johnson TM, et al, American Academy of Dermatology. Guidelines of care for the management of primary cutaneous melanoma. American Academy of Dermatology. J Am Acad Dermatol 2011;65(5):1032–47.
40. Geller AC, Swetter SM, Oliveria S, et al. Reducing mortality in individuals at high risk for advanced melanoma through education and screening. J Am Acad Dermatol 2011;65(5 Suppl 1):S87–94.
41. Swetter SM, Pollitt RA, Johnson TM, et al. Behavioral determinants of successful early melanoma detection: role of self and physician skin examination. Cancer 2012;118:3725–34.
42. Haigh P, DiFronzo L, McCready D. Optimal excision margins for primary cutaneous melanoma: a systematic review and meta-analysis. Can J Surg 2003;46:419–26.
43. Morton DL, Thompson JF, Cochran AJ, et al. Sentinel-node biopsy or nodal observation in melanoma. N Engl J Med 2006;355:1307–17.

44. Fukada H, Hiratsuka J, Kobayashi T, et al. Boron neutron capture therapy (BNCT) for malignant melanoma with special reference to absorbed doses to the normal skin and tumor. Australas Phys Eng Sci Med 2003;26(3):97–103.
45. Atkins MB, Kunkel L, Sznol M, et al. High-dose recombinant interleukin-2 therapy in patients with metastatic melanoma: long term survival update. Cancer J Sci Am 2000;6(Suppl 1):S11–4.
46. Jilaveanu LB, Aziz SA, Kluger HM. Chemotherapy and biologic therapies for melanoma: do they work? Clin Dermatol 2009;27(6):614–25.
47. Davis ID, Brady B, Kefford RF, et al. Clinical and biological efficacy of recombinant human interleukin-21 in patients with stage IV malignant melanoma without prior treatment: a phase IIa trial. Clin Cancer Res 2009;15(6):2123–9.
48. Williams P, Rafei M, Bouchentouf M, et al. A fusion of GMCSF and IL-21 initiates hypersignaling through the IL-21R alpha chain with immune activating and tumoricidal effects in vivo. Mol Ther 2010;18(7): 1293–301.
49. Szabolcs P, Moore MA, Young JW. Expansion of immunostimulatory dendritic cells among the myeloid progeny of human CD34+ bone marrow precursors cultured with c-kit ligand, granulocyte-macrophage colony-stimulating factor, and TNF-alpha. J Immunol 1995;154(11):5851–61.
50. Lawson DH, Lee SJ, Tarhini AA, et al. E4697: Phase III cooperative group study of yeast-derived granulocyte macrophage colony-stimulating factor (GM-CSF) versus placebo as adjuvant treatment of patients with completely resected stage III-IV melanoma. J Clin Oncol 2010;28:15s.
51. Weber RW, O'Day S, Rose M, et al. Low-dose outpatient chemobiotherapy with temozolomide, granulocyte-macrophage colony stimulating factor, interferon-alpha2b, and recombinant interleukin-2 for the treatment of metastatic melanoma. J Clin Oncol 2005;23(35):8992–9000.
52. Mansh M. Ipilimumab and cancer immunotherapy: a new hope for advanced stage melanoma. Yale J Biol Med 2011;84(4):381–9.
53. Chapman PB, Hauschild A, Rpbert C, et al. Improved survival with vemurafenib in melanoma with BRAF V600E mutation. N Engl J Med 2011; 364(26):2507–16.
54. Ribas A, Hauschild A, Kefford R, et al. Phase III, open-label, randomized, comparative study of tremelimumab (CP 675,206) and chemotherapy (temozolomide [TMZ] or dacarbazine [DTIC]) in patients with advanced melanoma. J Clin Oncol 2008;26:15s.
55. Tarhini AA, Cherian J, Moschos SJ, et al. Safety and efficacy of combination immunotherapy with interferon alfa-2b and tremelimumab in patients with stage IV melanoma. J Clin Oncol 2012;30(3):322–8.
56. MelaFind. Available at: http://www.melasciences.com. Accessed July 2, 2012.
57. Monheit G, Cognetta AB, Ferris L, et al. The performance of MelaFind: a prospective multicenter study. Arch Dermatol 2011;147(2):188–94.
58. Friedman RJ, Gutkowicz-Krusin D, Farber MJ, et al. The diagnostic performance of expert dermoscopists vs a computer-vision system on small-diameter melanomas. Arch Dermatol 2009;144(4):476–82.
59. Kirwood JM, Lee S, Moschos SJ, et al. Immunogenicity and antitumor effects of vaccination with peptide vaccine +/-granulocyte-monocyte colonocyte stimulating factor and/or IFN-alpha2b in advanced metastatic melanoma: Eastern Cooperative Oncology Group Phase II Trial E1696. Clin Cancer Res 2009;15:1443–51.
60. Adams S, O'Neill DW, Nonaka D, et al. Immunization of malignant melanoma patients with full-length NY-ESO-1 protein using TLR7 agonist imiquimod as vaccine adjuvant. J Immunol 2008;181(1):776–84.
61. Bogunovic D, Manches O, Godefroy E, et al. TLR4 engagement during TLR3-induced pro-inflammatory signaling in dendritic cells promotes IL-10-mediated suppression of anti-tumor immunity. Cancer Res 2011;71:5467–76.
62. Kefford RF, et al. Counseling and DNA testing for individuals perceived to be genetically predisposed to melanoma: a consensus statement of the Melanoma Genetics Consortium. J Clin Oncol 1999;17: 3245–51.

Nonmelanoma Skin Cancer

Lauren E. Dubas, MD[a], Adam Ingraffea, MD[b,*]

KEYWORDS

• Nonmelanoma skin cancer • Basal cell carcinoma • Squamous cell carcinoma
• Sebaceous carcinoma • Eccrine porocarcinoma • Merkel cell carcinoma • Atypical fibroxanthoma
• Microcystic adnexal carcinoma

KEY POINTS

- Nonmelanoma skin cancer (NMSC) is the most common form of malignancy in humans.
- The most common forms of NMSC include basal cell carcinoma, squamous cell carcinoma, sebaceous carcinoma, eccrine porocarcinoma, Merkel cell carcinoma, atypical fibroxanthoma, and microcystic adnexal carcinoma.
- Most NMSCs are related to ultraviolet light exposure; other predisposing factors include exposure to radiation, human papillomavirus, immunosuppression, and genetic predisposition.
- Surgery (Mohs micrographic surgery, standard excision, or curettage) remains the treatment of choice for most lesions, but other methods exist, including radiation, topical immunomodulators, photodynamic therapy, and new systemic medications.

INTRODUCTION

Nonmelanoma skin cancer (NMSC) is the most common form of malignancy in humans and represents nearly 95% of all cutaneous neoplasms.[1] The incidence of NMSC has increased yearly by 3% to 8% since 1960 worldwide.[2] Recent Medicare claims data revealed that more than 3.5 million people in the United States were diagnosed with NMSC in 2006.[3] Because of the current age shift of the US population, the incidence of NMSC may increase by an estimated 50% by 2030.[4] This increase is despite growing public awareness campaigns targeting the harmful effects of ultraviolet (UV) exposure.[5]

BASAL CELL CARCINOMA

Definition, Epidemiology, and Pathogenesis

Basal cell carcinoma (BCC) is a malignant neoplasm of keratinocytes that reside within the basal layer of the epidermis. There is some evidence that the malignant cells may be derived from immature pluripotent cells of the interfollicular epidermis and the outer root sheath of the hair follicle.[6] A definite correlation exists between UV exposure and the genesis of BCC, because there is a higher frequency of disease among patients with history of significant sun exposure. The pattern of exposure (intermittent and intense) and type of UV radiation (UVB) have also been linked to higher BCC rates.[7]

On the molecular level, nearly 90% of all sporadic BCCs have mutations in the hedgehog signaling pathway. The hedgehog pathway is an intracellular signaling cascade key to the regulation of cell growth and differentiation during embryogenesis.[8] The extracellular hedgehog protein binds to a transmembrane receptor, patched homolog 1 (PTCH1), and prevents downstream PTCH1-mediated inhibition of signaling by smoothened homolog (SMO). SMO signaling activates a family of transcription factors encoded by the GLI family zinc finger. Usually inactive in adult tissues, mutations to either PTCH-1 or SMO result in constitutive

[a] Department of Dermatology, University of Cincinnati College of Medicine, Hoxworth Building, Ground Floor, 3130 Highland Avenue, Cincinnati, OH 45267, USA; [b] Department of Dermatology, University of Cincinnati College of Medicine, 7690 Discovery Drive, West Chester, Cincinnati, OH 45069, USA
* Corresponding author. 7690 Discovery Drive, Suite 3100, West Chester, OH 45069.
E-mail address: ingrafam@ucmail.uc.edu

Facial Plast Surg Clin N Am 21 (2013) 43–53
http://dx.doi.org/10.1016/j.fsc.2012.10.003

activation of the hedgehog signaling pathway, thus allowing unrestricted proliferation of epidermal basal cells.[9]

Clinical Findings

BCC is divided clinically into 4 major subtypes: superficial (**Fig. 1**), nodular ulcerative (**Fig. 2**), pigmented (**Fig. 3**), and morpheaform (**Fig. 4**). The nodular ulcerative subtype is the most common, representing approximately 50% to 85% of all biopsied BCC lesions, followed by superficial, morpheaform, and pigmented forms.[10]

Classically nodular lesions appear as a pearly papule or nodule with visible telangiectasias and an elevated rolled border. As lesions progress, they can centrally ulcerate and, if left untreated, invade critical structures of the head and neck. Superficial BCC lesions present as erythematous smooth to finely scaling patches mainly on the neck and shoulders and are often confused for eczema, superficial squamous cell carcinoma (SCC), or dermatophytosis. Morpheaform lesions often pose the worst prognosis and mainly present on the face as depressed, indurated plaques with ill-defined borders. Pigmented BCCs appear similarly to malignant melanoma and benign pigmented seborrheic keratosis.

Histopathology

Histologic subtype is an important prognostic indicator and should be provided in all biopsy pathology reports. Nearly all clinical subtypes show the diagnostic finding of basaloid, basophilic staining cells budding downward from the epidermis with palisading of peripheral cells (**Fig. 5**). Tumors become infiltrative when basaloid islands lose their epidermal connections and invade the underlying dermis. Infiltrative growth and perineural invasion portends a more aggressive clinical behavior and increased risk of recurrence.[11]

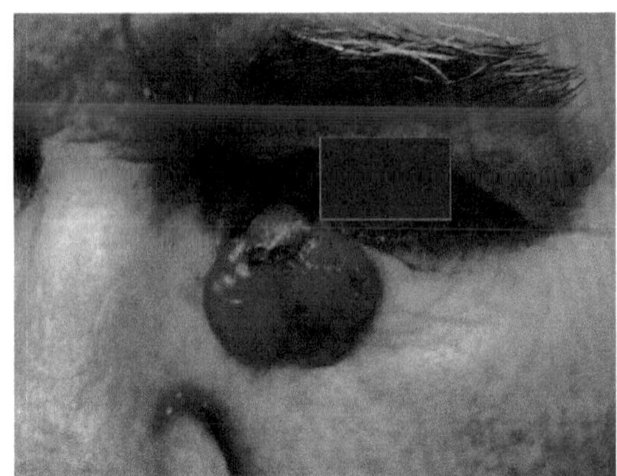

Fig. 2. Nodular ulcerative BCC.

Therapeutic Options

Management of BCC is determined by the lesion size, clinical and histopathologic subtype, depth, site, and patient comorbidities. The treatment of choice for lesions involving the head and neck is Mohs micrographic surgery (MMS), because it provides complete histopathologic examination of all margins of tissue removed. This procedure allows for preservation of healthy tissues in areas at high risk for recurrence (central, periauricular, and periorbital face). In addition, MMS offers the lowest 5-year recurrence rates of all treatment options: primary lesions (1%–2%), secondary lesions (4%–7%).[12] Multiple reviews of the literature support MMS as a more cost-effective treatment of NMSC (including BCC) than standard excision.[13,14] Other surgical options include standard wide local excision with 4-mm to 5-mm margins for nonaggressive BCC tumors in areas where tissue preservation is unessential. Curettage may be used to treat superficial lesions

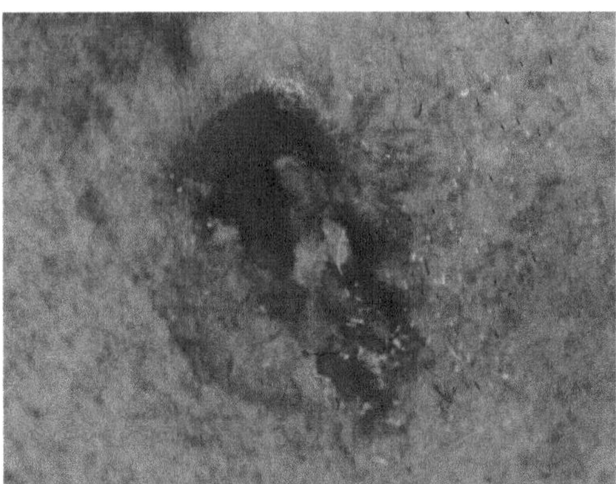

Fig. 1. Superficial BCC with focal ulceration.

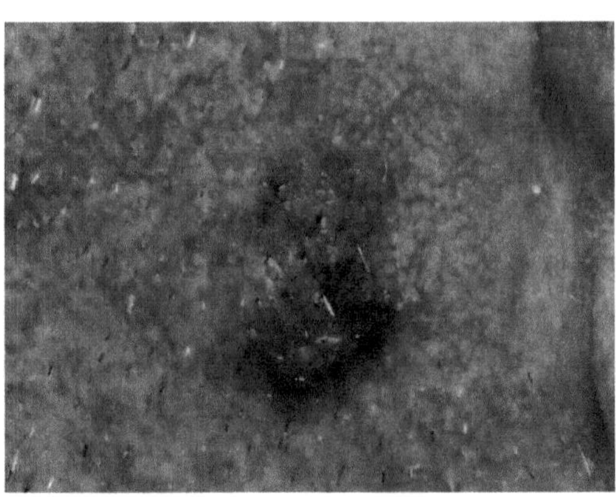

Fig. 3. Pigmented BCC.

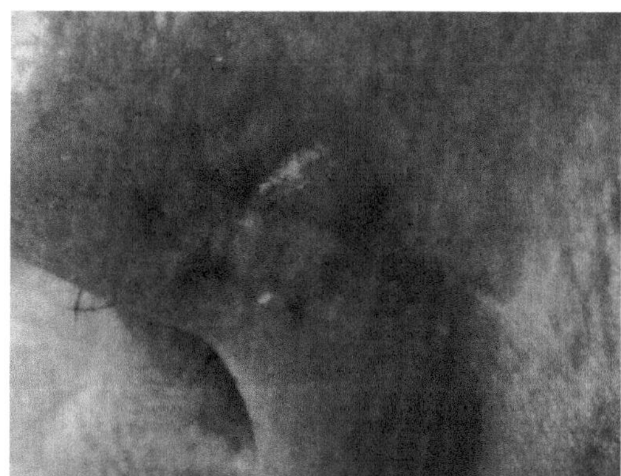

Fig. 4. Morpheaform BCC.

smaller than 2 cm or for patients who are poor surgical candidates.

Nonsurgical treatment options for BCC lesions include radiation, imiquimod, photodynamic therapy (PDT), ingenol mebutate (PEP005), and vismodegib.

External beam radiation

BCCs are relatively radioresponsive; therefore, radiotherapy can be used as a primary curative modality, surgical adjunctive therapy, or as palliative treatment.[15] Radiation is the primary treatment of choice for patients who are poor surgical candidates.[16]

Imiquimod

Topical imiquimod acts as an agonist of the toll-like receptor 7, which activates the cellular immune response to destroy dysplastic keratinocytes. Imiquimod 5.0% is approved by the US Food and Drug Administration (FDA) to treat nonfacial biopsy-confirmed superficial BCC.[17] Although the use of topical therapy does not confirm margin control, imiquimod monotherapy has shown a 5-year clearance rate as high as 80%.

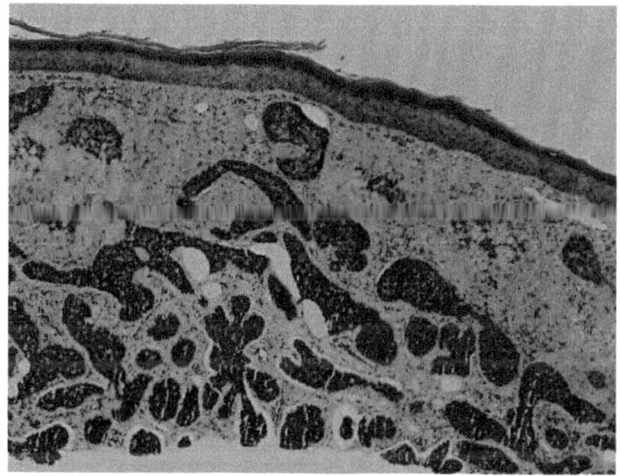

Fig. 5. Nodular BCC histopathology featuring basaloid, basophilic staining cells budding downward from the epidermis with palisading of peripheral cells and clefting.

PDT

PDT involves the activation of a photosensitizing drug (5-aminolevulinic acid, methyl ester form, methyl-5-aminolevulinate) by irradiation with light to create free radicals, resulting in highly targeted tumor cell destruction.[18] PDT is FDA approved only for the treatment of actinic keratoses (AKs); however, many clinical studies support PDT as an effective alternative treatment of superficial BCCs. A large multicenter study by Vinciullo and colleagues[19] showed a 92% response rate for superficial BCCs of the central face. Tumor thickness is a limiting factor for PDT, because the topical medication has limited absorption into the dermis. Therefore, nodular forms of BCC are best served by MMS or simple excision.

Ingenol mebutate (PEP 005)

A natural substance found in the sap of the plant *Euphorbia peplus*, ingenol mebutate has shown cytotoxic activity against AKs, SCC, and BCC lesions.[20] Recently (2012) approved by the FDA for the treatment of AKs, ingenol mebutate 0.05% gel offers a distinct advantage of shorter treatment duration (2–3 days) compared with imiquimod 5% cream (2–3 months). The proposed mechanism of action involves both neutrophil-mediated cytotoxicity and cellular necrosis of tumor cells. Early phase I/II trials show promising evidence for the use of ingenol mebutate in superficial BCCs.[21] One study reported complete clearance for 57% (16 of 28) of superficial BCC lesions after only 3 consecutive days of treatment. In addition, there were no recurring lesions over the study follow-up period (mean of 15 months).[18]

Vismodegib

Vismodegib was recently approved for the treatment of locally advanced and metastatic BCC. The medication targets gain-of-function mutations within the SMO protein, a member of the hedgehog intracellular signaling pathway. A phase I clinical trial showed an overall 54% response rate, both complete and incomplete, with the oral medication. Side effects are minor, including fatigue, hyponatremia, muscle spasm, and gastrointestinal upset.[22]

SCC

Epidemiology, Definition, and Pathogenesis

SCC is the second most common form of NMSC, with an estimated incidence of nearly 700,000 new cases annually in the United States.[3] SCC accounts for approximately 20% of all NMSC cases, and is the second most common form of cancer in the white population.[23]

A malignant neoplasm of keratinocytes, SCC lesions show full-thickness epidermal dysplasia. SCC may arise de novo or from AKs, promalignant precursor lesions that show partial-thickness epidermal dysplasia. AKs progress to full-thickness malignancy at an estimated rate of 0.025% to 16% for an individual lesion per year.[24] SCC lesions progress from in situ (Bowen disease) to invasive lesions once tumor cells invade the basement membrane of the dermal-epidermal junction.

UVB-induced inactivation of p53, a key tumor-suppressor gene, occurs in nearly 90% of all SCC lesions and 75% to 80% of premalignant AKs. p53 plays an important role in cell cycle arrest at the G1/S checkpoint. Normally the protein plays a fundamental role in the induction of apoptosis after UV light damage, thus preventing the development of malignant keratinocyte populations. Over time, keratinocytes acquire multiple UV-induced genetic mutations, leading to squamous cell dysplasia and subsequent in situ and invasive disease.

Clinical Findings

SCC typically develops on sun-exposed surfaces of the head and neck, including the scalp, ears, midface, lower lip, and neck.[25] AKs, precursor lesions of SCC, present as erythematous scaly or crusted macules and papules. AKs are important markers of UV-induced photodamage, and their presence generally signals an increased risk of NMSC.[26] SCC in situ (Bowen disease) presents as well-defined, erythematous, scaly papules and plaques (**Fig. 6**). More advanced lesions of SCC present with ill-defined, indurated, scaling papules, plaques, or nodules (**Fig. 7**). Ulceration and crusting may signal dermal invasion (**Fig. 8**); therefore, regional lymph nodes should be examined for signs of lymphadenopathy and metastatic disease.

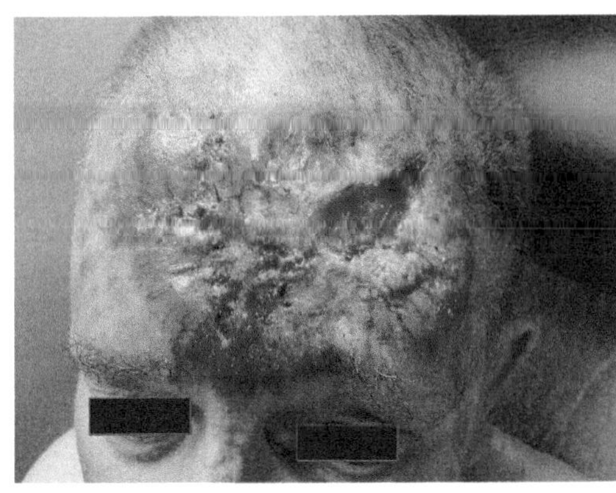

Fig. 7. Invasive SCC.

Histopathology

SCC is categorized by the thickness of epidermal invasion and degree of keratinocyte differentiation. In situ disease correlates with full-thickness epidermal involvement (**Fig. 9**), whereas invasive lesions show dermal invasion. Histologic grading is subdivided into 3 categories depending on the degree of keratinocyte keratinization: well-differentiated, moderately differentiated, and poorly differentiated. The degree of differentiation correlates with tumor aggressiveness, because poorly differentiated SCC lesions have higher recurrence (28.6%) and metastatic (32.8%) rates compared with rates of well-differentiated lesions (13.6%) and (9.2%), respectively.[27] Additional histopathologic features with poor prognostic implications include depth of invasion,

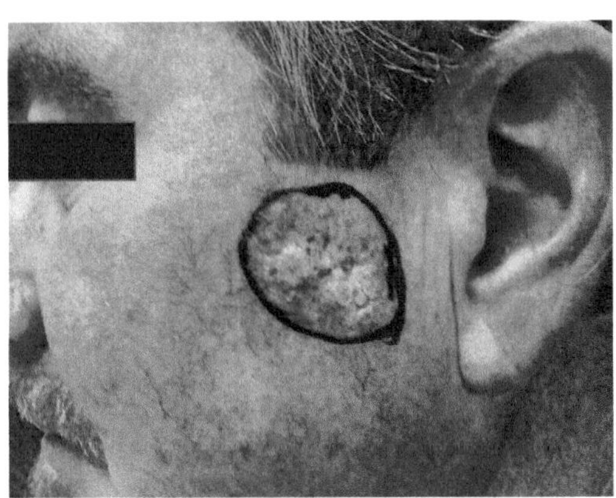

Fig. 6. SCC in situ.

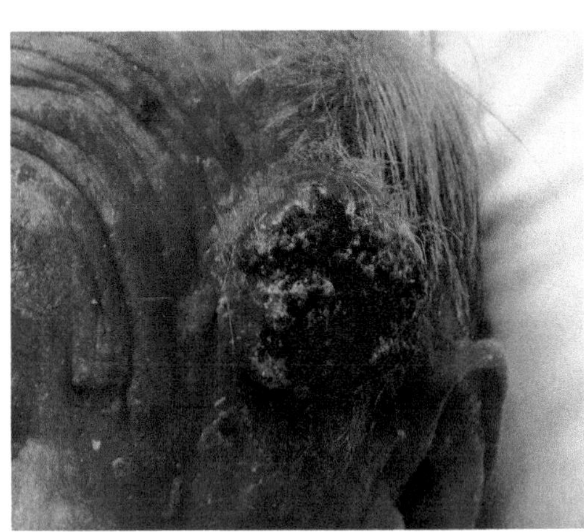

Fig. 8. Invasive SCC.

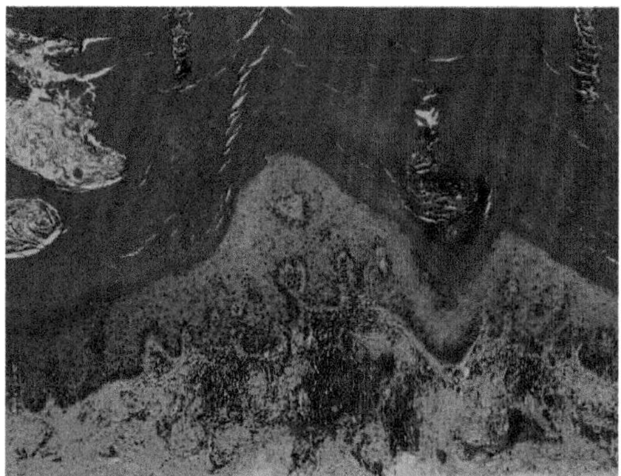

Fig. 9. SCC in situ histopathology featuring marked hyperkeratosis and full-thickness epidermal keratinocyte atypia.

desmoplastic reaction around infiltrating keratinocyte islands, and perineural or intravascular invasion.

Therapeutic Options

Multiple treatment modalities, both surgical and nonsurgical, exist for the treatment of SCC. The treatment of choice depends on the characteristics of the patient and their neoplasm. Considerations include the patient's age and functional status, surgical candidacy, lesion size, location, depth of invasion, level of differentiation, perineural or perivascular invasion, recurrence of previous SCC, and immunosuppression.[28]

Similar to BCC lesions, MMS is the treatment of choice for lesions involving the head and neck, most notably areas with a high risk of recurrence (central face, periorbital, periocular areas). Other indications for MMS include tumors larger than 2 cm, aggressive histology, recurrent tumors, lesions with ill-defined clinical margins, perineural or intravascular invasion, tumors arising in irradiated skin, and host immunosuppression. Other surgical options include simple excision, curettage, and cryosurgery.

Nonsurgical treatments for SCC may be used as a surgical adjuvant (decrease size of lesion before surgery or decrease recurrence rates after excision) or, in the case of superficial or in situ lesions, serve as the primary method of treatment. Current options for nonsurgical treatment include PDT, imiquimod, diclofenac, epidermal growth factor receptor (EGFR) inhibition (erlotinib, cetuximab), and external beam radiation.

PDT

PDT is a therapeutic option for SCC in situ lesions arising in patients who are poor surgical candidates or those who prefer noninvasive measures. Because of high recurrence rates and risk of metastatic disease, PDT is not a recommended treatment modality for invasive SCC tumors. A few case reports and series quote recurrence rates of 0% to 52% for SCC in situ and 82% for invasive SCC lesions.[29]

Imiquimod

Current evidence supports the limited use of topical imiquimod 5% cream in the treatment of SCC in situ lesions occurring in low-risk individuals or patients who are poor surgical candidates. A randomized, double-blind, placebo-controlled study[30] showed 73% (11 of 15) of biopsy-confirmed SCC in situ lesions achieved clearance after 16 weeks of therapy (applied once daily, 5 times a week). There were no documented cases of recurrence during a 9-month follow-up. Limitations to therapy include high rates of adverse effects (erythema, pruritus, and pain), lower clearance rates than other treatment modalities, and dependence on patient adherence to medication application.

Diclofenac

Diclofenac is a nonsteroidal antiinflammatory drug that works to inhibit the cyclooxygenase 2 enzyme, which is believed to be upregulated in NMSC lesions, thus promoting angiogenesis and impaired apoptosis.[31] Topical diclofenac 3% gel has been approved only for the treatment of AKs; however, a few case series showed clearance of SCC in situ lesions with daily treatment of 4 to 12 weeks.[32] One study showed no clinical evidence of SCC recurrence during a 10-month to 12-month follow-up period.[33] Further study is required to determine the optimum dosing regimen of diclofenac 3% gel, because this remains largely unknown.

EGFR inhibition

The EGFR is an extracellular signaling receptor within the ErbB tyrosine kinase receptor family. The extracellular binding domain found on keratinocytes is a target of multiple different ligands, including epidermal growth factor, epiregulin, and transforming growth factor α. Activation of the EGFR receptor by these various ligands stimulates keratinocyte proliferation, leading to increased cell survival and resistance to apoptosis. Keratinocytes within SCC lesions often show overexpression of the EGFR, leading to unrestricted cell growth. Advanced SCC lesions contain EGFR mutations in approximately 43% to 73% of cases, which may lead to a more aggressive tumor phenotype.[34]

Current treatment options for EGFR inhibition target either extracellular ligand binding inhibition or inactivation of intracellular tyrosine kinase signaling pathways. Cetuximab is a chimeric monoclonal antibody directed against the EGFR extracellular receptor domain and is FDA approved for the treatment of recurrent or metastatic SCC of the head and neck. A large study[35] comparing weekly cetuximab infusions with radiotherapy with radiotherapy alone showed improved locoregional control and overall survival rate in the cetuximab treatment group. The second method of EGFR is accomplished by erlotinib and gefitinib, which disrupt the intracellular signaling pathway of the tyrosine kinase domain. In a small case study, gefitinib was reported to have an 11% response rate and 53% control rate in patients with head and neck SCC.[36]

Radiotherapy

External beam radiation can function as both an adjunctive therapy to surgical excision or serve as primary treatment of head and neck SCC lesions in patients who are poor surgical candidates. Radiation may also play a role in palliative care for symptomatic relief of incurable skin cancers.[37] Adjunctive treatment of complex SCC lesions with high-risk factors for recurrence (desmoplastic features, perineural invasion) leads to a decreased local recurrence and increased overall disease-free survival rates.[38] One study of 167 patients with SCC and perineural invasion revealed a local recurrence rate of 43% with surgical excision alone compared with 20% with excision and adjunctive radiation. Likewise, disease-free survival increased from 53% to 73% in the 2 groups, respectively.[39] Radiotherapy may be considered for cases in which tumor cells are close to surgical margins or in which negative margin control is not possible.

SEBACEOUS CARCINOMA

Epidemiology, Definition, and Pathogenesis

Sebaceous carcinoma (SC), also known as sebaceous gland carcinoma, is a rare (0.5 cases per million patients) cutaneous neoplasm of sebaceous cells with a high rate of recurrence and metastasis to regional lymph nodes and distant organs.[40] The frequency of mortality from metastatic SC ranges from 9% to 50%, depending on disease progression at time of diagnosis.[41–43]

Risk factors for the development of SC include older age (median age at diagnosis is 72 years) and female sex (73% of patients are female).[44] Most lesions of SC arise de novo; however, some lesions have been shown to originate from preexisting sebaceous lesions (ie, sebaceous nevus).[45]

Clinical Findings

Most (~75%) SC lesions present on periocular skin, most commonly the eyelid.[46] SC typically presents as a painless round subcutaneous nodule (**Fig. 10**).[47] Other less common presentations include pedunculated lesions, diffuse thickening of the skin (pseudoinflammatory pattern), or as an irregular mass (signaling extensive tissue invasion). SC is often mistaken for BCC, SCC, or benign inflammatory conditions of the eye (ie, chalazia or blepharoconjunctivitis).[48]

Histopathology

SC lesions are classified based on level of differentiation and cell pattern of infiltration. Sebaceous cell differentiation is graded as well-differentiated, moderately differentiated, or poorly differentiated on histopathologic examination.[39] Undifferentiated sebaceous cells have eosinophilic cytoplasm with lipid granules, creating a frothy appearance (**Fig. 11**).[45] Four major patterns of infiltration are recognized: lobular, comedocarcinoma, papillary, and mixed.[39] SC lesions commonly have an irregular lobular pattern that stains with epithelial membrane antigen and Leu0M1 immunostains.[49]

Therapeutic Options

Surgical excision with 5-mm to 6-mm margins is standard of care for SC lesions with an associated mortality of 18% and recurrence rates of up to 36% at 5-year follow-up.[42,50] However, an improved recurrence rate of 11% was shown in a recent study using MMS for the removal of SC.[51] Exenteration is required for neoplasms infiltrating the orbit or when there is extensive bulbar conjunctival involvement.[52]

Nonsurgical therapeutic options include external beam radiation for advanced cases and palliative care. Radiation is frequently used in

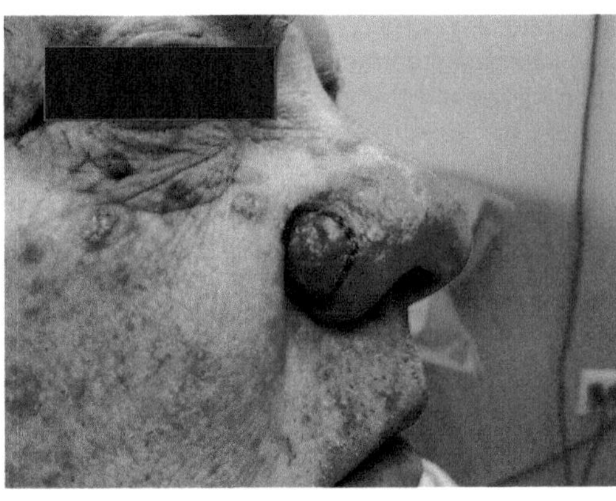

Fig. 10. Sebaceous carcinoma.

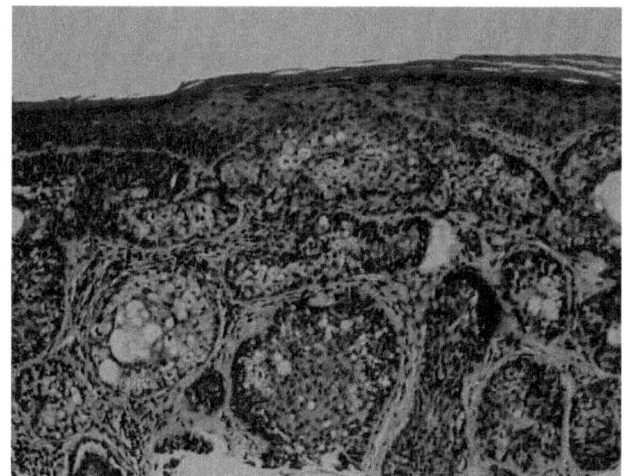

Fig. 11. Sebaceous carcinoma histopathology featuring well-differentiated lobules of sebaceous cells.

metastatic disease, most notably for patients who have orbital involvement but refuse exenteration.[53]

ECCRINE POROCARCINOMA

Epidemiology, Definition, and Pathogenesis

Eccrine porocarcinoma (EPC), also referred to as malignant eccrine poroma, is a rare malignancy arising from intraepidermal eccrine sweat ducts (acrosyringeum). Most commonly, lesions arise de novo; however, case reports exist of malignant degeneration of long-standing benign eccrine poromas.[54,55] EPC lesions occur most commonly on the lower extremities (60%), but are also found on the head and neck.[56] Patients are typically middle-aged, found equally between both genders, and have been documented in all races.[57]

Clinical Findings

Lesions of EPC present as firm, asymptomatic, erythematous to violaceous nodules usually smaller than 2 cm.[55] Signs or symptoms of malignant transformation include spontaneous bleeding, ulceration, pruritus or pain, and sudden increase in size.[58]

Histopathology

EPC neoplasms are characterized by glycogen-rich, clear-staining cells with large, hyperchromatic, and irregularly shaped (pleomorphic) nuclei.[59] EPC cells may be entirely contained within the epidermis or may extend into the dermis.[55] Dermally infiltrative lesions extend via asymmetric cords and lobules of polygonal cells, creating a characteristic cribriform pattern of proliferation. The connective tissue stroma surrounding dermal EPC may also take on myxoid, mucinous, or fibrotic features.[60]

Treatment Options

Primary surgical excision, the treatment of choice for EPC lesions, provides a curative rate of 70% to 80%.[61] Predictive factors for recurrence include tumors thicker than 7 mm, dermal infiltration, presence of lymphovascular invasion, and high number (>14) of mitoses per high-power field. High-risk tumors involving the head and neck may be best served by MMS. One case series of 5 primary EPC lesions treated by MMS showed no recurrence at 2 to 4 years' postoperative follow-up.[62]

No standard protocol exists for the treatment of recurrent or metastatic EPC tumors. Radiation therapy is reserved for palliative care, because tumor response is often partial or inconsistent.[63] Likewise, systemic chemotherapy (cyclophosphamide, bleomycin, cisplatin, and 5-fluorouracil) has shown limited effectiveness for metastatic EPC. Therefore, early detection and definitive excision provide the highest chances of survival.[64]

MERKEL CELL CARCINOMA

Epidemiology, Definition, and Pathogenesis

Merkel cell carcinoma (MCC), also known as neuroendocrine carcinoma, is a rare, aggressive, and often fatal cutaneous malignancy of epidermal neuroendocrine (mechanoreceptor) cells. The incidence of MCC has tripled over the past 15 years, with approximately 1500 new cases diagnosed each year.[65]

Recent research has shed light on a possible viral cause of MCC lesions. Feng and colleagues[66] identified a novel polyomavirus clonally integrated into approximately 80% of MCC tumors. These small double-stranded DNA viruses integrate into neuroendocrine cells, resulting in autonomous viral replication and malignant transformation.[67]

Risk factors for the development of MCC include immunosuppression, older age, and sun exposure. The average age of MCC diagnoses range from 67 to 69 years; only 5% of reported cases occur at less than 50 years of age.[68] Among immunosuppressed populations, the relative risk of MCC increases nearly 13-fold in patients with human immunodeficiency virus (HIV) and another 10-fold for patients who have had a solid-organ transplant.[69,70]

Clinical Findings

Most commonly found on the head, neck, and extremities (80%), MCC lesions tend to occur on sun-exposed skin surfaces.[71] Rarely suspected at the time of diagnosis, MCC lesions lack distinctive findings and are often mistaken for BCC, epidermoid cysts, or amelanotic melanoma.

MCC tumors typically present as rapidly enlarging asymptomatic red-blue dermal papules or nodules that develop over a course of weeks to months (**Fig. 12**).[71]

Histopathology

MCC tumors are dermally based neoplasms made up of small uniform round blue-staining cells that are arranged in cords, bands, or clusters. Individual Merkel cells have scant cytoplasm and a large, round vesicular nuclei with salt-and-pepper chromatin.[65] Immunohistochemistry is routinely used to confirm the diagnosis of MCC because cytokeratin 20 stains approximately 80% to 90% of MCC tumors with a diagnostic paranuclear dotlike pattern.[72]

Treatment Options

Surgical excision remains the mainstay of therapy for patients diagnosed with primary MCC. Margin size is based on the clinical size of the primary tumor: 1 cm for tumors smaller than 2 cm and 2 cm for tumors larger than 2 cm.[73] Because of the high propensity of MCC to metastasize to regional lymph nodes, sentinel lymph node (SLN) biopsy is recommended for all untreated primary tumors at the time of wide local excision.[74] SLN biopsy is included in the most recent American Joint Committee on Cancer staging guidelines, and is an important prognostic indicator for MCC.[75]

MCC is considered to be a radiosensitive neoplasm; therefore, radiation therapy plays a key role as both an adjunct to surgery and as primary therapy for inoperable lesions. Adjuvant radiation therapy to the primary site after wide local excision has shown a 3.7-fold decrease in MCC tumor recurrence.[76] Other considerations for targeted radiation include draining lymph node basins and in-transit lymphatics.[77]

ATYPICAL FIBROXANTHOMA

Epidemiology, Definition, and Pathogenesis

Atypical fibroxanthoma (AFX) is a rare neoplasm with intermediate malignant potential, which most commonly affects elderly white men.[70] Classified as a spindle cell tumor, AFX is a malignancy of dermal fibroblasts. Previously regarded as a low-grade malignancy, current case reports estimate an overall recurrence rate of approximately 6%. In addition, microsatellite and in-transit metastases have been reported, resulting in 5 patient deaths.[79]

UV light exposure is a major risk factor, because some AFX tumors have shown p53 gene mutations at dipyrimidine sites similar to SCC lesions.[80] Other possible risk factors include previous radiation exposure and immunosuppression.[81]

Clinical Findings

Lesions most commonly present on the head and neck in areas of chronic sun exposure. Tumors appear as rapidly enlarging skin colored to pink, dome-shaped papules and nodules that frequently ulcerate (**Fig. 13**).[82] AFX lesions may mimic nodular BCCs and inflamed dermal nevi.

Histopathology

AFX tumors are characterized by a pleomorphic spindle cell proliferation admixed with multinucleated giant cells within the dermis. Markers of aggressive tumor biology include infiltration into the subcutaneous fat and invasion of vascular structures. Immunohistochemical markers are essential for differentiating AFX from other cutaneous spindle cell neoplasms, including desmoplastic melanoma and the spindle cell variant of SCC. AFX lesions stain negative for cytokeratin, melan-A, and S-100 and strongly positive for CD10 (90% of cases).[77]

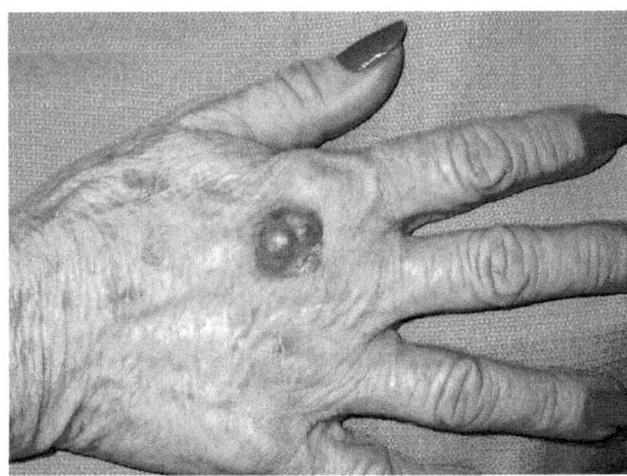

Fig. 12. Merkel cell carcinoma.

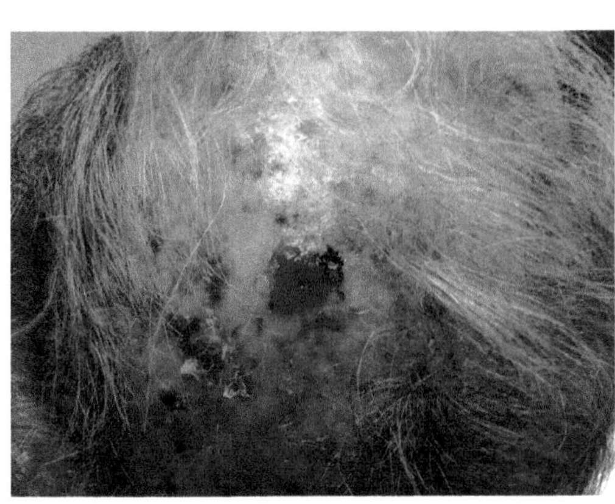

Fig. 13. Atypical fibroxanthoma.

Treatment Options

Previously, wide local excision with 2-cm margins served as standard of care for AFX lesions. However, recent studies have shown decreased recurrence rates with MMS. Ang and colleagues[83] reviewed the rate of recurrence for AFX lesions treated at the Mayo Clinic over a 15-year period. They found no cases of recurrence for MMS-treated lesions, versus 8.7% with wide local excision.

MICROCYSTIC ADNEXAL CARCINOMA

Microcystic adnexal carcinoma (MAC), also known as sclerosing sweat duct carcinoma, is a rare tumor with follicular and sweat gland differentiation.[84] MAC lesions typically present on the head, neck, or lips of older (medial age, 68 years) patients. Most cases have been noted in whites (90%).[85] Clinically, lesions appear as slow growing, skin colored to yellow, indurated plaques or cystic nodules. The average size of MAC lesions at diagnosis is 2 cm.[86] Tumors tend to be locally aggressive, with common perineural invasion and possible extension to underlying muscle and bone.[87] Treatment options include wide local excision, MMS, and radiation.

REFERENCES

1. Rubin AI, Chen EH, Ratner D. Basal-cell carcinoma. N Engl J Med 2005;353:2262–9.
2. Glass AG, Hoover RN. The emerging epidemic of melanoma and squamous cell skin cancer. JAMA 1989;262:2097–100.
3. Rogers HW, Weinstock MA, Harris AR, et al. Incidence estimate of nonmelanoma skin cancer in the United States, 2006. Arch Dermatol 2010;146(3):200–7.
4. Diffey BL, Langtry JA. Skin cancer incidence and the ageing population. Br J Dermatol 2005;153:679–80.
5. Diepgen TL, Mahler V. The epidemiology of skin cancer. Br J Dermatol 2002;146(Suppl 61):1–6.
6. Youseff KK, Van Keymeulen A, Lapouge G, et al. Identification of the cell lineage at the origin of basal cell carcinoma. Nat Cell Biol 2010;12:299–305.
7. Han J, Colditz GA, Hunter DJ. Risk factors for skin cancers: a nested case-control study within the Nurses' Health Study. Int J Epidemiol 2006;35:1514–21.
8. Ingham PW, McMahon AP. Hedgehog signaling in animal development: paradigms and principles. Genes Dev 2001;15:3059–87.
9. Xie J, Murone M, Luoh SM, et al. Activating smoothened mutations in sporadic basal-cell carcinoma. Nature 1998;391:90–2.
10. Chinem VP, Miot HA. Epidemiology of basal cell carcinoma. An Bras Dermatol 2011;86(2):292–305.
11. Rippey JJ. Why classify basal cell carcinomas? Histopathology 1998;32:393–8.
12. Leibovitch I, Huilgol SC, Selva D, et al. Basal cell carcinoma treated with Mohs surgery in Australia II. Outcome at 5-year follow-up. J Am Acad Dermatol 2005;53:452–7.
13. Tierney EP, Hanke CW. Cost effectiveness of Mohs micrographic surgery: review of the literature. J Drugs Dermatol 2009;8(10):914–22.
14. Rogers HW, Coldiron BM. A relative value unit-based cost comparison of treatment modalities for nonmelanoma skin cancer: effect of the loss of the Mohs multiple surgery reduction exemption. J Am Acad Dermatol 2009;61(1):96–103.
15. Hulyalkar R, Rakkhit T, Garcia-Auazaga J. The role of radiation therapy in the management of skin cancers. Dermatol Clin 2011;29:287–96.
16. National Comprehensive Cancer Network Clinical Practice Guidelines in Oncology. Basal cell and squamous cell skin cancers. V.1. 2010.
17. Gaspari AA, Tyring SK, Rosen T. Beyond a decade of 5% imiquimod topical therapy. J Drugs Dermatol 2009;8(5):467–74.
18. His RA, Rosenthal DI, Glatstein E. Photodynamic therapy in the treatment of cancer: current state of the art. Drugs 1999;57(5):725–34.
19. Vinciullo C, Elliott T, Francis D, et al. Photodynamic therapy with topical methyl aminolaevulinate for "difficult-to-treat" basal cell carcinoma. Br J Dermatol 2005;152:765–72.
20. Ramsay JR, Suhrbier A, Aylward JH, et al. The sap from *Euphorbia peplus* is effective against human NMSCs. Br J Dermatol 2011;164(3):633–6.
21. Siller G, Rosen R, Freeman M, et al. PEP (ingenol mebutate) gel for the topical treatment of superficial basal cell carcinoma: results of a randomized phase IIa trial. Australas J Dermatol 2010;51(2):99–105.
22. LoRusso PM, Rudin CM, Reddy JC, et al. Phase I trial of hedgehog pathway inhibitor vismodegib (GDC-0049) in patients with refractory, locally advanced or metastatic solid tumors. Clin Cancer Res 2011;17(8):2502–11.
23. Gloster HM, Brodland DG. The epidemiology of skin cancer. Dermatol Surg 1996;22(3):217–26.
24. Criscione VD, Weinstock MA, Naylor MF, et al. Actinic keratoses: natural history and risk of malignant transformation in the Veterans Affairs Topical Tretinoin Chemoprevention Trial. Cancer 2009;115(11):2523–30.
25. Madan V, Lear JT, Szeimies RM. Non-melanoma skin cancer. Lancet 2010;375:673–85.
26. Salasche SJ. Epidemiology of actinic keratoses and squamous cell carcinoma. J Am Acad Dermatol 2000;42:4–7.

27. Rowe DE, Carroll RJ, Day CL Jr. Prognostic factors for local recurrence, metastasis, and survival rates in squamous cell carcinoma of the skin, ear, and lip. Implications for treatment modality selection. J Am Acad Dermatol 1992;26:976–90.
28. Cherpelis BS, Marcusen C, Lang PG. Prognostic factors for metastasis in squamous cell carcinoma of the skin. Dermatol Surg 2002;28:268–73.
29. Marmur ES, Schmults CD, Goldberg DJ. A review of laser and photodynamic therapy for the treatment of nonmelanoma skin cancer. Dermatol Surg 2004; 30(2):264–71.
30. Patel GK, Goodwin R, Chawla M, et al. Imiquimod 5% cream monotherapy for cutaneous squamous cell carcinoma in situ (Bowen's disease): a randomized, double-blind, placebo-controlled trial. J Am Acad Dermatol 2006;54(6):1024–32.
31. Subbaramaiah K, Zakim D, Weksler BB, et al. Inhibition of cyclooxygenase: a novel approach to cancer prevention. Proc Soc Exp Biol Med 1997;216(2): 201–10.
32. Patel MJ, Stockfleth E. Does progression from actinic keratosis and Bowen's disease end with treatment: diclofenac 3% gel, an old drug in a new environment? Br J Dermatol 2007;156(3):53–6.
33. Dawe SA, Salisbury JR, Higgins E. Two cases of Bowen's disease successfully treated topically with 3% diclofenac in 2.5% hyaluronan gel. Clin Exp Dermatol 2005;30(6):712–3.
34. Uribe P, Gonzalez S. Epidermal growth factor receptor (EGFR) and squamous cell carcinoma of the skin: molecular bases for EGFR-targeted therapy. Pathol Res Pract 2011;207(6):337–42.
35. Bonner JA, Harari PM, Giralt J, et al. Radiotherapy plus cetuximab for squamous-cell carcinoma of the head and neck. N Engl J Med 2006;354: 567–78.
36. Glisson B, Kim S, Kies M, et al. Phase II study of gefitinib in patients with metastatic/recurrent squamous cell carcinoma of the skin. J Clin Oncol 2006;24(18):5331.
37. Han A, Ratner D. What is the role of adjuvant radiation therapy in the treatment of cutaneous squamous cell cancer with peri neural invasion? Cancer 2007; 30(1):93–6.
38. Garcia-Serra A, Hinerman RW, Mendenhall WM, et al. Carcinoma of the skin with perineural invasion. Head Neck 2002;24:78–83.
39. Veness MJ. High-risk cutaneous squamous cell carcinoma of the head and neck. J Biomed Biotechnol 2007;2007(3):80572.
40. Nelson BR, Hamlet KR, Gillard M, et al. Sebaceous carcinoma. J Am Acad Dermatol 1995;33:1–15.
41. Rao NA, Hidayat AA, McLean IW, et al. Sebaceous carcinomas of the ocular adnexa: a clincopathologic study of 104 cases with five-year follow-up data. Hum Pathol 1982;13:113–22.
42. Doxanas MT, Green WR. Sebaceous gland carcinoma. Review of 40 cases. Arch Ophthalmol 1984; 102:245–9.
43. Zurcher M, Hintschich CR, Garner A, et al. Sebaceous carcinoma of the eyelid: a clinicopathological study. Br J Ophthalmol 1998;82:1049–55.
44. Shields JA, Demirci H, Marr BP, et al. Sebaceous carcinoma of the eyelids: personal experience with 60 cases. Ophthalmology 2004;111:2151–7.
45. Matsuda K, Doi T, Kosaka H, et al. Sebaceous carcinoma arising in nevus sebaceous. J Dermatol 2005; 32:641–4.
46. Wick MR, Goellner JR, Wolfe JT 3rd, et al. Adnexal carcinomas of the skin. II. Extraocular sebaceous carcinomas. Cancer 1985;56:1163–72.
47. Buitrago W, Joseph AK. Sebaceous carcinoma: the great masquerader: emerging concepts in diagnosis and treatment. Dermatol Ther 2008;21: 459–66.
48. Ozdal PC, Codere F, Callejo S, et al. Accuracy of the clinical diagnosis of chalazion. Eye 2004;18:135–8.
49. Sinard JH. Immunohistochemical distinction of ocular sebaceous carcinoma from basal cell and squamous cell carcinoma. Arch Ophthalmol 1999; 117:776–83.
50. Snow SN, Larson PO, Lucarelli MJ, et al. Sebaceous carcinoma of the eyelids treated by Mohs micrographic surgery: report of nine cases with review of the literature. Dermatol Surg 2002;28:623–31.
51. Spencer JM, Nossa R, Tse DT, et al. Sebaceous carcinoma of the eyelid treated with Mohs micrographic surgery. J Am Acad Dermatol 2001;44: 1004–9.
52. Cook BE Jr, Bartley GB. Treatment options and future prospects for the management of eyelid malignancies: an evidence-based update. Ophthalmology 2001;108:2088–98.
53. Callahan EF, Appert DL, Roenigk RK, et al. Sebaceous carcinoma of the eyelid: a review of 14 cases. Dermatol Surg 2004;30:1164–8.
54. Gschanait F, Horn F, Lindlbauer R, et al. Eccrine porocarcinoma. J Cutan Pathol 1980;7:349.
55. Mohri S, Chika K, Saito I, et al. A case of porocarcinoma. J Dermatol 1980;7:431.
56. Penneys NS, Ackerman AB, Indgin SN, et al. Eccrine poroma. Br J Dermatol 1970;82:613.
57. Brown CW Jr, Dy C. Eccrine porocarcinoma. Dermatol Ther 2008;21:433–8.
58. Puttick L, Ince P, Comaish JS. Three cases of eccrine porocarcinoma. Br J Dermatol 1986;115:111–6.
59. Pinkus H, Mehregan AH. Epidermotropic eccrine carcinoma: a case combining features of eccrine poroma and Paget's disease. Arch Dermatol 1963; 88:597.
60. Yamamoto O, Haratake J, Yokoyama S, et al. A histopathological and ultrastructural study of eccrine porocarcinoma with special reference to its

subtypes. Virchows Arch A Pathol Anat Histopathol 1992;420:395–401.

61. Orella J, Peanalba A, San Juan C, et al. Eccrine porocarcinoma: report of nine cases. Dermatol Surg 1997;23:925–8.
62. Wittenberg G, Rovertson D, Solomon A. Eccrine porocarcinoma treated with Mohs micrographic surgery: a report of five cases. Dermatol Surg 1999;21:911–3.
63. Giorgi V, Sestini S, Massi D, et al. Eccrine porocarcinoma: a rare but sometimes fatal malignant neoplasm. Dermatol Surg 2007;33:371–7.
64. Goel R, Contos MJ, Wallace ML. Widespread metastatic eccrine porocarcinoma. J Am Acad Dermatol 2003;49:252–4.
65. Lemos B, Nghiem P. Merkel cell carcinoma: more deaths but still no pathway to blame. J Invest Dermatol 2007;127:2100–3.
66. Feng H, Shuda M, Chang Y, et al. Clonal integration of a polyomavirus in human Merkel cell carcinoma. Science 2008;319:1096–100.
67. Wang TS, Byrne PJ, Jacobs JK, et al. Merkel cell carcinoma: update and review. Semin Cutan Med Surg 2011;30:48–56.
68. Goessling W. Merkel cell carcinoma. J Clin Oncol 2002;20:588–98.
69. Engels EA, Frisch M, Goedert JJ, et al. Merkel cell carcinoma and HI infection. Lancet 2002;359:497–8.
70. Busam KJ, Jungbluth AA, Rekthman N, et al. Merkel cell polyomavirus expression in Merkel cell carcinomas and its absence in combined tumors and pulmonary neuroendocrine carcinomas. Am J Surg Pathol 2009;3:1378–85.
71. Hitchcock CL, Bland KI, Laney RG 3rd, et al. Neuroendocrine (Merkel cell) carcinoma of the skin. Its natural history, diagnosis, and treatment. Ann Surg 1988;207:201–7.
72. Bobos M, Hytiroglou P, Kostopoulos I, et al. Immunohistochemical distinction between Merkel cell carcinoma and small cell carcinoma of the lung. Am J Dermatopathol 2006;28:99–104.
73. Miller SJ, Alam M, Andersen J, et al. Merkel cell carcinoma. J Natl Compr Canc Netw 2009;7:322–32.
74. Gupta SG, Wang LC, Penas PF, et al. Sentinel lymph node biopsy for evaluation and treatment of patients with Merkel cell carcinoma: the Dana Farber experience and meta-analysis of literature. Arch Dermatol 2006;142:685–90.
75. Lemos BD, Storer BE, Iyer JG, et al. Pathologic nodal evaluation improves prognostic accuracy in Merkel cell carcinoma: analysis of 5823 cases as the basis of the first consensus staging system. J Am Acad Dermatol 2010;63:751–61.
76. Lewis KG, Weinstock MA, Weaver AL, et al. Adjuvant local irradiation for Merkel cell carcinoma. Arch Dermatol 2006;142:693–700.
77. Mojica P, Smith D, Ellenhorn JD. Adjuvant radiation therapy is associated with improved survival in Merkel cell carcinoma. J Clin Oncol 2007;25:1043–7.
78. Luzar B, Calonje E. Morphological and immunohistochemical characteristics of atypical fibroxanthoma with a special emphasis on diagnostic pitfalls: a review. J Cutan Pathol 2010;37:301–9.
79. Hollmig ST, Sachdev R, Cockerell CJ, et al. Spindle cell neoplasms encountered in dermatologic surgery: a review. Dermatol Surg 2012;1:1–26.
80. Dei Tos AP, Maestro R, Doglioni C, et al. Ultraviolet-induced p53 mutations in atypical fibroxanthoma. Am J Pathol 1994;145:11–7.
81. Hollstein M, Sidransky D, Vogelstein B, et al. p53 mutations in human cancers. Science 1991;253:49–53.
82. Fretzin DF, Helwig EB. Atypical fibroxanthoma of the skin. A histopathologic study of 140 cases. Cancer 1973;31:1541–52.
83. Ang GC, Roenigk RK, Otley CC, et al. More than 2 decades of treating atypical fibroxanthoma at the Mayo Clinic: what have we learned from 91 patients? Dermatol Surg 2009;35:765–72.
84. Goldstein DJ, Barr RJ, Santa Cruz DJ. Microcystic adnexal carcinoma: a distinct clinicopathologic entity. Cancer 1982;50(3):566–72.
85. Yu JB, Blitzblau RC, Patel SC, et al. Surveillance, epidemiology, and end results (SEER) database analysis of microcystic adnexal carcinoma (sclerosing sweat duct carcinoma) of the skin. Am J Clin Oncol 2010;33(2):125–7.
86. Leibovitch I, Huilgol SC, Selva D, et al. Microcystic adnexal carcinoma: treatment with Mohs micrographic surgery. J Am Acad Dermatol 2005;52(2):295–300.
87. Cooper PH, Mills SE. Microcystic adnexal carcinoma of the scalp. J Am Acad Dermatol 1984;10:908–14.

Effects of Topicals on the Aging Skin Process

J. Regan Thomas, MD[a], Tatiana K. Dixon, MD[b,*],
Tapan K. Bhattacharyya, PhD[a]

KEYWORDS

• Topicals • Skin aging • Retinoids • Retinoic acid • Glycolic acid • Ascorbic acid • Vitamin C • Peptides

KEY POINTS

- Retinoids are the most extensively studied skin topicals, and have been found to significantly improve the appearance of mild to moderate photodamage.
- Glycolic acid speeds up the process of exfoliation and skin cell turnover by weakening the intercellular cohesion of the stratum corneum, and appears to improve skin dyspigmenation better than fine wrinkles.
- Ascorbic acid is thought to act as an antioxidant and to also stimulate the production of procollagen types I and III.
- Peptides used in topical antiaging products have multiple applications and can be categorized into 4 groups based on their modes of action:
  - Carrier peptides
  - Signal peptides
  - Enzyme-inhibitor peptides
  - Neurotransmitter-inhibitor peptides

INTRODUCTION

Skin aging is a product of two processes:

1. Intrinsic, or chronologic aging, which is mainly genetic
2. Extrinsic aging from environmental stressors such as sun exposure or smoking

The resulting skin changes include dyschromia, roughness, and fine rhytids followed by persistent deeper folds. Structurally this is explained by dermal atrophy, decreased collagen, loss of subcutaneous fat, loss of inherent elasticity, and increased melanogenesis.[1]

Topical antiaging products were estimated to be a $2 billion industry in the United States in 2000,[2] largely due to people seeking to find cost-effective, noninvasive methods to reverse aging. However, the Food and Drug Administration (FDA) does not oversee these products, whose efficacy is largely unproved.

This article presents the supporting evidence for the some of the most popular topical antiaging products. The evidence is taken from the literature and the primary author's research, comprising previously published data and new results from ongoing projects.

RETINOIDS

The effect of retinoids has been extensively studied in humans and animals. Retinoic acids

Financial Disclosures: There is nothing to disclose.

[a] Department of Otolaryngology – Head and Neck Surgery, University of Illinois at Chicago, 1855 West Taylor, Suite 2.42, Chicago, IL 60611, USA; [b] Facial Plastic Surgery, Department of Otolaryngology – Head and Neck Surgery, University of Illinois at Chicago, 1855 West Taylor, Suite 2.42, Chicago, IL 60611, USA
* Corresponding author.
E-mail address: tfeuer1@uic.edu

Facial Plast Surg Clin N Am 21 (2013) 55–60
http://dx.doi.org/10.1016/j.fsc.2012.11.009
1064-7406/13/$ – see front matter

have specific retinoic acid receptors with DNA-binding domains, and accomplish their effects in the skin through regulated gene expression.[3] Retinoids are thought to increase fibroblast growth and procollagen synthesis, as well as inhibit the production of matrix-degrading metalloproteinases. These changes are made at the mRNA, protein, and enzyme activity levels.[4]

In the literature, there is conclusive evidence that retinoids improve the appearance of mild to moderate photodamage, thus giving the skin a more youthful appearance. A Cochrane review including 12 double-blind randomized controlled trials (RCTs) comparing tretinoin cream with placebo showed that tretinoin cream in concentrations of 0.02% or higher significantly improved fine and coarse wrinkles, roughness, freckles, and pigmentation.[5]

Tazarotene, a selective retinoic acid receptor agonist, and isotretinoin are less researched retinoids, but they have also been shown to significantly improve fine wrinkling and mottled hyperpigmentation. Kang and colleagues[6] compared the effect of 4 different concentrations of tazarotene with 0.05% tretinoin and placebo in an RCT. The investigators found that after 24 weeks of daily application, tazarotene of all concentrations (0.01%–0.1%) and 0.05% tretinoin cream showed significant improvement of fine wrinkling in comparison with the vehicle cream. However, for mottled hyperpigmentation, only 0.1% tazarotene cream and 0.05% tretinoin cream showed significant improvement over the vehicle cream. Isotretinoin 0.1%, when applied for 36 weeks, was also shown to significantly improve fine wrinkling and mottled pigmentation in patients with moderate to severe photodamaged skin when compared with placebo.[7]

Author Research on Topical Tretinoin

The authors' research evaluated the effects of topical 0.05% tretinoin cream on the dorsal skin of nonirradiated hairless mice. Profilometric evaluation showed significant effacement of wrinkles, with a decrease in roughness texture factor as well as a decrease in fine and coarse lines. Histologic evaluation showed significantly increased epidermal width and increased nuclear volume in the granular, spinous, and basal layers. An immunohistochemical evaluation of epidermal proliferating cell nuclear antigen (PCNA) showed an increased proliferation index of epidermal keratinocytes.[8,9]

Risks and Side Effects in Retinoid Use

Although the advantages of retinoids are well documented, the use of retinoids is not without risk. Adverse effects of retinoids include erythema, scaling, dryness, and irritation. Most adverse effects peak during the first 2 weeks of application and decrease with time. Of the 12 RCTs included in the evaluation of tretinoin cream the attrition rates were 7% to 25%, which is likely due to these undesirable side effects. Higher doses are associated with more adverse events, and the studies with the highest concentrations of tretinoin (0.1%) had the highest attrition rates.

Retinoids are also teratogens, and treatment of pregnant women with topical retinoids is not advised. However, the prevalence of anomalies in exposed women was not shown to be greater than the prevalence in nonexposed women. Topical tretinoin does not affect the endogenous levels of tretinoin or its metabolites, and no systemic adverse effects have been reported for topical tretinoin application.[10]

α-HYDROXYL ACIDS/GLYCOLIC ACID

α-Hydroxyl acids (AHAs), such as glycolic acid (GA) or lactic acid, are thought to speed up the process of exfoliation and skin cell turnover by weakening the intercellular cohesion of the stratum corneum.[11] At concentrations of 25%, AHAs are thought to promote increased epidermal thickness as well as increased production of collagen and hyaluronic acid. The FDA limits over-the-counter concentrations of AHAs to 10%, and peels containing 40% AHAs can only be applied by medical doctors.[12]

In the literature there is some evidence supporting the antiaging effects of AHAs. Stiller and colleagues[13] found 8% GA to significantly improve skin sallowness in an RCT after 22 weeks of daily treatment. Lactic acid 8% in this same trial was found to significantly decrease mottled hyperpigmentation, sallowness, and roughness compared with the vehicle control. In an RCT of 75 patients comparing 5% GA with placebo, Thibault and colleagues[14] found a significant change in general skin texture and discoloration, but no significant decrease in skin wrinkling. Application of a medical-strength 50% GA peel for 5 minutes weekly for 4 weeks was shown to improve mild photoaging of the skin in a double-blind, vehicle-controlled study of 41 patients.[15] This study showed significant improvement in fine wrinkling and solar keratoses. Histology showed thinning of the stratum corneum, granular layer enhancement, and epidermal thickening.

Author Research on AHAs

The senior authors evaluated the effect of 12% GA gel on the dorsal skin of nonirradiated hairless mice. Of 5 products tested (retinoic acid, GA, estrogen, vitamin C, and soy), GA caused the most dramatic thickening of the epidermis (**Fig. 1**). The epidermal thickness increased from an average of 18.3 μm to 55.5 μm, almost triple the thickness of the untreated skin. The nuclear volume of the basal layer and the spinous layer was also the highest in the GA group, and PCNA-positive cells were also markedly increased after treatment with GA.[9]

Risks and Side Effects in AHA Use

Skin erythema and flaking are listed as the major side effects of treatment with AHAs, the effects becoming more pronounced as the concentrations of the products increase. AHAs are also known to increase skin photosensitivity, and it has been shown that GA and ultraviolet-B (UVB) radiation inhibits proliferation and induces apoptosis in human keratinocytes.[16]

VITAMIN C/ASCORBIC ACID

Ascorbic acid is thought to affect skin aging by two mechanisms, the first of which is its antioxidant property. Ascorbic acid is an efficient water-soluble antioxidant, and is able to neutralize free radicals both intracellularly and extracellularly.[17] The second mechanism is collagen synthesis. Ascorbic acid has been shown to stimulate the synthesis of procollagen types I and III in cultured human skin fibroblasts.[18] Ascorbic acid is also necessary to form enzymes necessary for cross-linking collagen molecules, and therefore influences the quality of collagen produced.

In the literature, a few small RCTs support significant antiaging effects of ascorbic acid. In a double-blind study of 19 patients, Humbert and colleagues[19] found a significant improvement in roughness, suppleness, and small-wrinkle scores on comparing 5% ascorbic acid with placebo. Evaluation of skin biopsies of 10 of these patients showed evidence of repair of elastic tissue in the ascorbic acid group; however, there was no difference in melanocyte distribution. In a study of 10 patients comparing 10% ascorbic acid with placebo, Fitzpatrick and Rostan[20] showed a small significant decrease in the wrinkling scores of the treatment sides. However, there was no difference in pigmentation between the treated and untreated sides of the patients. Biopsies of the lateral cheeks of 4 of the patients showed increased Grenz zone collagen and increased staining for mRNA for type I collagen. A third trial including 19 patients showed significant improvement, with ascorbic acid better than the control for fine wrinkling, tactile roughness, coarse rhytids, skin laxity/tone, sallowness/yellowing, and overall features. Of all of the parameters measured, the greatest improvement was noted in the fine wrinkling.[21] Most recently, a split-face study of 20 patients with 23.8% ascorbic acid showed significant improvement in dyspigmentation, surface roughness, and fine lines.[22]

Author Research on Ascorbic Acid

In a comparison of the effects of 15% ascorbic acid with the effects of retinoic acid, GA, estrogen, and soy, ascorbic acid caused the smallest increase in epidermal thickness, the nuclear volumes of the different layers of the epidermis being the lowest among the 5 treatment groups. However, the expression of PCNA, which is described to play an important role in cytologic differentiation and growth, was still significantly increased in the skin of mice treated with ascorbic acid (**Fig. 2**).[9]

Risks and Side Effects in Topical Vitamin C Use

The adverse effects of topical ascorbic acid are mild compared with the effects of retinoic acid

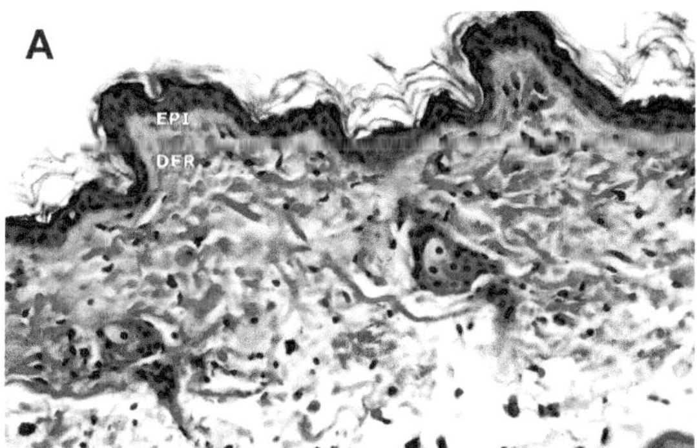

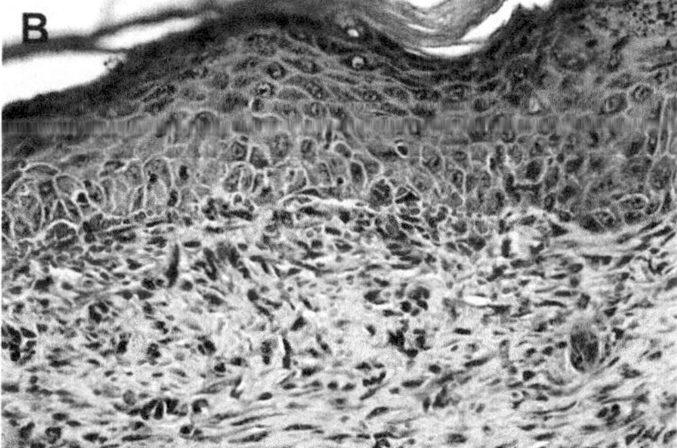

Fig. 1. (*A*) Histologic preparation of control mouse skin showing a thin epidermis (EPI). DER, dermis (original magnification ×200). (*B*) Mouse skin treated with glycolic acid for 2 weeks. The epidermis is highly differentiated and a profusion of fibroblasts is observed in the dermis (original magnification ×200).

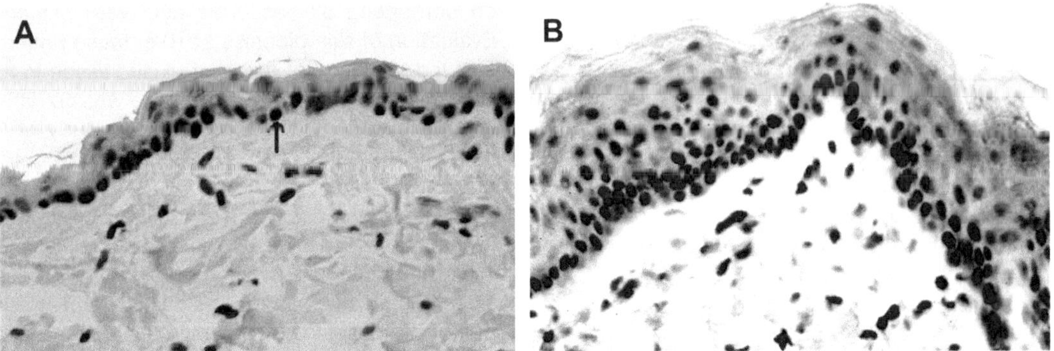

Fig. 2. (*A*) Control proliferating cell nuclear antigen (PCNA) reaction in mouse skin epidermis, showing dark positive cells (*arrow*) limited to the basal layer (original magnification ×200). (*B*) PCNA reaction in a mouse treated with topical vitamin C, showing proliferation of positive cells and peripheral spread. Nonreactive cells stained with hematoxylin (original magnification ×200).

and GA. Adverse effects include skin flaking and erythema. In one of the RCTs discussed earlier, patients described a unilateral stinging, making it difficult to keep the study blinded.[20]

PEPTIDES

Peptides used in topical antiaging products have multiple applications. Gorouhi and Maibach[23] categorized topical peptides into 4 groups based on their modes of action:

1. Carrier peptides
2. Signal peptides
3. Enzyme-inhibitor peptides
4. Neurotransmitter-inhibitor peptides

Carrier peptides are short chains of amino acids with a net positive charge, which cross the cell membrane in a receptor-independent and energy-independent manner.[24] Carrier peptides allow the transmembrane delivery of bioactive molecules as well as the delivery of collagen and elastin into the cell. The most common application has been for the delivery of trace elements such as copper and manganese into the cells. These elements are necessary for skin healing and enzymatic processes.

Signal peptides are aimed at stimulating matrix-protein production, collagen, and elastin synthesis. The effects of palmitoyl KTTKS (palmitoyl pentapeptide), a signal peptide, are documented in the literature. Palmitoyl pentapeptide is a subfragment of type I collagen, and is thought to promote synthesis of type I collagen by upregulating transforming growth factor β and maintaining the stability of mRNA.[25] In a double-blind RCT with 93 patients, topical 3 ppm palmitoyl pentapeptide was found to significantly reduce the length of fine wrinkles within 12 weeks.[26]

An example of an enzyme-inhibitor peptide is soy protein, which inhibits proteinases and is frequently used as an antiaging skin moisturizer. A double-blind, placebo-controlled study applying 2% soy extract to the forearms of 19 volunteers showed a significant increase in the papillae index (number of papillae per area) in the soy-extract group.[27] This increased interdigitation of the epidermis and dermis is thought to be a sign of rejuvenation, as the papillae index normally decreases with age.

Neurotransmitter-inhibitor peptides inhibit acetylcholine release at the neuromuscular junction. Subsequent paralysis of the muscles smoothes the overlying skin and prevents wrinkling secondary to facial animation. Botox is an example of such a neurotransmitter-inhibitor, and is also available as a topical gel. In a randomized, placebo-controlled study evaluating the effect of RT001 botulinum toxin type A topical gel on moderate to severe lateral canthal lines, 89% of 45 subjects achieved significant reduction in their lateral canthal lines at 4 weeks.[28]

Author Research on Peptides

The authors studied the effects of a peptide lotion with pentapeptides and hexapeptides. After daily application to the dorsal skin of the hairless mouse, the total dermis thickness was noted to be significantly higher than the control, with an almost equal effect as that with retinoic acid. A discernible improvement was also noted in the surface profile, with a pronounced reduction in surface-roughness factor. In further studies, a statistically significant reversal of epidermal edema caused by chronic UVB radiation with topical application of a peptide cream, and a vitamin C preparation was observed in an experiment with a mouse model (Bhattacharyya and colleagues, in preparation, 2012) (**Fig. 3**).

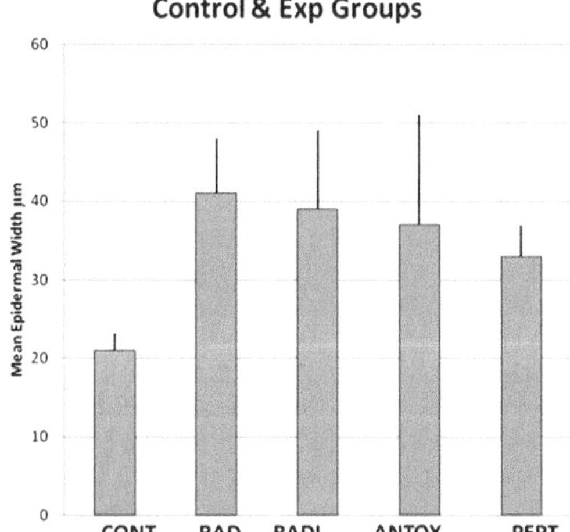

Fig. 3. Epidermal width in control (CONT) and experimental groups (mean ± SD). RAD, animals exposed to chronic ultraviolet-B radiation (8 weeks); ANTOX and PEPT, radiated skin topically treated with antioxidant solution and peptide cream, respectively, for 4 weeks; RADL, skin adjacent to treated areas and left alone for 4 weeks for comparison.

The authors also studied the effects of soy cream on the dorsal skin of the hairless mouse. The beneficial effect of soy on the skin microrelief (reduction of fine lines and wrinkles, roughness) was almost equal to that of retinoic acid. The total dermis thickness, however, did not increase as much as in the skin treated with retinoic acid.[8]

Risks and Side Effects in Topical Peptide Use

There are few data in the literature concerning adverse effects of topical peptides. Palmitoyl pentapeptide appears to be extremely well tolerated. In the study of 93 patients, there was no sign of irritation (erythema, skin flakiness, stinging) in any of the patients.[26] However, peptides should be used with caution, as there are conceivable grave consequences of introducing materials into cells and modulating transcription factors.

SUMMARY

Topical antiaging products are very popular because people are seeking cost-effective, noninvasive methods to improve their appearance. Retinoids are the most widely researched antiaging topicals, and there are several double-blind RCTs proving that they significantly improve fine and coarse wrinkles, roughness, freckles, and pigmentation.[5] GA also has evidence from large RCTs to support its efficacy. GA appears to be better for the reduction of pigmentation changes than reduction of fine wrinkles. Other products such as vitamin C and peptides show promise, but lack extensive data to support their efficacy.

REFERENCES

1. Glogau RG. Physiologic and structural changes associated with aging skin. Dermatol Clin 1997;15: 555–9.
2. Chiu A, Kimball AB. Topical vitamins, minerals and botanical ingredients as modulators of environmental and chronological skin damage. Br J Dermatol 2003; 49:681–91.
3. Kang S, Voorhees J. Photoaging therapy with topical tretinoin: an evidence-based analysis. J Am Acad Dermatol 1998;39(2):55–61.
4. Fisher GJ, Datta SC, Talwar HS, et al. Molecular basis of sun-induced premature skin aging and retinoid antagonism. Nature 1996;379:335–9.
5. Samuel M, Brooke R, Hollis S, et al. Interventions for photodamaged skin [review]. Cochrane Database Syst Rev 2005 Jan;55(1):CD001782.
6. Kang S, Leyden JJ, Lowe NJ, et al. Tazarotene cream for the treatment of facial photodamage: a multicenter, investigator-masked, randomized, vehicle controlled, parallel comparison of 0.01%, 0.025%, 0.05%, and 0.1% tazarotene creams with 0.05% tretinoin emollient cream applied once daily for 24 weeks. Arch Dermatol 2001;137:1597–604.
7. Maddin S, Lauharanta J, Agache P, et al. Isotretinoin improves the appearance of photodamaged skin: results of a 36-week, multicenter, double-blind, placebo-controlled trial. J Am Acad Dermatol 2000;42:56–63.
8. Bhattacharyya TK, Linton J, Mei L, et al. Profilometric and morphometric response of murine skin to cosmeceutical agents. Arch Facial Plast Surg 2009; 11(5):332–7.
9. Bhattacharyya TK, Higgins NP, Sebastian S, et al. Comparison of epidermal morphologic response to commercial antiwrinkle agents in the hairless mouse. Dermatol Surg 2009;35:1109–18.
10. Darlenski R, Surber C, Fluhr JW. Topical retinoids in the management of photodamaged skin: from theory to evidence-based practical approach. Br J Dermatol 2010;163(6):1157–65.
11. Fartasch M, Teal J, Menon GK. Mode of action of glycolic acid on human stratum corneum: ultrastructural and functional evaluation of the epidermal barrier. Arch Dermatol Res 1997;289:404–9.
12. Huang CK, Miller TA. The truth about over-the-counter topical anti-aging products: a comprehensive review. Aesthet Surg J 2007;27:402–13.
13. Stiller MJ, Bartolone J, Stern R, et al. Topical 8% glycolic acid and 8% L-lactic acid creams for the treatment of photodamaged skin. Arch Dermatol 1996; 132:631–6.

14. Thibault PK, Wlodarczyk J, Wenck A. Double-blind randomized clinical trial on the effectiveness of a daily glycolic acid 5% formulation in the treatment of photoaging. Dermatol Surg 1998;24:573–8.
15. Newman N, Newman A, Moy LS, et al. Clinical improvement of photoaged skin with 50% glycolic acid. A double-blind vehicle-controlled study. Dermatol Surg 1996;22(5):455–60.
16. Lai WW, Hsiao YP, Chung JG. Synergistic phototoxic effects of glycolic acid in human keratinocyte cell line (HaCaT). J Dermatol Sci 2011;64(3):191–8.
17. Colven RM, Pinnell SR. Topical vitamin C in Aging. Clin Dermatol 1996;14:227–34.
18. Geesin JC, Darr D, Kauffman R, et al. Ascorbic acid specifically increases type I and type III procollagen production messenger RNA levels in human dermal fibroblasts. J Invest Dermatol 1988;90:420–4.
19. Humbert PG, Haftek M, Creidi P, et al. Topical ascorbic acid on photoaged skin. Clinical, topographical and ultrastructural evaluation: double-blind study vs. placebo. Exp Dermatol 2003;12:237–44.
20. Fitzpatrick RE, Rostan EF. Double-blind, half-face study comparing topical vitamin C and vehicle for rejuvenation of photodamage. Dermatol Surg 2002;28:231–6.
21. Traikovich SS. Use of topical ascorbic acid and its effects on photodamaged skin topography. Arch Otolaryngol Head Neck Surg 1999;125:1091–8.
22. Xu TH, Chen JZ, Li YH, et al. Split-face study of topical 23.8% L-ascorbic acid serum in treating photo-aged skin. J Drugs Dermatol 2012;11(1):51–6.
23. Gorouhi F, Maibach HI. Role of topical peptides in preventing or treating aged skin. Int J Cosmet Sci 2009;31(5):327–45.
24. Nasrollahi SA, Fouladdel S, Taghibiglou C, et al. A peptide carrier for the delivery of elastin into fibroblast cells. Int J Dermatol 2012;51:923–9.
25. Samah NH, Heard CM. Topically applied KTTKS: a review. Int J Cosmet Sci 2011;33:483–90.
26. Robinson LR, Fitzgerald NC, Doughty DG, et al. Topical palmitoyl pentapeptide provides improvement in photoaged human facial skin. Int J Cosmet Sci 2005;27(3):155–60.
27. Sudel KM, Venzke K, Mielke H, et al. Novel aspects of intrinsic and extrinsic aging of human skin: beneficial effects of soy extract. Photochem Photobiol 2005;81(3):581–7.
28. Glogau R, Blitzer A, Brandt F, et al. Results of a randomized, double-blind, placebo-controlled study to evaluate the efficacy and safety of botulinum toxin type A topical gel for the treatment of moderate-to-severe lateral canthal lines. J Drugs Dermatol 2012;11(1):38–45.

Photodamage
Treatments and Topicals for Facial Skin

Marty O. Visscher, PhD[a,b,*], Brian S. Pan, MD[b,c], W. John Kitzmiller, MD[b,c]

KEYWORDS

• Facial skin • Photodamage • Facial restoration • Facial skin coloration

KEY POINTS

- Facial restoration uses a wide range of approaches albeit less technically effective than the gold standard of fully ablative laser modalities.
- Increasing the uniformity of facial skin coloration is an important treatment goal because it impacts the patient's perceived age.
- Topically applied facial cosmetic products (eg, combinations of skin lightening agents, vitamins, and sunscreens) produce measureable reductions in the characteristics associated with photodamage.
- The literature contains many reviews of facial restoration modalities but there is limited information on what the experienced, skilled facial plastic surgeon might achieve with a total treatment package. Of great interest is the magnitude of the reduction in perceived age that could be achieved.

INTRODUCTION

Perceived age is the marker for facial skin aging.[1] Treatments to reduce one's perceived age and restore facial skin condition are highly sought.[2] Surgeons have an armamentarium of methods for managing and optimizing facial skin color, uniformity, texture, and shape in restoring photodamaged skin. This article reviews the effectiveness of various treatment modalities including topicals (eg, cosmetics) in facial skin care. Studies are presented in the context of patient expectations for "decreasing perceived age." A particular area of concern is dark spots (eg, solar lentigines, hyperpigmentation). Postinflammatory hyperpigmentation can occur with UV exposure and resultant epidermal inflammation, generation of reactive oxygen species, and stimulation of melanocytes.[3] Solar lentigines (liver spots, age spots, actinic lentigines) are hyperpigmented spots caused by chronic UV exposure eventually becoming visible on the skin surface.[4] Because of their association with increased age, individuals seek treatments including laser resurfacing, chemical peels, dermabrasion, and topical agents.[5]

Treatments are designed to interact with the affected areas so as to change their characteristics or to "restore" the skin to a chronically earlier state at least temporarily and to prevent further damage. They may increase the levels of types I and II collagen or reorganize the collagen fibrils to decrease the severity of lines, reduce chronic

Funding Sources: None.
Conflict of Interest: None.

[a] Skin Sciences Program, Division of Plastic Surgery, Cincinnati Children's Hospital Medical Center, 3333 Burnet Avenue, Cincinnati, OH 45229, USA; [b] Division of Plastic, Reconstructive and Hand/Burn Surgery, Department of Surgery, College of Medicine, University of Cincinnati, 231 Albert Sabin Way, Cincinnati, OH 45267, USA; [c] Division of Plastic Surgery, Cincinnati Children's Hospital Medical Center, 3333 Burnet Avenue, Cincinnati, OH 45229, USA

* Corresponding author. Division of Plastic Surgery, Cincinnati Children's Hospital Medical Center, 3333 Burnet Avenue, Cincinnati, OH 45229.
E-mail address: Marty.visscher@cchmc.org

Facial Plast Surg Clin N Am 21 (2013) 61–75
http://dx.doi.org/10.1016/j.fsc.2012.10.004
1064-7406/13/$ – see front matter

inflammation, and smooth the surface (ie, reduce the observable features of photoaging, including wrinkling, dyschromia, dryness, rough surface texture, folds, and keratosis).[6]

Current trends in the treatment of photodamage have been published annually by the American Society for Aesthetic Plastic Surgery since 1997. A total of 22,700 surveys were mailed in 2011 and the 1015 respondents included 384 dermatologists, 211 otolaryngologists, and 420 plastic surgeons.[7] The procedures for photodamaged skin are chemical peels; laser resurfacing (ablative or nonablative); fraxel laser; intense pulsed light (IPL) laser; dermabrasion; microdermabrasion; and noninvasive tightening. Injections and fillers (ie, botulinum toxin, collagen, fat, hyaluronic acid, calcium hydroxylapatite, poly-L-lactic acid, and polymethyl methacrylate) have been excluded for the purposes of this discussion.

The total number of the procedures discussed here has increased since 1997 (**Fig. 1**A). The percentage of chemical peels decreased considerably between 1997 and 2005 and continues to decline (see **Fig. 1**B). Laser resurfacing accounted for 23% in 1997, decreased to 4.5% in 2002, then increased to 23% in 2004, where levels currently remain. Dermabrasion was at 6.5% initially, but now accounts for about 1%. In contrast, microdermabrasion rose sharply from 0% in 1998 to 22% in 1999 to 44% in 2000, peaking at 64% in 2002 before declining to 23% in 2011. Between 2008 and 2011, the percent of chemical peels, laser resurfacing, IPL laser, and microdermabrasion were comparable (see **Fig. 1**B,C). Between 2008 and 2011, the nonablative laser procedures increased to comparable levels as ablative procedures in 2001 (**Table 1**).

This article provides an overview of the current therapies for photodamaged facial skin and their efficacy, particularly the studies using the objective, quantitative evaluation methods discussed in the previous article. The role of topical treatments and cosmetics is discussed because they are not reported by the American Society for Aesthetic Plastic Surgery. A schema showing the relative effectiveness of various modalities in decreasing perceived age is presented.

LITERATURE REVIEW: TREATMENTS TO RESTORE FACIAL SKIN

There are a considerable number of reviews on therapeutic modalities for photoaged skin. For example, in 2009, an entire issue of *Facial Plastic Surgery* (volume 25, issue 2) was devoted to the topic of rejuvenation. **Table 2** lists several reviews and briefly describes the information provided in each. Next, the various modalities are discussed with the goal of addressing these questions: How effective are the treatments relative to each other? How much improvement can a consumer/patient expect against the goal of reducing perceived age? Can the treatment "tools" be combined to optimize outcomes? How much improvement could a patient potentially achieve on her or his own with commercially available facial skin care products?

For example, the effects of facial restoration procedures on perceived age were objectively determined from images of 75 patients.[8] Naive judges (198) evaluated before and after (6 months posttreatment) photographs presented individually but not in pairs. The mean decrease in perceived age was 6 years, with a range of 0.8 to 14.2. Reductions were 4.6 years for facelift; 2.5 for laser resurfacing; and 2 years each for fat injection, eyelid surgery, and forehead lift.

Therapeutic Modalities: Mechanism of Effects

Facial restoration procedures typically alter structures in the dermis, epidermis, and stratum corneum (SC) and vary by depth of effect. Fully ablative lasers (eg, CO_2, erbium:YAG [Er:YAG]) remove the entire epidermis, the papillary dermis, and part of the reticular dermis depending on energy settings and thermal effects. Removal of the epidermis and part of the dermis promotes collagen formation. Damage to the epidermis (eg, ablation and removal of the SC) produces inflammation whereby the fibroblasts are induced to produce collagen 1 and 4 and stimulates formation of keratinocytes.[9] Fractional ablative lasers apply energy in a grid pattern thereby preserving much of the epidermis and SC and destroying tissue in columnar patterns into the dermis.[10–12] In nonablative laser resurfacing, columns of thermal energy are directed into the dermis thereby using heat to create epidermal and dermal damage to levels of 300 to 400 μm.[11] The technique of dermabrasion penetrates into the dermis thereby stimulating collagen formation. In contrast, microdermabrasion is a more superficial technique and removes only the SC.[13] Depending on the technique and type of microdermabrasion, selective removal of the SC may occur. Partial SC loss enhances the penetration of topical agents and microdermabrasion may be performed for this purpose.[14]

Prevention: Photoprotection

Daily application of sun-protective agents (ie, UVA and UVB filters) reduced type I procollagen, increased extracellular matrix proteins, and

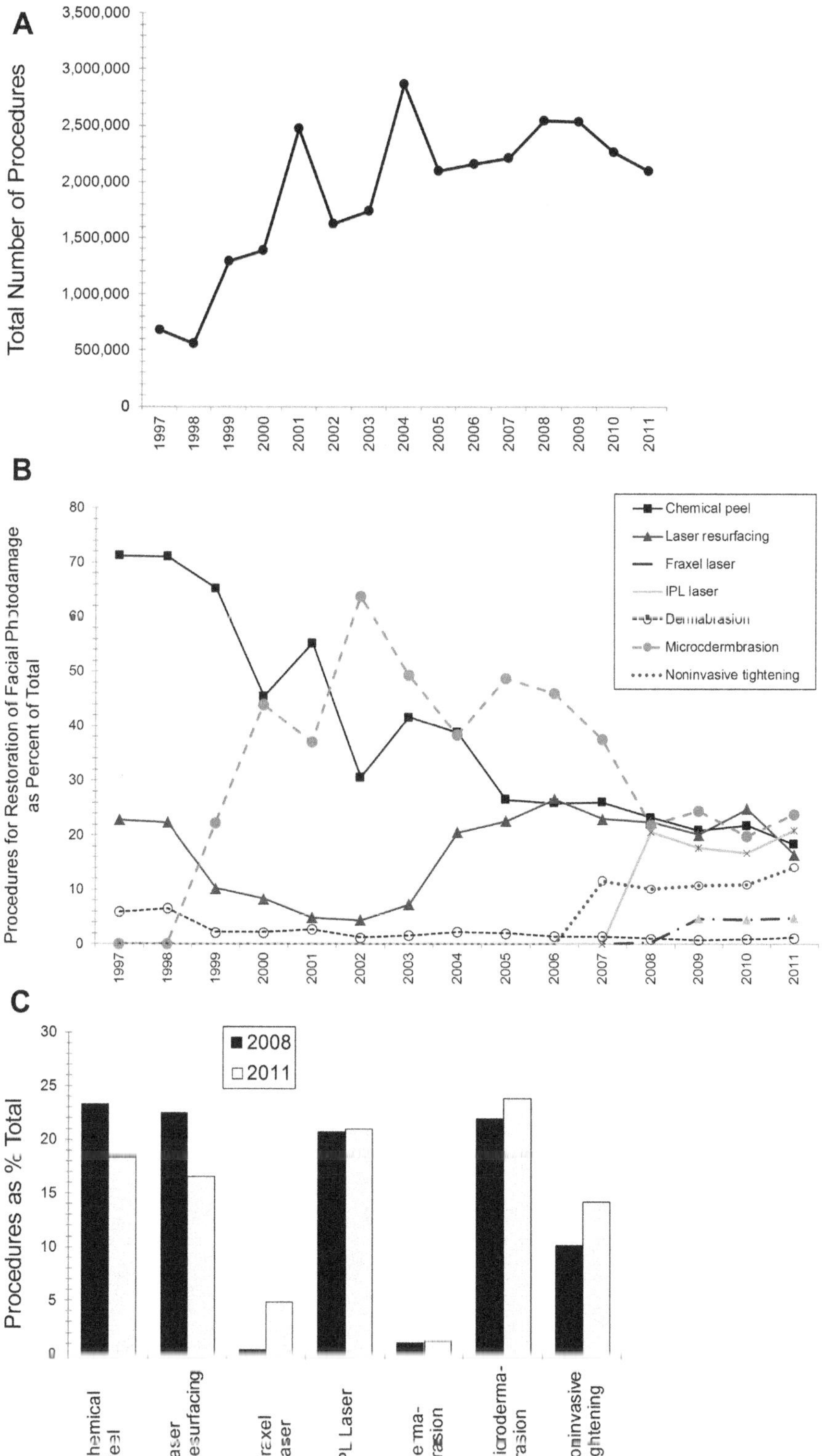

Fig. 1. (*A*) The total number of procedures for the restoration of facial photodamage has increased in the past 14 years. Specific procedures include chemical peels, laser resurfacing, fraxel laser, IPL laser, dermabrasion, microdermabrasion, and noninvasive tightening. (*B*) The percentage of chemical peels decreased considerably between 1997 and 2005 and continues to decline. Laser resurfacing decreased to 2002, then increased in 2004 where levels remained. Dermabrasion was at 6.5% initially but now accounts for about 1%. Microdermabrasion rose sharply peaking in 2002 before declining in 2011. (*C*) Between 2008 and 2011, the percent of facial procedures was at similar levels for chemical peels, laser resurfacing, IPL laser, and microdermabrasion.

Table 1
Between 2008 and 2011, the number of nonablative laser procedures increased and the ablative treatments decreased

	2008	2009	2010	2011
Ablative	18%	27%	36%	51%
Nonablative	82%	73%	64%	49%

prevented increases in the thickness of the SC and stratum granulosum.[15,16] The facial skin of females living in higher UV regions had significantly longer wrinkles, more wrinkles, more and larger hyperpigmented spots, more yellow coloration, and rougher surface texture by quantitative imaging and analysis than those with lower UV levels.[17,18] Regular, daily sunscreen use leads to reduced UV exposure, although the effects on facial skin characteristics have not yet been reported.[19] Protection of additional UV damage is an essential treatment component.

Laser Resurfacing

Ablative laser resurfacing

Ablative CO_2 lasers and ablative Er:YAG lasers are considered to be highly effective, "best in class" treatments for photodamage.[6] Examples of the results are discussed next.

Female subjects (n = 67) with periorbital rhytides were treated one time with a high-energy pulsed CO_2 laser (3 mm; fluence, 500 mJ/cm^2; 7-mW power) and evaluated at 1, 3, and 6 months.[20] Paired comparison evaluation of high-resolution photographs for severity (10-point scale: 1–3 mild, 4–6 moderate, 7–9 severe) showed significant improvement at 6 months. The extent of improvement was directly related to the pretreatment severity.

Subjects (n = 47) with periorbital, perioral, or glabella rhytides were treated once with a CO_2 laser with flashscanner (3-mm spot size; 7.5 W; 0.2-second pulse duration or 6-mm spot at 18–20 W). Pretreatment and posttreatment (mean, 9.7 weeks; range, 1–24) photographs were viewed together by five judges and evaluated for wrinkle improvement (0 = none, 1 = less than 25% improvement, 2 = 25%–50% improvement, 3 = 50%–75% improvement, 4 = greater than 75% improvement) and interpreted as none (0), poor (0.1–1), fair (1.1–2), good (2.1–3), and excellent (3.1–4). Mean scores after 1 month were 3.3 for periorbital, 3.1 for perioral, and 3.1 for glabella, indicating excellent improvement. Erythema was judged as none (0); mild (1); moderate (2); or severe (3). The highest mean erythema score was 1.27 at 4 to 12 weeks postsurgery and 0.9 at 12 to 24 weeks, indicating that visible redness lasted for up to 6 months.

The effects of treatment with ablative CO_2 lasers (pulse, 800 μs; fluence, 3.5–6.5 J/cm^2; 250–450 mJ pulse energy) and Er:YAG (300 μs; 5–8 J/cm^2; 1–1.5 J per pulse) were compared using a split face design in females (n = 21) with periorbital or perioral rhytides.[21] A panel of five physicians evaluated pretreatment and posttreatment photographs on a five-point scale (1 = poor improvement, 2 = fair, 3 = good, 4 = excellent, 5 = complete resolution of wrinkles). The improvement was significantly greater for the CO_2 laser versus the Er:YAG treatment. The occurrence of erythema was significantly lower for the Er:YAG side, as was the incidence of hyperpigmentation.

Ablative laser CO_2 resurfacing was compared with dermabrasion for perioral wrinkles with a split-face design (n = 20) using high-quality photographs, biophysical measures of skin color, hydration, and mechanical properties and patient assessment.[22] Masked evaluation of photographs by 10 plastic surgeons indicated that the laser treatment had a significantly higher erythema score at 1 month and a small but significantly greater improvement in perioral wrinkles at 6 months. Sixty-five percent of subjects believed the laser treatment to be more effective.

Fractional laser resurfacing

Subjects with moderate to severe photodamage were treated two to three times with ablative fractional therapy (10,600 nm; 30-W power; 500-μm pitch; 1000–1500 μs; forced cold air).[23] Photographs were evaluated 6 months after treatment for dyschromia, texture, and laxity using the grading scale of Alexiades-Armenakas.[24] Significant improvement was found for multiple characteristics of photoaging (ie, dyschromia [grade 1.5 after vs 3.2 before]; texture [grade 1.7 from 3.3]; laxity [grade 1.5 from 3.1]; and overall outcome [1.5 from 3.3]).

Two ablative fractional lasers (CO_2 and Er:YAG) were compared using a paired-comparison split-face design among 28 patients with mild to moderate periorbital wrinkles as judged with the Fitzpatrick Wrinkle Scale.[25] Both treatments produced a significant reduction in wrinkle score (4.8 before vs 4.3 after for CO_2; 4.6 before vs 4.3 after for Er:YAG), although the differences were small and the variability among the population seemed to be high. Wrinkle depth by optical profilometry was significantly reduced for both (2 mm before and 1.64 mm after for CO_2; 2 mm before and 1.6 mm after for Er:YAG). Interestingly, the variability was lower for the Er:YAG laser. The treatments were comparable and the investigators

Table 2
Reviews of therapeutic modalities for photodamaged skin

Category	Specific Modalities	Comments
Resurfacing, general[76]	Fully ablative treatments Fractional lasers Nonablative lasers Dermabrasion Chemical peels Microdermabrasion Topicals	Covers mode of interaction with skin and targets of laser energy, penetration depth, histologic effects, qualifications of practitioners, risks and side effects, types of ablative lasers Includes sample photographs Reports results from investigations
Laser resurfacing[74]	Ablative lasers	Provides a comprehensive, step-by-step review of procedures for the clinician, including patient assessment, preparation, postsurgery wound care, complications Emphasizes technique and asserts that skill in doing the procedure produces significant results
Laser resurfacing[77,78]	Ablative CO_2 lasers Ablative Er:YAG lasers Combined CO_2/Er:YAG Nonablative lasers	Reviews different types of lasers and mode of action, detailed description of settings and procedures, discusses efficacy
Laser resurfacing[6,26]	Ablative lasers Nonablative lasers Fractional ablative lasers	History, types of lasers, histology, patient characteristics for specific modalities, extent of improvement, complications (eg, scarring), management after procedures, shows examples
Laser resurfacing[79]	Fractional thermolysis	Reviews conditions, such as acne scars, fine wrinkles, dyschromia, melisma, hyperpigmentation, telangiectatic matting, residual hemangiomas, poikiloderma of Civatte, nevus of Ota Compares with fractional ablative treatment
Laser resurfacing[80]	Fractional ablative	Discusses complications vs fully ablative methods
Laser resurfacing[81]	Fractional ablative Fractional nonablative	Discusses history and uses for both Reports clinical findings and histology for multiple applications Comprehensive review of laser types, wavelengths, brands
Laser resurfacing[12]	Nonablative fractional laser	Discusses mode of action and use on Asian subjects with Fitzpatrick types III, IV
Laser resurfacing[27]	Nonablative	Provides an algorithm for treatment using nonablative methods
Chemical peels[9]	Glycolic acid Trichloroacetic acid Phenol Resorscinol α-Hydroxy acid β-Hydroxy acid	Reviews superficial, midlevel and deep peels, mechanisms, histology, frequency, agents used for each level, preprocedural and postprocedural care, side effects, application strategies
Chemical peels[41]	α-Hydroxy acid Trichloroacetic acid Baker-Gordon solution Phenol-Croton oil	Reviews history, patient selection criteria, skin classification scales, pretreatment and posttreatment, peel depth, peel agents, complications Compares with laser resurfacing Discusses application technique
Chemical peels[82]	Glycolic acid Jessner solution Pyruvic acid Resorcinol Salicylic acid Trichloroacetic acid Phenol	Discusses variables that impact penetration of peel agent, comprehensive list of peel agents, patient characteristics impacting selection of agent Describes visual appearance postapplication and interpretation of depth Comprehensive advantages and disadvantages for each agent
Microdermabrasion[36]	Crystals as agent	Describes equipment and operating premise Reviews current literature, describes the findings, comments on the quality of published literature Discusses safety

(*continued on next page*)

Table 2
(*continued*)

Category	Specific Modalities	Comments
Postinflammatory hyperpigmentation[5]	Chemical peels Laser treatment Hydroquinone Mequinol Retinoids Azelaic acid Kojic acid Arbutin Niacinamide *N*-acetylglucosamine Ascorbic acid (vitamin C) Licorice extract Soy Camouflage	Discusses epidemiology, etiology, visual characteristics, diagnosis, treatment with a variety of modalities and topical agents, adverse effects Presents clinical studies regarding outcomes of treatment Provides treatment algorithm
Photoprotection and topical agents[83]	Hormone therapy Sunscreens Antioxidants Cell regulators Vitamins Retinoic acid	Provides comprehensive discussion of the mechanisms of photodamage, genes and metabolic pathways Effects of hormones Comprehensive list of sunscreen actives Detailed discussion of objective quantitative methods to measure changes, biomechanical assessment of elastic properties, measurement of skin barrier function
Photoprotection and topical agents[50]	Sunscreens Retinoids Antioxidants: vitamin C, vitamin E, Idebenone α-Hydroxy acids	Discusses mechanisms of photoaging and the effects of each treatment on the skin biology Reviews literature and discusses results
Vitamins[84]	Retinoids Carotenoids Vitamins C, E, B_3, D, K	Review of the mechanisms of effect of UV radiation Comprehensive review of the literature for the effects of vitamins and discussion of the mechanisms of action
Over-the-counter skin care products[73]	Retinol, retinaldehyde, retinyl palmitate α-Hydroxy acids Ascorbic acid (vitamin C) Vitamin E Niacinamide (B_3) α-Lipoid acid *N*-acetylglucosamine Resveratrol Flavenoids, soy isoflavones Grape seed extract Coffea arabica	Discusses general effects and potential mechanisms for photodamaged skin Reviews results of studies on effectiveness Comments on the need for more rigorous and additional studies on over-the-counter products
Individual and combined treatments[85]	Injectables, side variety Chemical peels Ablative laser Nonablative laser	Comprehensive chart with methods, time to observable effect, mechanism of action, indications for use, benefits, adverse effects, length of time effects last (before repeat treatment is needed) Suggests combination of treatments

concluded that multiple treatments are probably needed thereby countering the benefit of reduced down time (vs conventional ablative therapy).

Compared with conventional ablative therapy, ablative fractional lasers are considered to be somewhat less effective for facial skin restoration but have fewer potential complications (eg, scarring, hypopigmentation, and higher recovery times).[6,26] In reviewing the literature, there appear to be no reports directly comparing the two methods.

Nonablative laser treatment

Nonablative laser treatments can generally target specific issues, such as hyperpigmentation of telangiectasia or diffuse redness.[27] They can also operate in the infrared wavelength region. Nonablative lasers are considered to be less effective than laser resurfacing for correction of photoaging.[25] However, a recent review indicated that there were no reports comparing the two methods.[23]

An Er:YAG laser in the thermal mode with 2.1 or 3.1 J/cm^2 and parallel air cooling was used to treat photodamaged skin (wrinkles) or scars in the periorbital or perioral regions.[28] The two treatments were 2 months apart with follow-up over 12 months. Good improvement was seen by 19% subjects with wrinkles and 31% reported no improvement. Of the subjects with scars, 50% reported good improvement and 100% had some improvement.

The effects of six mini-peels at 2-week intervals using an Er:YAG 2940-nm laser in the thermal mode (series of short pulses with energies of 2–3 J/cm^2 of 200–250 millisecond duration) were evaluated among six females.[29] The subjects reported an improvement in skin tightening, periorbital wrinkles, and appearance but the magnitude had decreased after 3 months, indicating the need for repeated treatments.

Nine patients with periorbital wrinkles were treated three times (at 3-week intervals) with a nonablative 1450-nm diode laser (4-mm spot size; 14–18 J/cm^2; cooling).[30] Pairs of pretreatment and posttreatment images were evaluated by 25 dermatologists and the posttreatment appearance was found to be superior (*P*<.05). Two physicians rated the posttreatment images higher. Seven subjects reported mild and two indicated moderate improvement. Note that the perceived outcomes differed for physicians versus patients.

IPL treatment

Treatment with an Er:YAG laser (micropeel) at 3.8 J/cm^2 and 15 μm per pass was compared with an IPL laser at 30 J/cm^2 with a 2.4- and 4-millisecond pulse (10-second delay, no cooling) in a split-face design among 10 patients.[31] Images collected with standard photography (VISIA) showed an improvement in dyschromia after one treatment for IPL and no change for the Er:YAG laser. No change in wrinkles was seen, perhaps because of the relatively low energy settings.

Korean subjects were treated with IPL in the range of 530 to 950 nm at 15.5 to 17.5 J/cm^2 (5 pulses, 20-second duration) three times at 4-week intervals.[32] Patient self-assessment showed that mottled pigmentation improved in 26.3% and slightly improved in 57.9%, skin tone improved in 15.8% and slightly improved in 57.9%, number of lesions improved in 31.6% and slightly improved in 36.8%, and lightening of lesions improved in 31.6% and slightly improved in 52.6%. For skin elasticity, wrinkles, and skin rejuvenation, at least some improvement was observed by 57.9%, 47.4%, and 63.2%, respectively. Melanin index and skin lightness by objective measurement were significantly reduced and skin elasticity was increased (*P*<.05).

A set of bipolar radiofrequency-based optical devices (IPL, infrared light, diode laser) was used to treat one side of the face at four 3-week intervals in Asian subjects.[33] Significant decreases were found for fine wrinkles and dyschromia from global assessment of photographs and instrumental measurement of melanin indices. Skin elasticity (objective assessment) increased with treatment and histology showed thicker collagen and more fine elastic fibers.

The effects of a long-pulse pulsed dye laser (595 nm; spot 7 mm; compression, 9–12 J/cm^2; duration 1.5 milliseconds for lentigines; 10–12 J/cm^2 and 20-millisecon duration, stacked methods for wrinkles) and IPL (fluence, 27–49 J/cm^2; duration 20 millisecond) were compared among 10 Asian females in a split-face design.[30] The improvement in lentigines was significantly greater for the long-pulse pulsed dye laser (81%) than the IPL (62.3%), as measured by evaluation of clinical photographs. The devices were comparable for the effects on wrinkles.

Home use nonablative laser

An over-the-counter home use 1410-nm midinfrared nonablative laser (12–15 mJ/μb) was evaluated among 124 subjects with periorbital wrinkles who had not had any type of facial resurfacing procedures for 2 years.[34] Treatments were daily for 4 weeks and twice weekly for 12 weeks, with evaluations at weeks 4, 12, 16, 20, and 28. Wrinkles were evaluated in live subjects or from high-resolution digital images using the 0 to 9 category

Fitzpatrick Wrinkle Scale (scores: 1–3 fine wrinkles, mild elastosis to 7–9 fine/deep wrinkles, severe elastosis).[35] The mean score reduction was 0.8 at 4 weeks and 1 at 8 weeks. The magnitude of the improvement could not be fully assessed because of the lack of a control group.

Microdermabrasion

Tissue removal with microdermabrasion was examined and differences were observed as a function of technique.[14] Specifically, (1) complete SC removal occurred with the mobile tip application procedure; (2) epidermal blistering and an intact SC with stationary application at 30 kPa (3 seconds) vacuum pressure; and (3) removal of the SC and much of the viable epidermis with the stationary procedure at 45 kPa.

This result confirms the experience of practitioners (i.e, that a resurfacing method may produce different effects or degrees of improvement based on operator technique). The finding may explain, in part, why microdermabrasion and light chemical peels are considered to produce a relatively small change in photoaged skin by physicians and patients.[36–38]

Treatment of photodamaged facial skin (n = 17) with serial (eight at 1-week intervals) microdermabrasion significantly improved skin coloration as judged by experts (plastic surgeons) and patients on a 0 to 5 scale.[39] Improvement in wrinkles was seen only by patients.

Six serial weekly microdermabrasion treatments (n = 16) significantly improved fine wrinkles, dullness, hyperpigmentation, blotchiness, milia, and pore size as judged by physicians on 0 (none) to 9 (severe) grading scales.[40] The lack of a control group limits the ability to determine the magnitude of the effects. Microdermabrasion is intended to remove the entire SC. Because treatment occurred at weekly intervals, it is unlikely that full restoration of the SC could occur before the next treatment and removal of any SC that had formed.

Chemical Peels

Over time, the types of facial skin restoration procedures have changed. The percentage of chemical peels has decreased because of development of laser resurfacing approaches, although some facial plastic surgeons believe the chemical peel continues to be an important tool.[41] Superficial chemical peels interact with and remove the SC only (ie, very superficial peels) and part of the epidermis.[9] Chemical peels of medium depth remove the epidermis and have effects into the reticular (upper part) of the dermis.[42] Mixtures of glycolic acid (70%) and trichloroacetic acid (35%) applied sequentially are considered to be effective because the glycolic prepared the skin to permit more uniform penetration of the trichloroacetic acid.[43] This combination peel reduced fine wrinkles but not deeper wrinkles.[40] Deep peels remove the SC, viable epidermis, reticular dermis, and part of the papillary dermis. The effectiveness of a given peel depends on preparation of the skin in advance. For example, topical application of retinoic acid before the peel (eg, 4 weeks) facilitates penetration of the peel agent.[9]

Five superficial peels (30% glycolic, 2-week intervals) were compared with single midlevel peel (35% trichloroacetic acid) in a split-face design using quantitative objective measurements of skin condition and actinic damage. Image analysis showed significantly greater improvement in wrinkles with the trichloroacetic acid but patients were more satisfied with the serial superficial peels. Both treatments increased skin elasticity and hydration.[44]

Topical Treatments

Definitions and regulations

Topically applied agents (ie, topicals) are widely defined in this section as being put on the skin surface. They are typically in the form of lotions, gels, creams, or ointments designed to be rubbed into the skin. They may include prescription drugs; over-the-counter products; cosmetics (including colorants); and "cosmeceuticals." Drugs are regulated by agencies, such as the Food and Drug Administration (FDA), and undergo a rigorous process to demonstrate safety and effectiveness. In general, cosmetics are developed, evaluated, and marketed by the skin care industry. In the United States, cosmetics are regulated by the FDA's Center for Food Safety and Applied Nutrition and must comply with safety and labeling guidelines. Cosmetic products are not allowed to make drug claims. Interestingly, most of the skin research is conducted by the skin care industry, as opposed to academic medical institutions.[45] The term "cosmeceutical" may be used to describe a topical product but cosmeceuticals are not recognized or regulated by the FDA. The term "cosmeceutical" was originally considered to describe something with the following characteristics[45,46]: (1) scientifically designed and intended for external application; (2) produces a useful, desired result; (3) has desirable aesthetic properties; and (4) meets rigid chemical, physical, and medical standards. The following sections include topicals that are prescription, cosmetic, or cosmeceutical.

Prescription topicals

Topical tretinoin (all-*trans*-retinoic acid, the acid form of vitamin A) is effective for the mitigation of mild to severe photodamage at levels of 0.02% and higher as demonstrated in multiple randomized controlled trials.[47] The clinical effects are caused by an increase in new collagen, restoration of normal elastic components, normalization of melanocyte structure, increased thickness of the epidermis and stratum granulosum, and increased denseness of the SC.[48,49] Because skin irritation (eg, erythema, stinging, burning, dryness) is a noted side effect,[50] doses must be titrated to determine tolerable levels.

Hydroquinone, a tyrosinase inhibitor, has been used extensively for hyperpigmentation at prescription levels of 3% to 10% and over-the-counter at 2%.[5,51] In 2001, the European Union banned the use of hydroquinone, as did authorities in Japan. In 2006, the US FDA proposed to remove hydroquinone from the generally recognized as safe list and require new drug applications for use. This proposal was based on newer reports describing carcinogenic and mutagenic effects.[52,53] At the request of the FDA, the National Toxicity Program is conducting specific studies to address the safety concerns.

Deoxyarbutin, a synthetic derivative of naturally occurring arbutin, has been synthesized and incorporated into a variety of formula matrices. Deoxyarbutin was less cytotoxic/cytostatic than hydroquinone in human melanocyte culture systems while effectively inhibiting tyrosinase activity and melanin content to a greater extent.[54] Skin lightening, following the development of postinflammatory hyperpigmentation caused by wounding, was demonstrated in a human xenograft model. Treatment of UV-induced pigmentation (tanning, human subjects) with deoxyarbutin led to significantly greater skin lightening that was reversible when treatment was discontinued.[55] In contrast, hydroquinone initially lightened the skin but darkening occurred with additional treatment, presumably caused by irritation and the resulting postinflammatory hyperpigmentation. Two other skin lightening agents, kojic acid and native arbutin, were ineffective in this model. There are currently very few published human trials of deoxyarbutin and evaluation of its effectiveness for solar lentigines and postinflammatory hyperpigmentation are warranted. An extensive human safety assessment indicated that deoxyarbutin does not seem to pose the risks identified for hydroquinone and some believe it to be the most effective skin lightening compound.[56]

Two skin care systems for hyperpigmentation were evaluated in parallel groups of females with at least mild photodamage over 12 weeks.[57] Products were SkinMedica Hyperpigmentation System (SkinMedica, Inc., Carlsbad, CA, USA) (n = 17) with cleanser, 4% microentrapped hydroquinone with retinol and antioxidants, sunscreen of SPF 30 and tri-retinol at 1.5%; and Obagi Nu-Derm System (Obagi Medical Products, Inc., Long Beach, CA, USA) with cleanser, toner, clear hydroquinone at 4%, exfoliant, blender hydroquinone at 4%, sunscreen of SPF 35 and tretinoin at 0.025% (n = 18).

Relative to the starting condition, both systems resulted in significant reduction of hyperpigmentation, global photoaging, sallowness, and scores of "marked improvement" and "almost cleared" as judged by physicians. There was no change in fine wrinkles. Burning-stinging scores were higher at Week 8 for the Obagi system and peeling was higher at Week 12 for the SkinMedica system. The subject evaluations paralleled the physician assessment. No other differences between the systems were noted.

Nonprescription topical treatments: cosmetics

Antioxidants: vitamin C Topical daily application vitamin C (10% ascorbic acid and 7% tetrahexyldecyl ascorbate in an anhydrous polysilicone vehicle) was compared with the vehicle in a split-face study among 10 subjects with moderate photodamage for 12 weeks.[58] Significant improvements in wrinkles were noted for the treatment in the periorbital, perioral, and cheek regions relative to baseline and for the placebo in the periorbital sites. Overall, the vitamin C treatment produced a directional improvement in wrinkles versus the vehicle (P = .08). The treatments did not impact skin pigmentation. Four of 10 subjects judged the treatment side to be improved.

Vitamins and mixtures Topical application of 2% niacinamide significantly reduced the percent area of hyperpigmentation after 4 and 8 weeks of treatment relative to baseline and the vehicle control in a split-face trial.[59] Relative to a vehicle control, the use of 5% niacinamide for 12 weeks led to significant reductions in percent area of hyperpigmentation (image analysis), red blotchiness (expert evaluation), total wrinkle line length (image analysis), and yellow skin color (analysis of b* channel images), and increases in skin elasticity (biomechanical measures) and elastic recovery.[60] A combination of 5% niacinamide (vitamin B_3) and 1% *N*-undecylenol phenylalanine, shown in vitro to reduce melanin production by melanocytes, was compared with niacinamide alone and vehicle among groups of Asian (Japanese) and white subjects with photodamage in a split-face design.[61] The combination treatment reduced the percent area of hyperpigmentated spots to a greater extent than niacinamide alone or the vehicle in both groups after 8 weeks. A lotion containing 4% niacinamide, 0.5% panthenol (provitamin B_5), and 0.5% tocopherol acetate (vitamin E acetate) was compared with a moisturizer vehicle among 207 women aged 30 to 60 years from India (baseline skin lightness greater than 51 from the L scale of a standardized color image) over 10 weeks.[62] These features of photoaging were reduced: percent area of hyperpigmented spots; percent area of melanin-specific spots (measured using spectrophotometric intracutaneous analysis); fine lines/wrinkles (expert visual assessment); and skin texture (expert assessment). Skin lightness (L value) and evenness of skin tone both increased with treatment. Importantly, the use of moisturizer (ie, a cosmetic) without sunscreen also reduces the features associated with photodamaged facial skin.[58,59]

Prescription versus cosmetics

Tretinoin at 0.02% (Renova; Ortho Dermalogics, Los Angeles, CA, USA) and an SPF 30 moisturizing sunscreen (Neutrogena Healthy Defense Daily Moisturizer SPF; Neutrogena Corporation, Los Angeles, CA, USA) both applied daily were compared with a cosmetic regimen for 8 weeks among 197 females (40–65 years, parallel groups) with moderate to moderately severe periorbital wrinkles.[63] A subset of 25 subjects from each group continued treatment for another 16 weeks. The cosmetics were three commercially available products each containing niacinamide (vitamin B_3), palmitoyl-lysine-threonine and palmitoyl-lysine-threonine-threonine-lysine-serine and carnosine. Product 1: daytime lotion with additional ingredients for SPF 30, vitamin C, and vitamin E (Olay Professional Pro-X Age Repair Lotion SPF 30, Procter & Gamble Company, Cincinnati, OH, USA). Product 2: a night cream with the four ingredients (Olay Professional Pro-X Wrinkle Smoothing Cream, Procter & Gamble Company, Cincinnati, OH, USA). Product 3: a wrinkle treatment with the four components plus retinyl propionate (Olay Professional Pro-X Deep Wrinkle Treatment, Procter & Gamble Company, Cincinnati, OH, USA) twice a day. After 8 weeks, the appearance of fine lines and wrinkles was judged by experts to be improved for both treatments. A higher number of subjects on the cosmetic regimen had a minimum positive grade of +1 and more had improvements two grades or greater. By image analysis, the cosmetic group had a significantly greater reduction in periorbital wrinkle area fraction. Both groups had improvements in deep wrinkles. The subject assessments of eye lines and wrinkles, overall skin feel, and overall appearance were larger for the cosmetics. The SC barrier integrity was poorer for the tretinoin group, measured as transepidermal water loss (TEWL), compared with baseline and unchanged for the cosmetics. For the 25 subjects per group who continued, there were no treatment differences at Weeks 16 and 24.

Combinations: Skin Resurfacing and Topical Treatments

The effects of topical vitamin C applied after fraxel laser treatment of photodamage were evaluated among 44 Korean women.[33] Subjects received two treatments 4 weeks apart with power of 26 to 27 W, duration of 500 to 800 μs, and spacings of 400 to 650 μm. One group applied a vitamin C–containing treatment three times daily. Both groups used SPF 30 sunscreen and moisturizer use was permitted. Measures of SC barrier integrity differed significantly for the two groups (ie, increases in TEWL were lower [less compromise] and pH changes higher for the vitamin C group). At posttreatment week 4, TEWL had not returned to prelaser treatment values indicating ongoing restoration of epidermal barrier function. The conclusion was that vitamin C assisted in skin recovery but it was not clear whether these effects could be attributed to difference in moisturizer or vehicle effects between the groups.

IPL treatment alone was compared with IPL treatment in combination with injected treatments (ie, vitamin C, hyaluronic acid [low molecular weight], and β-glucan) and the combination was found to produce more positive results.[64] One hundred women (56.3 years median) were divided into two groups (matched for age, skin type, and photodamage) and treated as follows. Treatment 1 (n = 40) consisted of seven sessions of IPL of three to four passes at 550-nm cutoff at 2-week intervals. Treatment 2 (n = 60) consisted of with IPL (same settings) seven times at 2-week intervals and low-intensity diode light (623 nm and 40 mW/cm^2) nine times (alternating weeks of IPL) and 10 to 15 injections into the superficial and deep dermis. Patients and physicians (from photographs) rated satisfaction on a 0 (none) to 5 (excellent) scale. The patients scored the combination treatment significantly higher for positive results than the IPL treatment along. The physicians judged the combination significantly higher for facial skin texture and firmness (**Table 3**). No differences were observed between the treatments for hyperpigmentation and telangiectasia by physicians but both received a high percent of positive results.

The effects of methyl aminolevulinate and red light (8 minutes, 37 J/cm^2) were compared with placebo and red light in a split-face study among

Table 3
IPL treatment alone compared with IPL treatment in combination with injected treatments vitamin C, hyaluronic acid (low molecular weight), and β-glucan

Rating	Patients		Physicians Hyperpigmentation and Telangectasia		Physicians Texture and Firmness	
Treatment	1	2	1	2	1	2
Positive	35%	70%	70%	75%	30%	70%
Poor	65%	30%	30%	25%	70%	30%
Significance	$P<.05$ favors treatment 2		Not different		$P<.05$ favors treatment 2	

Data from Mezzana P. Multi light and drugs: a new technique to treat face photoaging. Comparative study with photo-rejuvenation. Lasers Med Sci 2008;23(2):149–54.

48 subjects with photodamage.[65] Subjects were treated twice (15-day interval) and evaluated 1 month later. The combination treatment resulted in significant improvement in global photodamage, fine lines, coarse lines, mottled pigmentation, tactile roughness, sallowness, erythema, and sebaceous hyperplasia as judged by subjects. Physician assessment from photographs was consistent with subject findings. Pain occurred in the combination treatment and impacted satisfaction in 20% of subjects.

DEVELOPMENTS IN PROGRESS

Significant contributions to the scientific literature on the subject of skin photoaging have been made by the skin care industry, either in their own laboratories or through collaborations with clinicians in academic settings or private practice. Genomics research, including advances in analytical methods (ie, gene array technology) and statistical methods for interpreting complex data sets, is a promising approach for understanding changes at the molecular level and identifying targets for intervention.[66–68] Specifically, transcriptomic analysis of chronically young versus old skin in UV-exposed and UV-protected areas showed downregulation of genes responsible for synthesis of the SC barrier lipids cholesterol, fatty acids, and sphingolipids in both types of aging.[66] Genes for epidermal differentiation (eg, transglutaminase 5 and keratinocyte transcription factor p63) were downregulated for both types but more so for intrinsic aging. Genes involved with inflammation and wound healing were upregulated. Genes for elastic fiber components including elastin, fibulins (1, 2, and 5), and elastic microfibril protein fibrillin 1 were increased in photoaged skin. Genes for collagen type 1 $\alpha1$, type 1 $\alpha2$, type III $\alpha1$, type V $\alpha1$, and type V $\alpha2$ genes were significantly decreased only for intrinsic aged skin. Tissue samples from solar lentigenes and uninvolved (UV protected) skin in the same subjects were analyzed by transcriptomic analysis.[67] Levels of β-adrenergic receptor 1 (ADRB1) were 14 times higher in the hyperpigmented lesion suggesting that they were involved in pigmentation as propigmentation receptors. This hypothesis was confirmed when transfection of siRNA against ADRB1 into cell cultures substantially reduced melanin generation. When the cosmetic ingredient undecylenoyl phenylalanine was added to cell cultures, melanin levels were also reduced suggesting potential use in reduction of hyperpigmented spots. Application of an undecylenoyl phenylalanine-containing moisturizer significantly reduced the percent area of facial hyperpigmented spots relative to placebo after 4 weeks.[67]

In another example of application of gene expression methods to the problem of photoaging, human keratinocytes and fibroblasts were treated with *Aframomum angustifolium* seed extract and the response evaluated using low-density DNA arrays.[69] Increased expression of the antioxidant genes metallothionein 1, metallothionein 2, and thioredoxin and genes for epidermal renewal, keratinocyte differentiation, and dermal-epidermal junction was observed in keratinocytes. The effects of a topical skin care product containing *A angustifolium* seed extract were evaluated among 100 females with photodamage for 8 weeks using photographic images and subject self-assessment. The improvement in fine lines, pigmentation, and erythema was comparable with that achieved with IPL treatment, although data for the light treatment were not shown.

OPTIMIZATION, SUMMARY, AND PERSPECTIVE

Optimal treatment of photodamage is a multistep process and may require combination of modalities. A comprehensive strategy would be pretreatment with retinoic acid (at sufficient levels to avoid irritation); selection of the resurfacing laser to maximize dermal effects (eg, collagen remodeling), and postsurgical products and procedures to accelerate wound healing and minimize complications.[70] For example, treatment of facial skin with platelet-rich plasma after ablative CO_2 fractional laser resurfacing accelerated healing relative to no postsurgical treatment.[71] Postsurgical wound care with Aquaphor (Beiersdorf, Inc., Hamburg, Germany) after fractional CO_2 laser resurfacing resulted in less erythema and crusting than treatment with a Biafine topical emulsion (water, liquid paraffin, ethylene glycol monostearate, stearic acid, propylene glycol, paraffin wax, squalane, avocado oil, trolamine/sodium alginate, triethanolamine, cetyl palmitate, methylparaben, sorbic acid, propylparaben, and fragrance, Ortho Dermalogics, Los Angeles, CA, USA).[72]

In preparing this article, the authors noted a recurring theme in the discussion sections of publications. It stated that there are few studies, a limited number of controlled studies, and a need for rigorous studies for topical products and facial resurfacing procedures.[73] However, the information synthesized for this and the previous article suggests a schema to describe the relative effectiveness of therapeutic modalities in reducing perceived age, shown in **Fig. 2**. Some elements are based on actual clinical studies. Others are suggested from physician experience, consumer preference, and success in the marketplace. Unfortunately, the relative comparison among modalities is only approximate. There is substantial variation in the treatment features (eg, dose, duration, multiple vs single) and the methods of evaluation (eg, grading scales, objective image analysis, biomechanical properties). Note that increasing the uniformity of facial skin coloration is an important treatment goal because it substantially impacts the patient's perceived age.

The question remains: What is the maximum reduction in perceived age that can be achieved with a "total package" including (1) early daily sunscreen use and continuation after restoration procedures; (2) preprocedure treatment with retinoic acid; (3) laser resurfacing or chemical peeling combined with nonablative modes; (4) additional

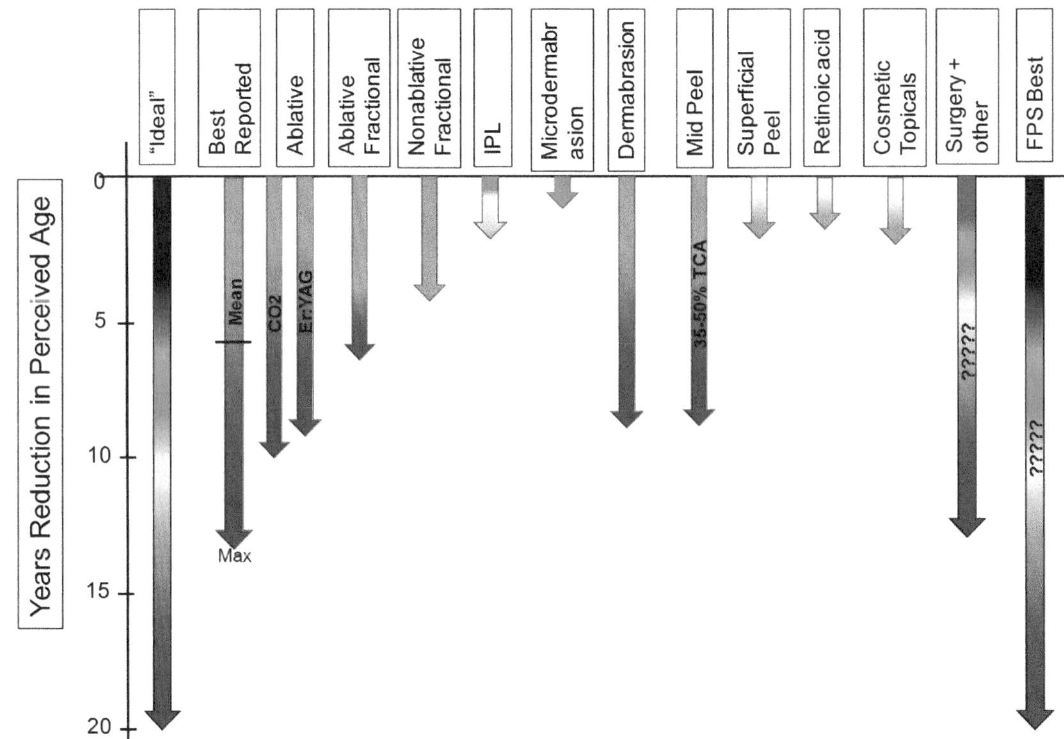

Fig. 2. Relative performance of treatment modalities for facial photodamage. The "ideal" of 20 years reduction in perceived age refers to the fact that facial coloration can reduce perceived age by as much as 20 years.[86,87] The reported best is from Swanson.[8] The "surgery + other" is hypothetical for a combination of surgical techniques or topicals. The "FPS best" is the facial plastic surgeon's treatment scheme combined with experience and skilled technique.

of topicals including vitamins and skin lightening agents; (5) best-in-class wound care postsurgery; (6) maintenance with multicomponent cosmetics (skin lighteners, vitamins, sunscreens); and (7) effective use of color cosmetics. Perhaps future publications will include "face offs" where physicians propose and evaluate their best combinations and objectively quantify the outcomes for patient review.

As one surgeon (D. Railand, MD) stated, "the benefits of laser skin resurfacing in trained hands remains unequaled."[74] Facial plastic surgeons are likely to achieve optimum benefits by combinations of products, their knowledge of the science, their experience, and their art.[75]

REFERENCES

1. Gunn DA, Rexbye H, Griffiths CE, et al. Why some women look young for their age. PLoS One 2009; 4(12):e8021.
2. Mayes AE, Murray PG, Gunn DA, et al. Ageing appearance in China: biophysical profile of facial skin and its relationship to perceived age. J Eur Acad Dermatol Venereol 2009;24(3):341–8.
3. Gilchrest BA. Skin aging and photoaging: an overview. J Am Acad Dermatol 1989;21(3 Pt 2):610–3.
4. Ortonne JP, Pandya AG, Lui H, et al. Treatment of solar lentigines. J Am Acad Dermatol 2006; 54(5 Suppl 2):S262–71.
5. Callender VD, St Surin-Lord S, Davis EC, et al. Postinflammatory hyperpigmentation: etiologic and therapeutic considerations. Am J Clin Dermatol 2011; 12(2):87–99.
6. Alexiades-Armenakas MR, Dover JS, Arndt KA. The spectrum of laser skin resurfacing: nonablative, fractional, and ablative laser resurfacing. J Am Acad Dermatol 2008;58(5):719–37 [quiz: 738–40].
7. Cosmetic Surgery National Data Bank statistics. Garden Grove (CA): The American Society for Aesthetic Plastic Surgery; 2011.
8. Swanson E. Objective assessment of change in apparent age after facial rejuvenation surgery. J Plast Reconstr Aesthet Surg 2011;64(9):1124–31.
9. Fischer TC, Perosino E, Poli F, et al. Chemical peels in aesthetic dermatology: an update 2009. J Eur Acad Dermatol Venereol 2010;24(3):281–92.
10. Hantash BM, Mahmood MB. Fractional photothermolysis: a novel aesthetic laser surgery modality. Dermatol Surg 2007;33(5):525–34.
11. Manstein D, Herron GS, Sink RK, et al. Fractional photothermolysis: a new concept for cutaneous remodeling using microscopic patterns of thermal injury. Lasers Surg Med 2004;34(5):426–38.
12. Sachdeva S. Nonablative fractional laser resurfacing in Asian skin: a review. J Cosmet Dermatol 2010; 9(4):307–12.
13. Alkhawam L, Alam M. Dermabrasion and microdermabrasion. Facial Plast Surg 2009;25(5):301–10.
14. Gill HS, Andrews SN, Sakthivel SK, et al. Selective removal of stratum corneum by microdermabrasion to increase skin permeability. Eur J Pharm Sci 2009;38(2):95–103.
15. Seite S, Fourtanier AM. The benefit of daily photoprotection. J Am Acad Dermatol 2008;58(5 Suppl 2): S160–6.
16. Sambandan DR, Ratner D. Sunscreens: an overview and update. J Am Acad Dermatol 2011;64(4):748–58.
17. Akiba S, Shinkura R, Miyamoto K, et al. Influence of chronic UV exposure and lifestyle on facial skin photo-aging: results from a pilot study. J Epidemiol 1999;9(Suppl 6):S136–42.
18. Hillebrand GG, Miyamoto K, Schnell B, et al. Quantitative evaluation of skin condition in an epidemiological survey of females living in northern versus southern Japan. J Dermatol Sci 2001;27(Suppl 1): S42–52.
19. Diffey BL. The impact of topical photoprotectants intended for daily use on lifetime ultraviolet exposure. J Cosmet Dermatol 2011;10(3):245–50.
20. Alster TS, Bellew SG. Improvement of dermatochalasis and periorbital rhytides with a high-energy pulsed CO2 laser: a retrospective study. Dermatol Surg 2004;30(4 Pt 1):483–7 [discussion: 487].
21. Khatri KA, Ross V, Grevelink JM, et al. Comparison of erbium:YAG and carbon dioxide lasers in resurfacing of facial rhytides. Arch Dermatol 1999;135(4):391–7.
22. Kitzmiller WJ, Visscher M, Page DA, et al. A controlled evaluation of dermabrasion versus CO2 laser resurfacing for the treatment of perioral wrinkles. Plast Reconstr Surg 2000;106(6):1366–72 [discussion: 1373–4].
23. Tierney EP, Hanke CW. Fractionated carbon dioxide laser treatment of photoaging: prospective study in 45 patients and review of the literature. Dermatol Surg 2011;37(9):1279–90.
24. Alexiades-Armenakas M. A quantitative and comprehensive grading scale for rhytides, laxity, and photoaging. J Drugs Dermatol 2006;5(8):808–9.
25. Karsai S, Czarnecka A, Junger M, et al. Ablative fractional lasers (CO(2) and Er:YAG): a randomized controlled double-blind split-face trial of the treatment of peri-orbital rhytides. Lasers Surg Med 2010;42(2):160–7.
26. Brightman LA, Brauer JA, Anolik R, et al. Ablative and fractional ablative lasers. Dermatol Clin 2009; 27(4):479–89, vi–vii.
27. Weiss RA, McDaniel DH, Geronemus RG. Review of nonablative photorejuvenation: reversal of the aging effects of the sun and environmental damage using laser and light sources. Semin Cutan Med Surg 2003;22(2):93–106.
28. Kunzi-Rapp K, Dierickx CC, Cambier B, et al. Minimally invasive skin rejuvenation with Erbium: YAG

laser used in thermal mode. Lasers Surg Med 2006;38(10):899–907.

29. El Domyati M, El-Ammawi TS, Medhat W, et al. Multiple minimally invasive erbium: yttrium aluminum garnet laser mini-peels for skin rejuvenation: an objective assessment. J Cosmet Dermatol 2012;11(2):122–30.
30. Kopera D, Smolle J, Kaddu S, et al. Nonablative laser treatment of wrinkles: meeting the objective? Assessment by 25 dermatologists. Br J Dermatol 2004;150(5):936–9.
31. Hantash BM, De Coninck E, Liu H, et al. Split-face comparison of the erbium micropeel with intense pulsed light. Dermatol Surg 2008;34(6):763–72.
32. Shin JW, Lee DH, Choi SY, et al. Objective and non-invasive evaluation of photorejuvenation effect with intense pulsed light treatment in Asian skin. J Eur Acad Dermatol Venereol 2011;25(5):516–22.
33. Kim JE, Chang S, Won CH, et al. Combination treatment using bipolar radiofrequency-based intense pulsed light, infrared light and diode laser enhanced clinical effectiveness and histological dermal remodeling in Asian photoaged skin. Dermatol Surg 2012;38(1):68–76.
34. Leyden J, Stephens TJ, Herndon JH Jr. Multicenter clinical trial of a home-use nonablative fractional laser device for wrinkle reduction. J Am Acad Dermatol 2012;67(5):975–84.
35. Fitzpatrick RE, Goldman MP, Satur NM, et al. Pulsed carbon dioxide laser resurfacing of photo-aged facial skin. Arch Dermatol 1996;132(4):395–402.
36. Bhalla M, Thami GP. Microdermabrasion: reappraisal and brief review of literature. Dermatol Surg 2006;32(6):809–14.
37. Grimes PE. Microdermabrasion. Dermatol Surg 2005;31(9 Pt 2):1160–5 [discussion: 1165].
38. Pozner JN, Goldberg DJ. Superficial erbium:YAG laser resurfacing of photodamaged skin. J Cosmet Laser Ther 2006;8(2):89–91.
39. Coimbra M, Rohrich RJ, Chao J, et al. A prospective controlled assessment of microdermabrasion for damaged skin and fine rhytides. Plast Reconstr Surg 2004;113(5):1438–43 [discussion: 1444].
40. Spencer JM, Kurtz ES. Approaches to document the efficacy and safety of microdermabrasion procedure. Dermatol Surg 2006;32(11):1353–7.
41. Mangat DS, Tansavatdi K, Garlich P. Current chemical peels and other resurfacing techniques. Facial Plast Surg 2011;27(1):35–49.
42. Brody H. Chemical peeling. 1st edition. St Louis (MO): 1997.
43. Coleman WP III, Futrell JM. The glycolic acid trichloroacetic acid peel. J Dermatol Surg Oncol 1994;20(1):76–80.
44. Kitzmiller WJ, Visscher MO, Maclennan S, et al. Comparison of a series of superficial chemical peels with a single midlevel chemical peel for the correction of facial actinic damage. Aesthet Surg J 2003;23(5):339–44.
45. Saint-Leger D. Cosmeceuticals. Of men, science and laws. Int J Cosmet Sci 2012;34(5):396–401.
46. Reed RE. The definition of cosmeceuticals. J Soc Cosmet Chem 1962;13:103–10.
47. Samuel M, Brooke RC, Hollis S, et al. Interventions for photodamaged skin. Cochrane Database Syst Rev 2005;(1):CD001782.
48. Bhawan J. Short- and long-term histologic effects of topical tretinoin on photodamaged skin. Int J Dermatol 1998;37(4):286–92.
49. Bhawan J, Olsen E, Lufrano L, et al. Histologic evaluation of the long term effects of tretinoin on photodamaged skin. J Dermatol Sci 1996;11(3):177–82.
50. Antoniou C, Kosmadaki MG, Stratigos AJ, et al. Photoaging: prevention and topical treatments. Am J Clin Dermatol 2010;11(2):95–102.
51. Levitt J. The safety of hydroquinone: a dermatologist's response to the 2006 Federal Register. J Am Acad Dermatol 2007;57(5):854–72.
52. Department of Health and Human Services FDA, editor. Federal Register. Washington, DC: National Archives and Records Administration; 2006. 21 CFR part 358 subpart A: Miscellaneous External Drug Products for Over-the-Counter Human Use: Skin Bleaching Drug Products.
53. McGregor D. Hydroquinone: an evaluation of the human risks from its carcinogenic and mutagenic properties. Crit Rev Toxicol 2007;37(10):887–914.
54. Hamed SH, Sriwiriyanont P, deLong MA, et al. Comparative efficacy and safety of deoxyarbutin, a new tyrosinase-inhibiting agent. J Cosmet Sci 2006;57(4):291–308.
55. Boissy RE, Visscher M, DeLong MA. DeoxyArbutin: a novel reversible tyrosinase inhibitor with effective in vivo skin lightening potency. Exp Dermatol 2005;14(8):601–8.
56. Draelos ZD. Skin lightening preparations and the hydroquinone controversy. Dermatol Ther 2007;20(5):308–13.
57. Fabi S, Massaki N, Goldman MP. Efficacy and tolerability of two commercial hyperpigmentation kits in the treatment of facial hyperpigmentation and photo-aging. J Drugs Dermatol 2012;11(8):964–8.
58. Fitzpatrick RE, Rostan EF. Double-blind, half-face study comparing topical vitamin C and vehicle for rejuvenation of photodamage. Dermatol Surg 2002;28(3):231–6.
59. Hakozaki T, Minwalla L, Zhuang J, et al. The effect of niacinamide on reducing cutaneous pigmentation and suppression of melanosome transfer. Br J Dermatol 2002;147(1):20–31.
60. Bissett DL, Oblong JE, Berge CA. Niacinamide: a B vitamin that improves aging facial skin

appearance. Dermatol Surg 2005;31(7 Pt 2):860–5 [discussion: 865].
61. Bissett DL, Robinson LR, Raleigh PS, et al. Reduction in the appearance of facial hyperpigmentation by topical N-undecyl-10-enoyl-L-phenylalanine and its combination with niacinamide. J Cosmet Dermatol 2009;8(4):260–6.
62. Jerajani HR, Mizoguchi H, Li J, et al. The effects of a daily facial lotion containing vitamins B3 and E and provitamin B5 on the facial skin of Indian women: a randomized, double-blind trial. Indian J Dermatol Venereol Leprol 2010;76(1):20–6.
63. Fu JJ, Hillebrand GG, Raleigh P, et al. A randomized, controlled comparative study of the wrinkle reduction benefits of a cosmetic niacinamide/peptide/retinyl propionate product regimen vs. a prescription 0.02% tretinoin product regimen. Br J Dermatol 2010;162(3):647–54.
64. Mezzana P. Multi light and drugs: a new technique to treat face photoaging. Comparative study with photorejuvenation. Lasers Med Sci 2008;23(2): 149–54.
65. Sanclemente G, Medina L, Villa JF, et al. A prospective split-face double-blind randomized placebo-controlled trial to assess the efficacy of methyl aminolevulinate + red-light in patients with facial photodamage. J Eur Acad Dermatol Venereol 2011;25(1):49–58.
66. McGrath JA, Robinson MK, Binder RL. Skin differences based on age and chronicity of ultraviolet exposure: results from a gene expression profiling study. Br J Dermatol 2012;166(Suppl 2):9–15.
67. Osborne R, Hakozaki T, Laughlin T, et al. Application of genomics to breakthroughs in the cosmetic treatment of skin ageing and discoloration. Br J Dermatol 2012;166(Suppl 2):16–9.
68. Kimball AB, Grant RA, Wang F, et al. Beyond the blot: cutting edge tools for genomics, proteomics and metabolomics analyses and previous successes. Br J Dermatol 2012;166(Suppl 2):1–8.
69. Talbourdet S, Sadick NS, Lazou K, et al. Modulation of gene expression as a new skin anti-aging strategy. J Drugs Dermatol 2007;6(Suppl 6): s25–33.
70. Lupo M, Jacob L. Cosmeceuticals used in conjunction with laser resurfacing. Semin Cutan Med Surg 2011;30(3):156–62.
71. Lee JW, Kim BJ, Kim MN, et al. The efficacy of autologous platelet rich plasma combined with ablative carbon dioxide fractional resurfacing for acne scars: a simultaneous split-face trial. Dermatol Surg 2011; 37(7):931–8.
72. Sarnoff DS. A comparison of wound healing between a skin protectant ointment and a medical device topical emulsion after laser resurfacing of the perioral area. J Am Acad Dermatol 2011; 64(Suppl 3):S36–43.
73. Nolan KA, Marmur ES. Over-the-counter topical skincare products: a review of the literature. J Drugs Dermatol 2012;11(2):220–4.
74. Railan D, Kilmer S. Ablative treatment of photoaging. Dermatol Ther 2005;18(3):227–41.
75. Gold M. The science and art of hyaluronic acid dermal filler use in esthetic applications. J Cosmet Dermatol 2009;8(4):301–7.
76. Doherty SD, Doherty CB, Markus JS, et al. A paradigm for facial skin rejuvenation. Facial Plast Surg 2009;25(4):245–51.
77. Goldberg DJ. Lasers for facial rejuvenation. Am J Clin Dermatol 2003;4(4):225–34.
78. Papadavid E, Katsambas A. Lasers for facial rejuvenation: a review. Int J Dermatol 2003;42(6):480–7.
79. Tierney EP, Kouba DJ, Hanke CW. Review of fractional photothermolysis: treatment indications and efficacy. Dermatol Surg 2009;35(10):1445–61.
80. Tajirian AL, Goldberg DJ. Fractional ablative laser skin resurfacing: a review. J Cosmet Laser Ther 2011;13(6):262–4.
81. Bogdan Allemann I, Kaufman J. Fractional photothermolysis: an update. Lasers Med Sci 2010; 25(1):137–44.
82. Fabbrocini G, De Padova MP, Tosti A. Chemical peels: what's new and what isn't new but still works well. Facial Plast Surg 2009;25(5):329–36.
83. Elsner P, Fluhr JW, Gehring W, et al. Anti-aging data and support claims: consensus statement. J Dtsch Dermatol Ges 2011;9(Suppl 3):S1–32.
84. Zussman J, Ahdout J, Kim J. Vitamins and photoaging: do scientific data support their use? J Am Acad Dermatol 2010;63(3):507–25.
85. Beer KR. Combined treatment for skin rejuvenation and soft-tissue augmentation of the aging face. J Drugs Dermatol 2011;10(2):125–32.
86. Fink B, Grammer K, Matts PJ. Visual skin color distribution plays a role in the perception of age, attractiveness, and health of female faces. Evol Hum Behav 2006;27(6):433–42.
87. Matts PJ, Fink B. Chronic sun damage and the perception of age, health and attractiveness. Photochem Photobiol Sci 2010;9(4):421–31.

Stem Cells and Molecular Advances in the Treatment of Facial Skin

Anthony P. Sclafani, MD[a,b,*]

KEYWORDS

• Stem cells • Fibrin mesh • Growth factors • Neovascularization • Angiogenesis • Vasculogenesis • Stromal vascular fraction

KEY POINTS

- Stem cells are capable of self-replication and differentiation into various cell lines. Embryonic stem cells can differentiate into all cells lines, whereas adult stem cells can differentiate into cells types within their cell line. Treatment with certain transcription factors can induce adult cells to revert to induced pleuripotent stem cells.
- Mesenchymal stem cells tolerate ischemia and respond by replication.
- Adipose-derived stem cells (ADSCs) can affect local tissues both through differentiation and release of growth factors.
- ADSCs can stimulate the growth of existing capillaries and the development of new capillaries.
- Platelet-rich plasma and platelet-rich fibrin matrix, through the release of platelet growth factors, can induce local cellular changes.
- ADSCs and platelet preparations have been described for use in aesthetic surgery; however, optimal delivery and application is still being defined.

CLINICAL REVIEW OF THE LITERATURE

Restoration of the skin's normal architecture, contours, and physical characteristics is currently addressed with a variety of chemical, mechanical, and energy-based technologies. However, beyond the concept of wound contracture followed by wound healing, little is currently known about the process. At best, created wounds will heal naturally.

As our understanding of the cellular and biochemical milieu of the skin wound becomes more robust and thorough, attempts to enhance the clinical response to wounding based on these laboratory findings have been made, however, these are often shotgun approaches, and interpreting the results of some of these studies can be challenging and difficult to reconcile.[1,2]

A more thorough grasp of the nature of autologous stem cells and the growth factors to which they respond and secrete is now emerging, providing a framework on which more rational treatment strategies can be built.

Classic wound healing occurs in 3 overlapping phases: the inflammatory, proliferative, and remodeling phases. During the inflammatory phase, platelets aggregate on a fibrin clot and achieve active hemostasis, whereas acute inflammatory cells remove debris and create a favorable environment for the proliferative phase to occur. The proliferative phase is characterized by the formation of granulation tissue, collagen deposition, angiogenesis, epithelial migration, and wound coverage. Remodeling occurs with collagen resorption and replacement.

[a] Division of Facial Plastic Surgery, Department of Otolaryngology, The New York Eye & Ear Infirmary, 310 East 14th Street, New York, NY 10003, USA; [b] New York Medical College, Valhalla, NY, USA
* Division of Facial Plastic Surgery, Department of Otolaryngology, The New York Eye & Ear Infirmary, 310 East 14th Street, New York, NY 10003.
E-mail address: asclafani@nyee.edu

Facial Plast Surg Clin N Am 21 (2013) 77–80
http://dx.doi.org/10.1016/j.fsc.2012.10.005
1064-7406/13/$ – see front matter

However, it is now known that fibrin does more than serve as a binding site for platelets. The fibrin mesh that forms acts as scaffolding for subsequent cell binding and cellular activity (including collagen deposition), and provides binding sites for growth factors. A principal source of growth factors is the platelet, which releases stored growth factors from alpha granules on activation and continues to synthesize and secrete these growth factors for the rest of the lifespan of the platelets (5–10 days). These growth factors are chemoattractive, mitogenic, and angiogenic; of these, vascular endothelial growth factor (VEGF) and transforming growth factor-beta (TGF-β) are the best characterized.

During the proliferative phase, collagen is deposited, new blood vessels are formed and epithelial continuity is reestablished. Neovascularization occurs both by angiogenesis (blood vessel development from existing capillaries) and vasculogenesis (generation of new capillaries de novo). Vasculogenesis requires the presence of stem cells, which serve not only as progenitor cells but also regulate tissue growth through the release of growth factors. Resident tissue-specific stem cells in the hair follicle bulge out of the outer root sheath and in the basal layer of the interfollicular epidermis, they respond to injury by expansion to reepithelialize the wound.

Stem cells are characterized by their ability to replicate as well as differentiate under specific conditions into specific cell lines. Pluripotent cells, such as embryonic stem cells, are capable of differentiating into every cell in the body, whereas mesenchymal stem cells (MSCs), such as bone-marrow-derived (BMDSCs) or adipose-derived stem cells (ADSCs), can differentiate into cells in the mesenchymal line. ADSCs are an attractive source of MSCs as the fat can be easily harvested via a liposuction procedure. Differential centrifugation isolates the stromal vascular fraction (SVF), containing white and red blood cells, endothelial cells, fibroblasts, pericytes, and ADSCs.[3] Jurgens and colleagues[4] have argued that abdominal fat harvesting yields higher SVF and ADSC cell counts than other donor areas, although several other studies have failed to demonstrate significant differences in recovery of viable adipocytes from various donor sites.[5] Although the SVF can be added to adipocytes and injected in the technique of cell-assisted lipotransfer[6] (CAL), ADSCs can also be isolated and expanded in vitro before use.

MSCs, such as ADSCs, possess many interesting and exploitable properties in terms of wound healing. In addition to their capacity for self-renewal and differentiation, MSCs are known to better tolerate ischemia[7] and proliferate under ischemic conditions.[8–11] MSCs migrate to areas of ischemia, injury and inflammation.[12] MSCs secrete a variety of growth factors, including VEGF, TGF-β, hepatocyte growth factor, platelet-derived growth factor (PDGF), basic fibroblast growth factor, and placental growth factor, and stimulate a proangiogenic, immunotolerant, and antioxidative environment through cytokine release.[3,11,12] Analysis of critical length skin flaps treated with injections of radiolabeled ADSCs demonstrated that, in addition to the proangiogenetic effects mediated by VEGF and PDGF (among other growth factors), new capillaries are formed directly from the ADSCs.[13] However, by virtue of the numbers of cells involved as well as the positive effect seen with the application of MSC culture media,[13] it is clear that a significant degree of MSC activity is via a paracrine effect.

Numerous animal studies have been performed to examine the effect of MSCs/ADSCs on wound healing, and have included application of stem cells topically or by local injection. Steinberg and colleagues[14] found no difference in healing of ischemic wounds between groups treated with topically applied ADSCs or dermal fibroblasts in fibrin sealant, but many studies have shown a positive therapeutic effect.[15–19] Clinically, there are number of case reports describing stem cell use, including a report by Rigotti and colleagues[20] of subjective improvement in 20 patients with severe radiodermatitis and osteoradionecrosis treated with ADSCs. CAL as described by Yoshimura[6] is probably the best known application of stem cells in aesthetic plastic surgery.

Although stem cells can provide both the cellular proliferative engines and paracrine stimuli to enhance wound healing, platelets can provide the necessary stimuli for the wound-healing response through the release of growth factors. Topical PDGF (becaplermin 0.01%, Regranex, OMJ Pharmaceuticals, Inc, San German, Puerto Rico) and keratinocyte growth factor (KGF, palifermin, Kepivance, Biovitrum AB, Stockholm, Sweden) are approved by the US Food and Drug Administration (FDA) for diabetic foot ulcers and oral mucositis, respectively, but prolonged use has been associated with an increase in cancer mortality.

Platelet-rich plasma (PRP) seeks to amplify the body's normal wound response. PRP has traditionally been defined as a preparation with at least a 5- to 6-fold increase in platelet concentration (compared with peripheral blood) in plasma; fibrin is not concentrated and limited due to the low plasma volume. Platelets are activated with bovine thrombin and (usually) supraphysiologic concentrations of calcium. Red blood cells are generally limited, but white cells are generally increased. An alternative preparation, platelet-rich fibrin matrix

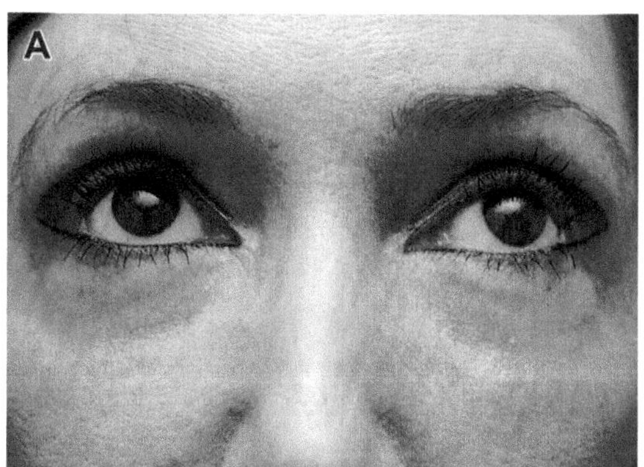

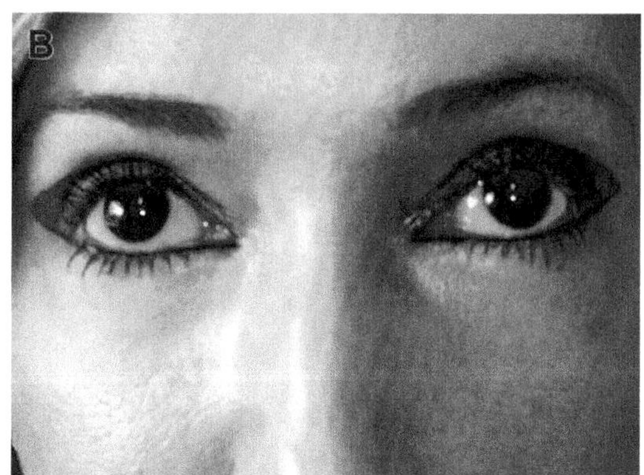

Fig. 1. (*A*) Involutional changes leading to infraorbital hollowing and exposure of early orbital fat pseudoherniation. (*B*) Photograph of same patient 6 months after 2 treatments of PRFM injected subdermally; the hollows are well effaced and the pseudoherniated fat is camouflaged.

(PRFM), is a less concentrated platelet preparation, but includes plasma proteins, especially fibrinogen/fibrin, providing a more physiologic milieu for platelet function. PRFM has been shown to release bioactive platelet growth factors for up to 7 days after activation.

PRP has been shown to accelerate experimental[2] as well as chronic nonhealing wounds.[21,22] The cellular effects of PRP seem to occur early and be short-lived.[1] However, the stimulation of cells can begin a reparative process. PRP injections into ischemic skin flaps decrease skin necrosis and are associated with increased mRNA for VEGF, PDGF, and endothelial growth factor.[23]

PRFM has also been shown to be effective in chronic nonhealing lower extremity ulcers.[24] Sclafani first described the aesthetic use of PRFM in 2010, demonstrating significant improvement in deep nasolabial folds in as little as 2 weeks and persisting for 12 weeks (the duration of the study) after dermal and subdermal injections of PRFM.[25] Histologically, intradermal PRFM injection is associated with activation of fibroblasts with collagen deposition, development of new blood vessels, and adipogenesis.[26] PRFM has been used in a variety of applications in aesthetic facial plastic surgery (**Fig. 1**), both by dermal and subdermal injection or mixed with autologous fat before injection.[27,28] In addition to the effects of the growth factors released from the platelets, fibrin mesh binding of the harvested fat lobules may provide additional structural integrity to support the clinical observation of enhanced fat survival when mixed with PRFM. This result contrasts with the mixed results of PRP treatment of fat grafts.[29,30]

SUMMARY

Aesthetic facial plastic surgery is entering new territory, as our understanding of regenerative medicine is increasingly defined and techniques refined. No automated system for the isolation of stem cells for clinical use has received FDA approval. Centrifugation to isolate the SVF from lipoaspirate can be performed if the cells are not isolated or expanded. For the latter, formal FDA approval of an investigational new drug application is necessary. PRP and PRFM systems are currently FDA approved and clinically available. Platelet growth factors, when released in a physiologic fashion, can induce accelerated wound healing, and PRFM alone or mixed with autologous fat has been described for facial soft tissue augmentation.

REFERENCES

1. Sclafani AP, Romo T, Ukrainsky G, et al. Modulation of wound response and soft tissue ingrowth in synthetic and allogeneic implants with platelet concentrate. Arch Facial Plast Surg 2005;7:163–9.
2. Hom DB, Linzie BM, Huang TC. The healing effects of autologous platelet gel on acute human skin wounds. Arch Facial Plast Surg 2007;9:174–83.
3. Gir P, Oni G, Brown SA, et al. Human adipose stem cells: current clinical applications. Plast Reconstr Surg 2012;129:1277–90.
4. Jurgens WJ, Oedayrajsingh-Varma MJ, Helder MN, et al. Effect of tissue-harvesting site on yield of stem cells derived from adipose tissue: implications for cell-based therapies. Cell Tissue Res 2008;332: 415–26.
5. Ullmann Y, Shoshani O, Fodor A, et al. Searching for the favorable donor site for fat injection: in vivo study using the nude mice model. Dermatol Surg 2005;31: 1304–7.
6. Yoshimura K, Sato K, Aoi N, et al. Cell-assisted lipotransfer for facial lipoatrophy: efficacy of clinical use of adipose-derived stem cells. Dermatol Surg 2008; 34:1178–85.

7. Ko SH, Nauta A, Wong V, et al. The role of stem cells in cutaneous wound healing: what do we really know? Plast Reconstr Surg 2011;127(Suppl 1): 10S–20S.
8. Lee EY, Xia Y, Kim WS, et al. Hypoxia-enhanced wound-healing function of adipose-derived stem cells: increase in stem cell proliferation and up-regulation of VEGF and bFGF. Wound Repair Regen 2009;17:540–7.
9. Grayson WL, Zhao F, Bunnell B, et al. Hypoxia enhances proliferation and tissue formation of human mesenchymal stem cells. Biochem Biophys Res Commun 2007;358:948–53.
10. Ren H, Cao Y, Zhao Q, et al. Proliferation and differentiation of bone marrow stromal cells under hypoxic conditions. Biochem Biophys Res Commun 2006;347:12–21.
11. Kilroy GE, Foster SJ, Wu X, et al. Cytokine profile of human adipose-derived stem cells: expression of angiogenic, hematopoietic, and pro-inflammatory factors. J Cell Physiol 2007;212:702–9.
12. Hanson SE, Gutowski KA, Hematti P. Clinical applications of mesenchymal stem cells in soft tissue augmentation. Aesthet Surg J 2010;30:838–42.
13. Gnecchi M, Zhang Z, Ni A, et al. Paracrine mechanisms in adult stem cell signaling and therapy. Circ Res 2008;103:1204–19.
14. Steinberg JP, Hong SJ, Geringer MR, et al. Equivalent effects of topically-delivered adipose-derived stem cells and dermal fibroblasts in the ischemic rabbit ear model for chronic wounds. Aesthet Surg J 2012;32:504–19.
15. Hanson SE, Bentz ML, Hematti P. Mesenchymal stem cell therapy for non-healing cutaneous wounds. Plast Reconstr Surg 2010;125:510–6.
16. Badiavas EV, Falanga V. Treatment of chronic wounds with bone marrow-derived cells. Arch Dermatol 2003;139:510–6.
17. Badiavas EV, Ford D, Liu P, et al. Long-term bone marrow culture and its clinical potential in chronic wound healing. Wound Repair Regen 2007;15: 856–65.
18. Ichioka S, Kouraba S, Sekiya N, et al. Bone marrow-impregnated collagen matrix for wound healing: experimental evaluation in a microcirculatory model of angiogenesis, and clinical experience. Br J Plast Surg 2005;58:1124–30.
19. Yoshikawa T, Mitsuno H, Nonaka I, et al. Wound therapy by marrow mesenchymal cell transplantation. Plast Reconstr Surg 2008;121:860–77.
20. Rigotti G, Marchi A, Galie M, et al. Clinical treatment of radiotherapy tissue damage by lipoaspirate transplant: a healing process mediated by adipose-derived adult stem cells. Plast Reconstr Surg 2007; 119:1409–22.
21. Knighton DR, Fiegel VD, Doucette M, et al. The use of topically applied platelet growth factors in chronic non-healing wounds; a review. Wounds 1989;1:71–8.
22. Margolis DJ, Kantor J, Santanna J, et al. Effectiveness of platelet releasate for the treatment of diabetic neuropathic foot ulcers. Diabetes Care 2001; 24:483–8.
23. Li W, Enomoto M, Ukegawa M, et al. Subcutaneous injections of platelet-rich plasma into skin flaps modulate proangiogenic gene expression and improve survival rates. Plast Reconstr Surg 2012;129:858–66.
24. O'Connell SM, Impeduglia T, Hessler K, et al. Autologous platelet-rich fibrin matrix as cell therapy in the healing of chronic lower extremity ulcers. Wound Repair Regen 2008;16:749–56.
25. Sclafani AP. Platelet-rich fibrin matrix for improvement of deep nasolabial folds. J Cosmet Dermatol 2010;9:66–71.
26. Sclafani AP, McCormick SA. Induction of dermal collagenesis, angiogenesis, and adipogenesis in human skin by injection of platelet-rich fibrin matrix. Arch Facial Plast Surg 2012;14:132–6.
27. Sclafani AP. Applications of platelet-rich fibrin matrix in facial plastic surgery. Facial Plast Surg 2009;25: 270–6.
28. Sclafani AP, Saman M. Platelet-rich fibrin matrix for facial plastic surgery. Facial Plast Surg Clin North Am 2012;20:177–86.
29. Por YC, Yeow VK, Louri N, et al. Platelet-rich plasma has no effect on increasing free fat graft survival in the nude mouse. J Plast Reconstr Aesthet Surg 2009;62:1030–4.
30. Nakamura S, Ishihara M, Takikawa M, et al. Platelet-rich plasma (PRP) promotes survival of fat-grafts in rats. Ann Plast Surg 2010;65:101–6.

Approaching Delayed-Healing Wounds on the Face and Neck

Jeffrey J. Houlton, MD[a], David B. Hom, MD[b,*]

KEYWORDS

• Wound healing • Skin • Wound-bed preparation • Dermal • Delayed healing • Growth factor • Hyperbaric oxygen • Platelet-rich plasma

KEY POINTS

- Excellent dermal blood supply to the head and neck allow for these wounds to heal more rapidly and with fewer complications compared to wounds in other areas of the body.
- When poor healing does occur in this area, common causes are from previous irradiation, smoking, ischemia, chronic steroid use, or diabetes.
- The goal of wound treatment is to identify and remove the barriers that keep it in the delayed healing state so that the wound is able to transform into an acute healing state.
- Wounds that exhibit signs of persistent inflammation lasting more than 7 days signifies a prolonged inflammatory phase, constituting a sign of wound complication.

INTRODUCTION

Dermal wounds of the face and neck are known to heal more rapidly and with fewer complications in comparison with wounds in other areas of the body. This fact is generally attributed to the excellent blood supply and increased dermal perfusion to the head and neck. Nevertheless, when poorly healing wounds do occur they can be extremely debilitating, both functionally and cosmetically. Poorly healing wounds can lead to facial dysfunction, social stigma, dysphagia, loss of oral competence, and, at times, life-threatening exposure of major blood vessels (carotid artery). When poor healing does occur, it generally results from an underlying impediment to healing (ie, irradiation, smoking, ischemia, chronic steroid use, diabetes). Because of the impact these wounds have on patients, it is imperative that facial surgeons possess a framework for their treatment. This knowledge must be based on the basic tenets of maintaining adequate blood supply, infection control, and wound debridement. In addition, surgeons must be able to identify the local and systemic factors that contribute to poor healing, intervene on the variables that can be altered, and be familiar with the adjuvant techniques for treating recalcitrant wounds.

This review provides a general approach to assess and treat delayed and poor skin-wound healing to the face and neck. The factors that contribute to poor healing are identified, the circumstances of the particularly challenging irradiated dermal wounds are described, and recent

This paper was supported by a research grant by the Cincinnati Children's Hospital Medical Center.

[a] Department of Otolaryngology - Head & Neck Surgery, University of Cincinnati College of Medicine, P.O. Box 670528, 231 Albert Sabin Way, Cincinnati, OH 45267-0528, USA; [b] Division of Facial Plastic & Reconstructive Surgery, Department of Otolaryngology – Head & Neck Surgery, Cincinnati Children's Hospital Medical Center, University of Cincinnati College of Medicine, P.O. Box 670528, 231 Albert Sabin Way, Cincinnati, OH 45267-0528, USA

* Corresponding author.

E-mail address: david.hom@uc.edu

Facial Plast Surg Clin N Am 21 (2013) 81–93
http://dx.doi.org/10.1016/j.fsc.2012.11.003

modalities to treat refractory skin wounds are presented.

PHASES OF NORMAL SKIN HEALING: A BRIEF SYNOPSIS

Acute healing involves a highly complex biological cascade that requires coordination of a variety of cytokines, growth factors, structural elements, and cell types (**Fig. 1**).[1] This process is simplified by dividing acute healing into 4 phases: coagulative phase, inflammatory phase, proliferative phase, and remodeling phase. These phases need to occur in a well-ordered sequence. If any delay in these healing phases occurs the entire healing process will be prolonged, thus increasing the risk of developing a chronic wound. The goal of treatment of a chronic wound is to actively identify and remove the barriers that keep it in the chronic healing state. By removing the impediments of healing, the wound will be able to reengage into the acute healing phases, thus transforming the wound into an acute healing state.[2] The overall phases of normal healing are briefly described here.

Coagulative Phase (Minutes)

The first phase of wound healing begins with a hemostatic cascade that is initiated within seconds of injury.[3] Thrombocytes are activated by exposed collagen, and activated platelets adhere to the collagen. The extrinsic clotting cascade is activated, and a fibrin-platelet matrix is formed. This matrix not only provides clot formation but also acts as a scaffold, which concentrates growth factors.[4] Platelets, mast cells, and fibrin-split products release factors that incite inflammation and edema.

Inflammatory Phase (2–5 Days)

As a result of platelet degranulation and cytokine cascade, capillaries vasodilate and become

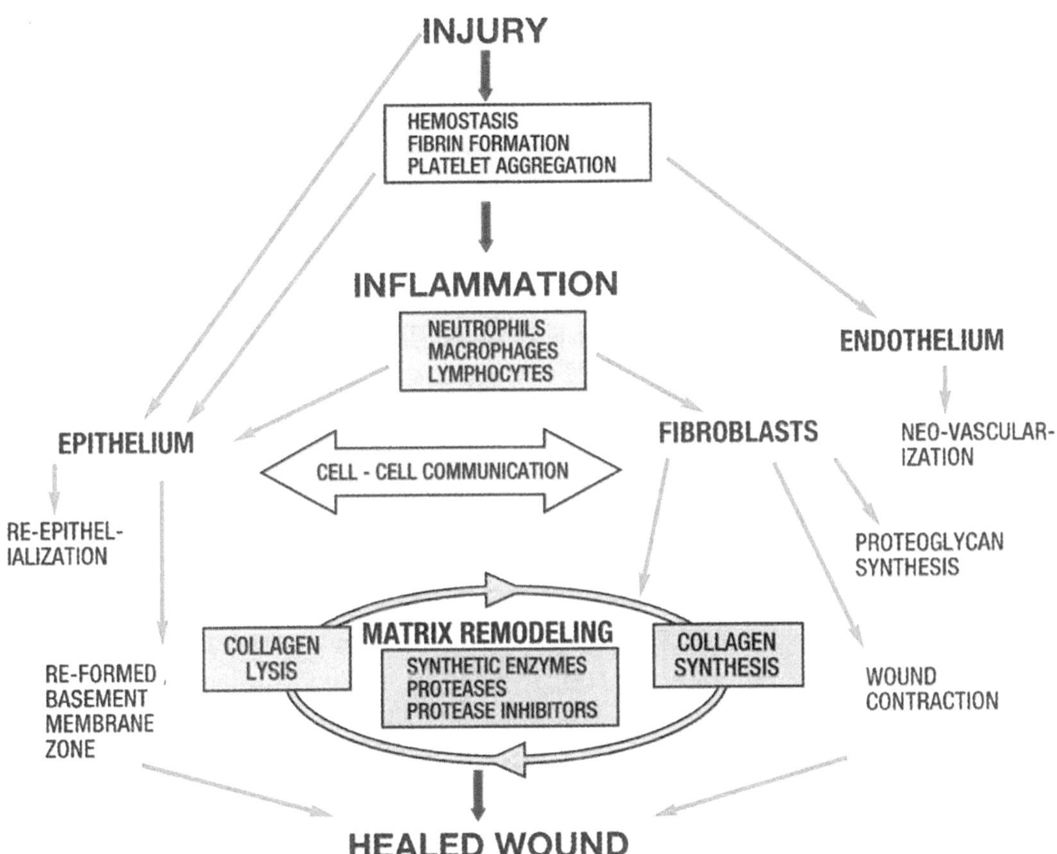

Fig. 1. Normal wound healing of skin consists of a complex and coordinated response involving multiple cellular and matrix tissue components. (*Adapted from* Hunt TK, Knighton DR, Thakral KK, et al. Cellular control of repair. In: Hunt TK, Heppenstall RB, Pines E, et al, editors. Soft and hard tissue repair: biological and clinical aspects. New York: Praeger; 1984. p. 3–19; and *From* Hebda PA. Wound healing of the skin. In: Hom DB, Hebda PA, Gosain A, et al, editors. Essential tissue healing of the face and neck. Shelton, CT: BC Decker and PMPH; 2009; with permission.)

permeable, which results in induration and hyperemia. Circulating neutrophils are recruited by chemokines to the wound to phagocytose bacteria and other foreign-body material. Similarly, circulating monocytes appear at approximately day 3, as a result of chemokines, and transform into macrophages. Macrophages are critical in amplifying, coordinating, and sustaining the healing response, releasing numerous growth factors, cytokines, and chemokines.[5] The wound remains in the inflammatory phase as long as bacterial burden or other inflammatory nidus is present. Data suggest that the amount of inflammation that occurs during the inflammatory phase is directly proportional to the amount of scarring that will ultimately result.[6]

Proliferative Phase (3–14 Days)

Neovascularization, angiogenesis, and reepithelialization occur in the proliferative phase.[7] Fibroblasts deposit disorganized type III collagen during the formation of granulation tissue. This granulating tissue replaces the fibrin-platelet matrix as the second provisional matrix for wound healing. After adequate wound-bed granulation tissue has emerged, reepithelialization initiated by keratinocytes occurs from the wound edge and adnexal structures (hair follicles, sebaceous glands, sweat glands). Myofibroblasts contract the wound.[8]

Remodeling Phase (3 Weeks to 1 Year)

Fibroblasts and collagen matrix represent the third scaffold for dermal repair. This extracellular matrix matures as fibroblast and capillary density decreases. Extracellular matrices remodel as a result of regulated proteases, and become more similar to normal skin. The wound continues to mature and contract for up to 1 year. Type III collagen is remodeled and replaced by the stronger and more organized type I collagen.[8] Wound strength plateaus at 80% of its original strength 3 months following injury.[9]

APPROACHING DELAYED-HEALING WOUNDS

The initial step in approaching wounds with delayed healing is to recognize the parameters contributing to its poorly healing state. The microenvironment of a normal acutely healing wound differs from a chronic poorly healing wound, as depicted in **Fig. 2.** Armed with knowledge of the phases of acute healing, one should recognize that wounds that exhibit signs of persistent inflammation (redness, swelling, warmth, pain) for more than 7 days are prolonging the inflammatory phase. Prolonged inflammation is a frequent first sign of wound complications. In addition, during the proliferative phase, epithelialization should occur within 2 to 3 weeks. If epithelialization does not occur within this time span, wound healing is delayed. This clinical relevance is especially applicable to monitoring postprocedure partial-thickness wounds that have been subjected to dermabrasion, laser resurfacing, and chemical peels. In addition, the wound should be monitored closely in the postoperative period for evidence of dehiscence, malodor, necrosis, and increased exudate, as these signs also herald poor healing.

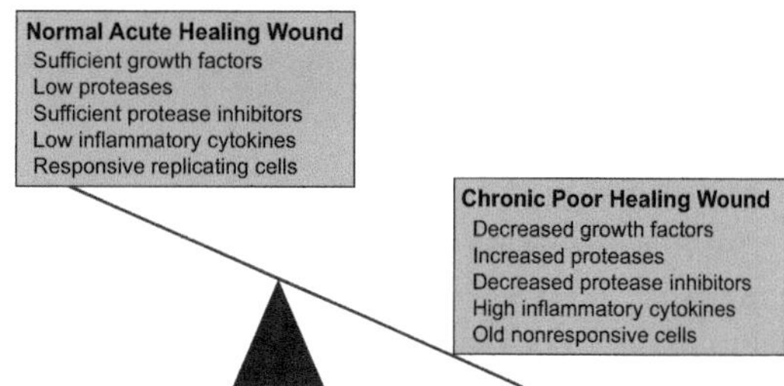

Fig. 2. Balanced comparisons of microenvironment between a normal acute wound and a chronic poorly healing wound. (*Adapted from* Mast B, Schultz G. Interactions of cytokines, growth factors and proteases in acute and chronic wounds. Wound Rep Reg 1996;4:411–20; and *From* Hom DB, Dresser H. General approach to a poor healing wound—a practical overview. In: Hom DB, Hebda PA, Gosain A, et al, editors. Essential tissue healing of the face and neck. Shelton, CT: BC Decker and PMPH; 2009; with permission.)

After a poorly healing wound is recognized, it is important to thoughtfully consider and identify all factors that are contributing to its delay. These factors include systemic comorbidities that affect the wound environment as well as local tissue factors, explained here in more detail.

Systemic Factors

The most frequent systemic factors that affect wound healing include conditions that impair tissue oxygenation such as cigarette smoking, anemia, chronic obstructive pulmonary disease, congestive heart failure, and vascular disease. Furthermore, common factors that impair the wound-healing cascade are chronic steroid use, hypothyroidism, malnutrition, and renal failure. A more complete list of these systemic factors is displayed in **Table 1**. It is important to evaluate for these systemic comorbidities when treating a delayed-healing wound or, more importantly, before initial surgical intervention. A history and physical examination identifies most comorbid conditions. In addition,

Table 1
Systemic factors that contribute to poor healing

Diabetes mellitus
Cigarette smoking
Anemia
Congestive heart failure
Vascular disease
Chronic obstructive pulmonary disease
Renal failure
Immune deficiency
Alcoholism
Prolonged steroid use
Hypothyroidism
Malnutrition
Malignancy
Medications

the authors recommend a laboratory workup during treatment of a chronic wound to identify any unrecognized conditions. Workup includes a complete blood count, renal panel, serum glucose, hemoglobin A1c (HbA1c), nutritional panel (albumin, prealbumin, transferrin), and thyroid-stimulating hormone (particularly for irradiated patients). A rheumatologic workup (erythrocyte sedimentation rate, rheumatoid factor, antinuclear antibodies) and testing for human immunodeficiency virus may be ordered if an immune disorder is suspected.

Collaboration with a primary medical physician is highly desirable when treating a poorly healing wound, as every effort should be made to optimize comorbid conditions. In the authors' experience diabetes, hypothyroidism, chronic steroid use, and malnutrition seem to be the most commonly modifiable comorbidities that impair healing. Diabetes causes vascular and neurologic impairment, which affects tissue perfusion. In addition, glycosylation impairs inflammatory and cellular processes in the healing cascade.[10] Data suggest that diabetic patients with higher levels of HbA1c are more prone to wound complications than those with more controlled blood-sugar levels.[11] This risk increases proportionally with each percentage point that HbA1c rises above the abnormal range (HbA1c >6.5%).[12] Hypothyroidism impairs wound healing by inhibiting anabolic processes and reducing collagen metabolism.[13] Chronic corticosteroid users are prone to poor healing as a result of impairment of the inflammatory phase of healing, angiogenesis, and collagen deposition.[14] In addition to corticosteroids, a variety of other medications can impair healing and may be modifiable, as displayed in **Table 2**.

Malnutrition

It has long been accepted that malnourishment leads to delayed skin healing. Like other wound impairments, recognition of malnutrition is the most important initial step in treatment. A thorough history and physical examination is accurate in predicting malnutrition 80% to 90% of the time.[15] If the patient has muscle wasting, cachexia, a history of significant weight loss (>20% signifies severe malnutrition), or gastrointestinal malabsorption (such as history of Crohn disease or gastric bypass), malnourishment is likely.[16] In addition to the history and physical examination, a laboratory workup can be used to evaluate signs of malnutrition such as low serum albumin (<3.0 mg/dL), prealbumin (<15 mg/dL), and transferrin (<200 mg/dL). Albumin has a half-life of 20 days and reflects long-term protein stores. Prealbumin has a shorter half-life of 3 days and can reflect response to treatment.

The best specific nutrient supplementation to address poorly healing wounds has not been universally agreed on. Protein malnutrition is the most recognized form of malnourishment. However, protein depletion rarely occurs as an isolated deficiency and most typically occurs in a globally malnourished state whereby multiple nutrients are diminished. Lipids, amino acids arginine and glutamine, vitamins A and C, and the trace element zinc all may play an important role in wound impairment.[16]

All patients at risk for malnutrition should be treated with protein/multinutrient supplementation as early as possible before surgery. If it is predicted that a patient will not be able to eat for at

Table 2
Medications that impair healing

Steroids
Chemotherapeutic agents
Aspirin
Penicillamine
Cyclosporin
Colchicine
Phenylbutazone
Nicotine
Other antirheumatic drugs
Other vasoconstricting drugs

least 2 weeks, enteral nutrition should be initiated. If enteral feeds cannot be initiated or tolerated, parenteral nutrition should be strongly considered. However, parenteral nutrition does carry an increased risk of sepsis, pneumonia, and other infections.[17] The goals of supplementation are to avoid weight loss, alleviate vitamin and amino acid deficiency, and to maintain a positive nitrogen balance.

Local Tissue Factors

Whereas medical personnel are a helpful adjunct in treating systemic healing impairments, the surgeon should be an expert in clinically optimizing the healing environment of local tissue. Local tissue factors that impair healing include ischemia, venous congestion, wound dehiscence, infection, excessive exudate, desiccation, foreign bodies, irradiated tissue, and necrosis/eschar, as displayed in **Table 3**. Treatment begins by assessing the physical characteristics of the wound.

- What are the wound dimensions and depth?
- Are any underlying vascular structures exposed?
- What is the moisture balance of the wound?
- Is there excessive exudate or is the wound desiccated?
- Are there significant necrotic tissues that require debriding?
- Are the wound edges healthy and epithelializing?
- Are there increased inflammatory changes?
- Is purulence present to suggest infection?

Taking into account these clinical findings, the wound is classified as healing, delayed healing, or in a chronic poorly healing state. The impediments to the healing are identified and the impairments systematically treated. In the setting of infection, a wound culture is mandatory. However, in the setting of bacterial colonization a wound culture is not as relevant, because a colonized wound does not have bacterial invasion into viable tissue. A tissue biopsy is important to rule out malignancy in a chronically nonhealing ulcer, bleeding scar, or an otherwise suspicious persistent wound.

Table 3 Local factors contributing to poor healing
Tissue ischemia
Venous insufficiency
Foreign body
Necrotic tissue
Dehiscence
Shearing forces
Infection
Excessive exudates

Crucial is the institution of the key tenets of local wound care: proper wound debridement, controlling infection, and maintaining adequate blood supply. These concepts culminated in a systematic approach for wound-bed preparation developed by the Wound Consensus Panel in 2003.[2] Wound-bed preparation represents the concept that a poorly healing wound must be adequately prepared to "jump-start" it back into the acutely healing phases. This goal is achieved by methodically identifying the barriers that delay its healing to promote its endogenous healing. The tenets of wound-bed preparation are depicted in **Table 4** and are represented by the acronym TIME[2]:

Tissue
Infection/Inflammation
Moisture imbalance
Edge

In summarizing this very informative table, wound-bed preparation is divided into 4 steps[18]:

1. Proper debridement of the wound
2. Controlling infection/inflammation
3. Maintaining a properly moist environment while avoiding excessive exudates
4. Evaluating wound edges for proper reepithelialization

Debridement

Effective debridement is the essential first step for wound-bed preparation. Necrotic tissue prolongs inflammation, presents a nidus for infection, inhibits epithelialization, and impairs phagocytosis. Therefore, necrotic tissue and eschar should be removed from the chronic wound before it can be transformed to an acute healing state and before reconstructive coverage is performed. A variety of debridement methods can achieve this goal, including surgical debridement, mechanical debridement, autolytic debridement, and enzymatic debridement.

The ideal form of debridement would remove all necrotic tissue from the wound while avoiding damage to delicate healing tissue. However, these two goals are generally at odds with one another. Specifically, the methods that debride most aggressively also cause the most damage to underlying tissue, a tradeoff that generally guides decisions on which debridement method to

Table 4
Wound-bed preparation (WBP) using the TIME principle

TIME Acronym	Clinical Observations	Proposed Pathophysiology	WBP Clinical Actions	Effect of WBP Actions	Clinical Outcomes
T	Tissue nonviable or deficient	Defective matrix and cell debris impair healing	Debridement (episodic or continuous) Autolytic, sharp surgical, enzymatic, mechanical, or biological Biological agents	Restoration of wound base and functional extracellular matrix proteins	Viable wound base
I	Infection or inflammation	High bacterial counts or prolonged inflammation ↑ Inflammatory cytokines ↑ Protease activity ↓ Growth factor activity	Remove infected foci topical/systemic Antimicrobials Anti-inflammatories Protease inhibition	Low bacterial counts or controlled inflammation: ↓ Inflammatory cytokines ↓ Protease activity ↑ Growth factor activity	Bacterial balance and reduced inflammation
M	Moisture imbalance	Desiccation slows epithelial cell migration. Excessive fluid causes maceration of wound margin	Apply moisture-balancing dressings, compression, negative pressure, or other methods of removing fluid or surgical skin coverage	Restored epithelial cell migration, desiccation avoided, edema and excessive fluid controlled, maceration avoided	Moisture balance
E	Edge of wound, nonadvancing or undermined	Nonmigrating keratinocytes, nonresponsive wound cells, and abnormalities in extracellular matrix, or abnormal protease activity	Reassess cause or consider corrective therapies Debridement Skin grafts, skin flaps Biological agents Adjunctive therapies	Migrating keratinocytes and responsive wound cells. Restoration of appropriate protease profile	Advancing edge of wound

From Schultz GS, Sibbald RG, Falanga B, et al. Wound bed preparation: a systematic approach to wound management. Wound Repair Regen 2003;11:S1–28; with permission.

choose. Frequently more than one method of debridement is used. Typically a wound will require an initial aggressive method of debridement followed by a gentler method for maintenance. A general description of the types of debridement is given here.

Surgical debridement describes a method of removing necrotic debris with sharp surgical excision, generally with cold instruments. This type of debridement can be performed at the bedside or in the operating room. It is generally appropriate for the removal of a large burden of necrotic tissue or when infection is severe and needs to be controlled in an expeditious fashion (necrotizing fasciitis). This form of debridement is the most effective, but results in the most underlying tissue damage.

Mechanical debridement describes the removal of debris by physical force. The most common form of mechanical debridement is wet-to-dry dressings. This method is fairly effective, but still results in a moderate amount of tissue damage. Wet-to-wet dressing changes are also effective and may be slightly gentler to the healing wound. Wound cleansing is a key component to wet-dressing treatments, and is generally achieved with normal saline or antibiotic irrigations. Wound cleansers should be differentiated from skin cleansers (ie, povidone-iodine, sodium hypochlorite, hydrogen peroxide, acetic acid), which can be cytotoxic with repetitive use in a wound.[19,20] A general dictum in choosing the best wound-irrigation fluid to use is "you should not put in a chronic wound what you would not put in the eye," thus avoiding damage to healing tissues with repetitive irrigation fluid over time. However, the harsher preparations may be appropriate in the setting of actively infected wounds.

Autolytic debridement takes advantage of the body's naturally occurring proteolytic enzymes to break down and liquefy necrotic debris. This goal is achieved by placing an occlusive or semiocclusive dressing over the wound for 2 to 3 days while enzymatic processes ensue. Autolytic debridement is the gentlest to underlying tissues but debrides fairly slowly. It is not appropriate for highly exudative, infected, or deep wounds. Hydrogels can be used in combination with occlusive dressings to soften the wound and expedite debridement.

Enzymatic debridement takes advantage of exogenous topically applied enzymes to digest and break down debris. The 2 most common preparations are papain-urea cream and collagenase ointment. Collagenase debrides more slowly than papain-urea preparations, but is more selective in avoiding underlying tissue.[21] This form of debridement is slightly harsher than autolytic debridement, but is generally faster.

Infection

Active bacterial infection leads to prolonged inflammation, delayed healing, increased exudative drainage, and ultimately increased fibrosis and scar formation.[22] Wound infection should be recognized as prolonging the inflammatory phase of healing (redness, warmth, and induration >5–7 days from injury). When a wound infection is recognized, it should be treated immediately and aggressively.

The wound is opened to allow an oxygenated environment to impair obligate anaerobic bacterial growth, obtain wound cultures, and effectively remove necrotic debris. The mainstay of therapy is local treatment with aggressive debridement to decrease exudate. Topical antibiotics or skin-cleansing solutions can be used with dressing changes, as infection control takes precedence over tissue preservation. When necessary, the patient should be started empirically on antibiotics, which should eventually be tailored to culture results. As the infection resolves, gentler maintenance debridement methods should be instituted.

The optimal treatment for surgical site infection is avoidance, which is achieved through meticulous sterility, avoiding wound tension, maintaining adequate tissue perfusion, and using the appropriate prophylactic antibiotics.

Antibiotic prophylaxis has been shown to reduce wound infection by 44% in clean-contaminated cases.[23] Prophylaxis should be administered just before incision (no more than 1 hour) to reduce bacterial burden at the surgical site. No evidence suggests that the use of antibiotics for greater than 24 hours reduces surgical-site infections in clean-contaminated cases.[24] Conversely, the overuse of antibiotics may lead to unnecessary pharmacologic complications. Clean cases in the head and neck have an extremely low rate of infection, therefore prophylaxis is not necessary.[25]

Moisture balance

Data originating in the 1960s suggest that keeping a moist wound bed doubles the speed of epithelialization.[26] Likewise, dry wounds and desiccation should be avoided, as epithelial migration is impaired by dry devitalized tissue. Moisture-retentive ointments and dressings (ie, hydrogels) can be helpful in maintaining this moist environment. Alternatively, excessive fluid in the wound should be removed with absorbent dressings (ie, calcium alginate) to avoid maceration, which also impairs wound healing.[27]

A GENERALIZED APPROACH TO THE POORLY HEALING WOUND

1. Determine if surgical debridement and skin coverage is needed; this is especially important when structures (joints, nerves, carotid artery) are exposed or if aggressive surgical excision is needed (necrotizing fasciitis). Ideally tissue coverage should be delayed until the wound is cleared of infection.
2. Identify the systemic factors that are contributing to poor healing and consult with a multidisciplinary team as needed (internist, nutritionist, wound-care nurse).
3. Perform initial debridement. Surgical debridement may be needed if the necrotic burden is high.

4. Control the Infection. Open and lightly pack the wound. Tailor antibiotic treatment to wound cultures.
5. Divert salivary flow if present and loosely pack dead spaces.
6. Maintain moisture balance by using hydrogel ointments to prevent desiccation or absorbent dressings to avoid maceration. A moist environment will assist in formation of granulation tissue.
7. Ensure fresh wound edges to further promote reepithelialization.
8. Determine a reconstructive plan. Allow the wound to heal by secondary intention, rearrangement of local tissue, skin grafting, or transfer of free tissue.
9. Reassess the wound-healing state at 2 to 4 weeks and adjust wound treatments accordingly. Consider other adjuvant therapies if continued poor healing exists. A delayed-healing wound should begin to show signs of healing within 2 to 4 weeks. If healing does not occur by this time, the patient must be reevaluated and a new treatment approach instituted.

Using these wound-healing principles in patients who are at high risk for poor healing early on during the treatment course will optimize surgical repair (**Fig. 3**).

THE IRRADIATED WOUND

Radiation therapy is commonly used to treat patients with head and neck cancer. In soft tissue, delayed wound healing often results after surgery, with an increased incidence of wound complications, which can manifest as poorly healing ulceration, wound infection, tissue ischemia, or salivary fistula. Up to 60% of previously irradiated patients who have surgery following irradiation suffer a wound complication (**Fig. 4**).[28] This scenario is most evident when reviewing the laryngectomy literature, in which there is a 33% to 66% increase in wound complications when surgical intervention is preceded by irradiation.[29,30] These complications include fistula formation, skin atrophy, soft-tissue fibrosis, desquamation, and epithelial ulceration.[28–30] In addition to the increased risk for poor healing, open wounds can result in life-threatening exposure of the carotid artery requiring reconstructive coverage.[31,32]

Radiation damage to skin can be classified as either early or late injury. Early radiation injury can occur in as little as 2 weeks after the initiation of radiotherapy. Early injury is the result of DNA damage to rapidly dividing skin cells undergoing mitoses. Stem cells divide to replace the damaged skin. If these stem cells are injured an acute injury occurs, resulting in ulceration and necrosis. Similar to burn injuries, acute skin toxicity is graded in various degrees of severity, as listed in **Table 5**. The minimum tolerance dose (the dose that will result in ulceration for 5% of patients) for skin is 55 Gy and the maximum tolerance dose (the dose that will result in symptoms for 50% of patients) is 70 Gy.[33] This risk of injury increases in patients with anemia, smoking, vascular disease, diabetes, or malnutrition.[34]

Radiation disrupts wound healing by causing obliterative endarteritis, excessive fibrosis, and aberrant cellular replication.[35] Current understanding infers that the healing pathophysiology of irradiated tissue may be related to the microenvironment and its interaction with its cells.

In the early phases of healing, the cytokines, transforming growth factor β (TGF-β), vascular endothelial growth factor (VEGF), tumor necrosis factor α, interferon-γ, and proinflammatory cytokines such as interleukin-1 and interleukin-8 are overexpressed after the radiation injury, leading to uncontrolled matrix accumulation and fibrosis.[35] During the proliferative phase of healing, the major cytokines are TGF-β, VEGF, epidermal growth factor, fibroblast growth factor (FGF), and platelet-derived growth factor (PDGF).[35] In normal wounds, nitric oxide (NO) promotes wound healing by inducing collagen deposition.[36] In irradiated wounds of experimental animals, NO levels are reduced.[37]

During the remodeling phase, matrix metalloproteinases (MMPs) and their tissue inhibitors play a key role.[38,39] MMP-1 has been found to be decreased after radiation therapy.[39] These enzymes regulate extracellular matrix synthesis.[40,41] TGF-β may play an important detrimental role in causing fibrosis in irradiated tissue.

Late radiation injury can occur months to years following treatment. Such injury is due to radiation damage to vascular and connective tissues, and results in permanently impaired tissue ischemia and progressive fibrosis. The key mechanism of injury is damage to the microvascular endothelium.[34]

The management of irradiated wounds follows principles similar to those for generalized wound care. Early ulceration should be cleansed to avoid infection, and ointment should be applied to protect the skin and promote epithelialization. Wound desiccation should be avoided. If wet desquamation or deep ulceration develops, cessation of radiotherapy is probably necessary, and the wound should be treated with wet-to-wet dressings.

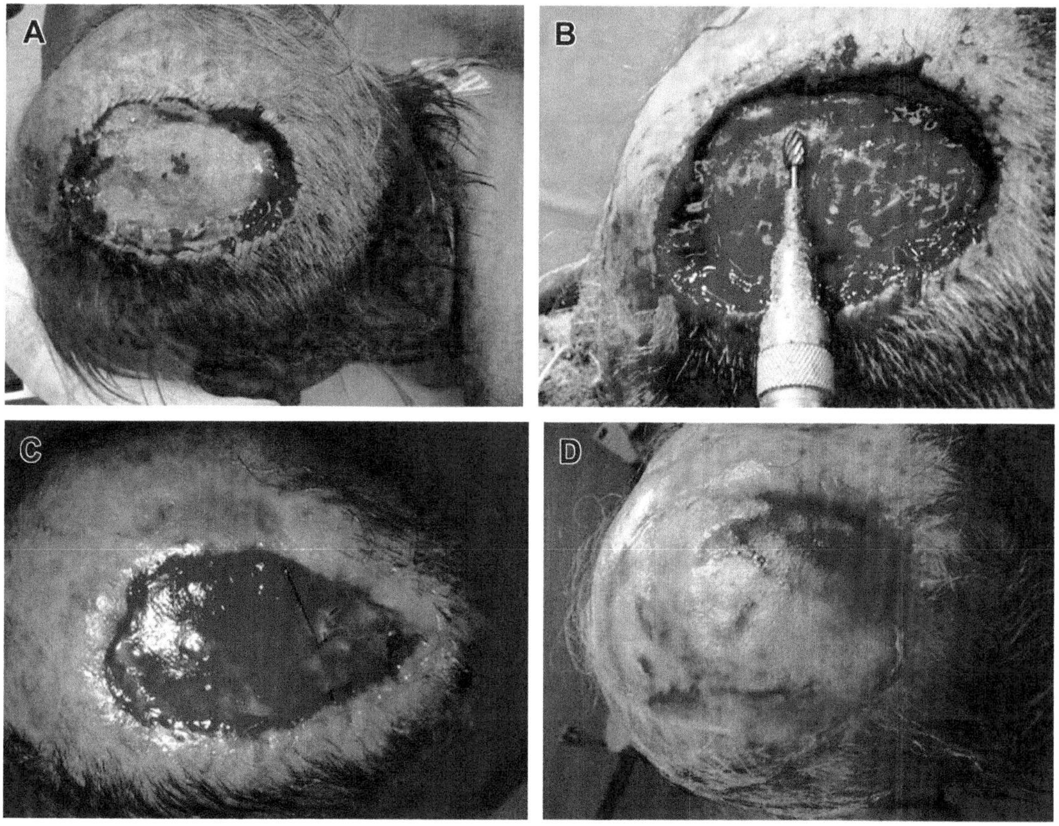

Fig. 3. (*A*) A 75-year-old man with a history of type 1 diabetes, on methotrexate for severe rheumatoid arthritis with previous multiple recurrent basal cell carcinomas excised, resulting in a severely scarred scalp. The patient required extensive Moh micrographic surgery, resulting in a full-thickness scalp wound down to bare bone without periosteum. (*B*) Because of the patient's medical condition and request, he was not amenable for free-flap coverage. To induce formation of granulation tissue on this bare bone, the outer table of the calvarial bone was burred down to the diploic layer to jump-start the wound. (*C*) Formation of granulation tissue after 2 months with moisture-retentive dressings to allow for future split-thickness coverage. (*D*) The new granulation tissue bed was covered with a skin graft. The defect is shown 1 year following the graft.

Once skin has been irradiated it will never behave normally. It will always remain fibrotic and ischemic to some degree. This consideration is important when surgical procedures are planned (local skin flaps) within the previous radiation field. A very conservative approach to maximize blood supply to tissue should be used when operating in the irradiated field. Patients should be

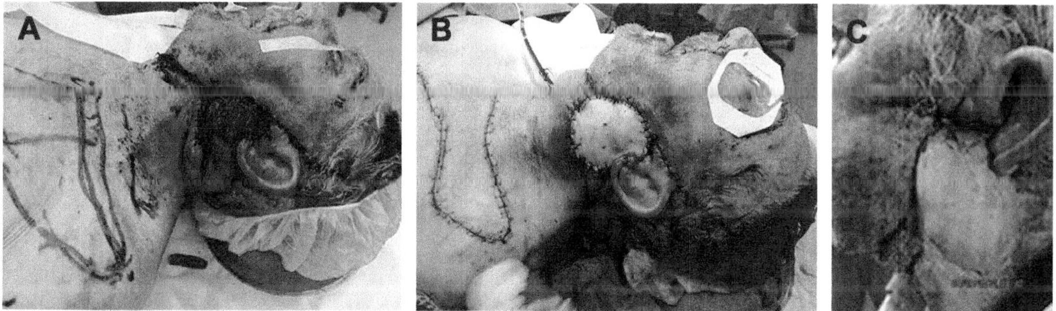

Fig. 4. (*A*) An 81-year-old man with a prior 2-year history of previous irradiation to the face requiring surgical excision of preauricular skin and a radical parotidectomy. For coverage, a posterior auricular skin flap was attempted, which became ischemic, resulting in skin-flap necrosis. (*B, C*) Debridement of the soft tissue was required, followed by coverage with a more robust vascular pectoralis major myocutaneous paddle flap.

Table 5
Types of radiation toxicity to skin

Symptom/Sign	Degree 1	Degree 2	Degree 3	Degree 4
Erythema	Minimal, transient	Moderate	Marked	Severe
		<10% body surfacc area (BSA)	10% 40% BSA	>40% BSΛ
Sensation/itching	Pruritus	Slight intermittent plain	Moderate persistent pain	Severe persistent pain
Blistering	Rare	Rare	Bullae	Bullae
		Hemorrhage		Hemorrhage
Desquamation	Absent	Patchy, dry	Patchy, moist	Confluent, moist
Ulcer/necrosis	Epidermal only	Dermal	Subcutaneous	Muscle or bone
Onycholysis	Absent	Partial	Partial	Complete

Data from Waselenko JK, MacVittie TJ, Blakely WF, et al. Medical management of the acute radiation syndrome: recommendations of the Strategic National Stockpile Radiation Working Group. Ann Intern Med 2004;140:1039.

counseled about the increased risks of wound complications. Thyroid function should be assessed, as hypothyroidism is a common complication of irradiation, which itself impairs wound healing. A chronic nonhealing wound in an irradiated patient should be biopsied to rule out neoplastic recurrence.

REFRACTORY WOUNDS

Data have shown that if a chronic wound heals by 20% or more over a 2- to 4-week period, it will likely continue to improve (**Fig. 5**).[2] However, if the wound fails to respond over this time frame, nonhealing will likely continue. In this scenario, a complete reassessment of the wound and its treatment are warranted by 2 weeks. Local and systemic factors should be evaluated, which should include a laboratory workup. A biopsy should be obtained to rule out neoplasia. A multidisciplinary team should be assembled and should include the surgeon, a medical physician, a wound-care specialist, the nursing team, and a nutritionist. A speech pathologist may be helpful when swallowing or nutrition is impaired.[42]

Questions to be addressed by the team should include:

- Is the diagnosis of the wound-healing barriers correct?
- Are there any contributing local or systemic factors that are unrecognized?
- Is wound care being carried out as prescribed?

POSSIBLE ADJUVANT THERAPIES FOR CHRONIC WOUNDS

Vacuum-Assisted Closure Devices

Vacuum-assisted closure devices (VAC) have gained popularity in the treatment of chronic

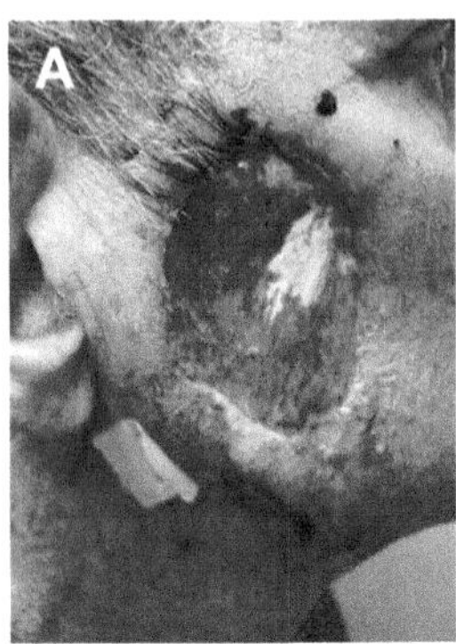

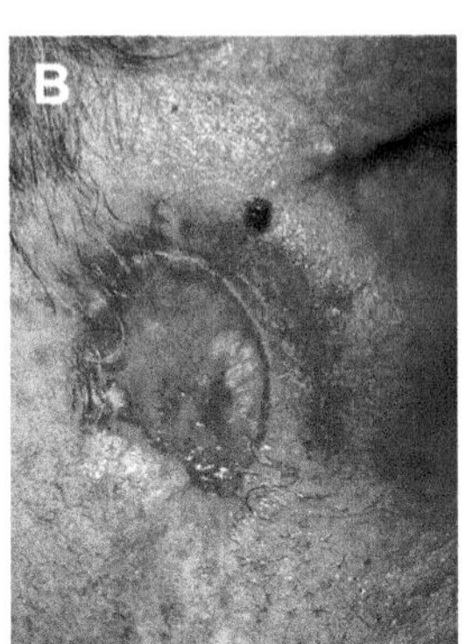

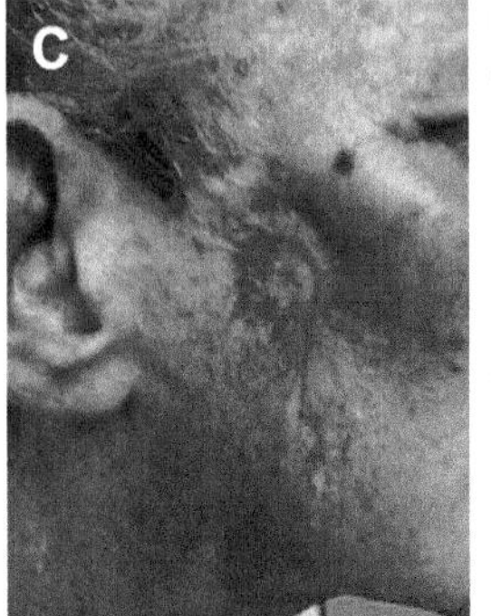

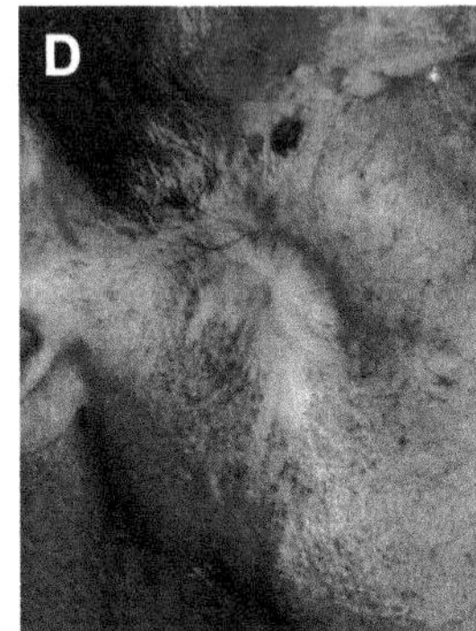

Fig. 5. (*A*) An 85-year-old man with a history of diabetes, severe coronary disease and on Coumadin, with an open wound after surgical resection of skin and radical parotidectomy. Coronoid bone is exposed. Because of his multiple medical comorbidities, the patient chose to let the wound heal by secondary intention with moisture-retentive dressings, using the wound-healing principles described. (*B*) Granulating wound 3 weeks later. (*C*) Reepithelialized wound 7 weeks later. (*D*) Mature wound 6 months later.

wounds over the last several decades. A VAC consists of a polyurethane sponge held in place by an adhesive dressing, kept under negative pressure with a vacuum pump. This negative pressure is thought to improve healing by inducing granulation tissue, removing excess fluid (thus maintaining moisture balance), and improving blood supply.[43]

Initially the use of the VAC in the head and neck region was limited in comparison with its use other body sites, because of its cumbersome nature of application to this area. More specifically, the challenge was the inability for the VAC to hold suction around the nose, mouth, or stoma. However, several reports using the VAC for facial wounds and the irradiated neck have shown benefits in treating refractory wounds.[44] The VAC is discussed in more detail in an article by Strub and colleagues in this issue.

Hyperbaric Oxygen

The use of hyperbaric oxygen (HBO) to treat necrotizing soft-tissue infections is controversial. It remains even more controversial in how it may influence dermal wound healing. Some studies using animal data have shown that HBO may improve the survival of flaps and grafts.[45] The principle of HBO is to subject the wound to elevated oxygen concentrations at supra-atmospheric pressures. This exposure causes vasoconstriction and increased partial pressures of oxygen in the blood. This higher oxygen gradient in tissue stimulates angiogenesis and fibroblast proliferation.[46] For bone healing, HBO is used to treat osteoradionecrosis.[47] An HBO "dive" of 2.4 atm will induce a higher partial pressure of oxygen to 800 to 1100 mm Hg in the wound.[47] However, the side effects of HBO include barotrauma and exacerbation of congestive heart failure, as well as the requirement for highly specialized equipment with increased costs. More clinical studies are needed to further establish its utility in improving dermal wound healing.

Growth Factors

The use of topical growth factors in the treatment of chronic wounds represents a different approach to wound-bed preparation. In wound-bed preparation clinicians attempt to identify and remove the impediments to healing and, by doing so, passively reinitiate the endogenous healing pathways. Instead, topical growth factor therapy aims to artificially enhance the endogenous healing phases with recombinant or autologous growth factors. Recombinant forms of multiple factors have been developed over the last 15 years (PDGF, keratinocyte growth factor, FGF, bone morphogenetic protein, TGF-β).[48] While many have shown promise, the results remain inconsistent and the indications limited.

The first growth factor to be approved by the United States Food and Drug Administration was recombinant human platelet-derived growth factor (rhPDGF).[49] It was initially approved based on its efficacy in the treatment of nonischemic, diabetic foot ulcers,[49] and was shown to be most effective in inducing the formation of granulation tissue. Since that time, rhPDGF has been reported for the treatment of a variety of off-label chronic wounds, including its use in previously irradiated wounds of the head and neck.[50]

The off-label use of growth factors has been reported to attempt to improve the healing of poorly healing wounds.[51] On the other hand, it must be remembered that adding growth factors to a wound is an adjunctive method of jump-starting a healing wound, and is not a replacement for standard wound care. The key principles of wound management still hold true (ie, minimize infection, maximize tissue oxygenation, ensure adequate nutrition, debridement, institute proper wound care) in allowing a problem wound to properly heal.

One limitation of growth factor therapy, including PDGF, is the theoretical risk of inducing a malignancy. This risk should always be discussed with the patient before use and appropriate informed consent should be obtained. This situation is particularly limiting for surgeons of the face and neck, as a significant number of chronic wounds in the head and neck region are a result of the irradiation of malignancies. A biopsy should be considered before instituting growth factor therapy to ensure that a local neoplastic process is not present.

Platelet-Rich Plasma

Various studies have reported the controversial use of concentrated platelets to increase hemostasis and possibly promote dermal healing.[52,53] Platelet-rich plasma (PRP) is a blood product processed to concentrate the patient's own platelets. Commercial devices are available to concentrate the platelets from the patient severalfold. Over a 10-year period, a systemic meta-analysis of published literature regarding PRP on cutaneous wounds was conducted.[54] The skin-wound types were classified into chronic wounds, acute secondary closure wounds, and acute primary closure wounds. From the meta-analysis the investigators concluded that in chronic wounds, PRP favored healing. For acute wounds, PRP appeared to reduce infection. The challenge in analyzing these multiple published clinical studies is that different methods and definitions were used to measure the healing parameters.

SUMMARY

Poorly healing wounds in the head and neck can lead to debilitating functional and cosmetic outcomes. The goal of treating a poorly healing wound should be to remove the barriers that impair its healing, thus transforming the wound into a state of acute healing. In addition, one must identify and address the local and systemic factors that contribute to the poor healing. Wound-bed preparation involves the principles of debridement, infection control, moisture balance, and maintaining fresh wound edges. When a wound is refractory to its initial treatment, a multidisciplinary approach is very helpful. Adjunctive measures such as vacuum-assisted closure devices, HBO, and topical growth factor therapy can be considered in the appropriate setting. However, it must be remembered that adjunctive treatments are not a replacement for standard wound care. The key principles for treating poorly healing dermal wounds (reduce infection, increase tissue oxygenation, maximize nutrition, debride the wound when necessary, institute proper wound care) are the essential components of optimizing the healing process.

REFERENCES

1. Mast B, Schultz G. Interaction of cytokines, growth factors and proteases in acute and chronic wounds. Wound Repair Regen 1996;4:411–20.
2. Schultz GS, Sibbald RG, Falang B, et al. Wound bed preparation: a systematic approach to wound management. Wound Repair Regen 2003;11:S1–28.
3. Furie B, Furie BC. Mechanisms of thrombus formation. N Engl J Med 2008;359:938–49.
4. Robson MC, Steed DL, Franz MG. Wound healing: biologic features and approaches to maximize healing trajectories. Curr Probl Surg 2001;38:72–140.
5. Eming SA, Krieg T, Davidson JM. Inflammation in wound repair: molecular and cellular mechanisms. J Invest Dermatol 2007;127:514–25.
6. Redd MJ, Cooper L, Wood W, et al. Wound healing and inflammation: embryos reveal the way to perfect repair. Philos Trans R Soc Lond B Biol Sci 2004;359:777–84.
7. Bauer SM. Angiogenesis, vasculogenesis, and induction of healing in chronic wounds. Vasc Endovascular Surg 2005;39:293–306.
8. Arnold F, West DC. Angiogenesis in wound healing. Pharmacol Ther 1991;52:407–22.
9. Levenson SM, Geever EF, Crowley LV, et al. The healing of rat skin wounds. Ann Surg 1965;161:293–308.
10. Huijberts MS, Schaper NC. Advanced glycation end products and diabetic foot disease. Diabetes Metab Res Rev 2008;24:S19–24.
11. Boulton AJ. The diabetic foot: an update. Foot Ankle Surg 2008;14:120–4.
12. Selvin E, Margolis DJ. Hemoglobin A1c predicts healing rate in diabetic wounds. J Invest Dermatol 2011;131:2121–7.
13. Ekmektzoglou KA, Zografos G. A concomitant review of the effects of diabetes mellitus and hypothyroidism in wound healing. World J Gastroenterol 2006;12(17):2721–9.
14. Cohen IK, Diegelmann RF, Johnson ML. Effect of corticosteroids on collagen synthesis. Surgery 1977;82:15–20.
15. Jeejeebhoy KN, Detsky AS, Baker JP. Assessment of nutritional status. JPEN J Parenter Enteral Nutr 1990;14:S193–6.
16. Mazzotta MY. Nutrition and wound healing. J Am Podiatr Med Assoc 1994;84:156–62.
17. Saluja SS. Enteral nutrition in surgical patients. Surg Today 2002;32:672–8.
18. Falanga V. Classification for wound bed preparation and stimulation of chronic wounds. Wound Repair Regen 2000;8:347–52.
19. Bergstrom N, Allman RM, Alvarez OM, et al. Treatment of pressure ulcers: clinical practice guideline. Rockville (MD): US Department of Health and Human Services, Public Health Service, Agency for Health Care Policy and Research; 1994.
20. Sibbald RG. Preparing the wound bed-debridement, bacterial balance, and moisture balance. Ostomy Wound Manage 2000;46:14–22.
21. Hebda PA, Lo C. Biochemistry of wound healing: the effects of active ingredients of standard debriding agents—papain and collagenase—on digestion of native and denatured collagenous substrates, fibrin, and elastin. Wounds 2007;13:190–4.
22. Robson MC, Stenberg BD, Heggers JP. Wound healing alterations caused by infection. Clin Plast Surg 1990;17:485–92.
23. Velanovich V. A meta-analysis of prophylactic antibiotics in head and neck surgery. Plast Reconstr Surg 1991;87:429–35.
24. Johnson JT, Schuller DE, Silver F, et al. Antibiotic prophylaxis in high-risk head and neck surgery; one day vs. five day therapy. Otolaryngol Head Neck Surg 1986;95:554–7.
25. Johnson JT, Wagner RL. Infection following uncontaminated head and neck surgery. Arch Otolaryngol Head Neck Surg 1987;113:368–9.
26. Winter G. Formation of the scab and the rate of epithelialization of superficial wounds in the skin of the young domestic pig. Nature 1962;193:293–4.

27. Brown CD, Zitelli JA. Choice of wound dressing and ointments. In: Hom DB, Hebda PA, Gosain AK, Friedman CD, editors. Essential tissue healing of the face and the neck. Shelton (CT): PMPH and BC Decker; 2009. p. 224–38.
28. Girod DA, McCulloch TM, Tsue TT, et al. Risk factors for complications in clean-contaminated head and neck surgical procedures. Head Neck 1995;17:7–13.
29. Habel D. Surgical complications in irradiated patients. Arch Otolaryngol 1967;82:382–6.
30. Genden EM, RInaldo A, Shaha AR, et al. Pharyngocutaneous fistula following laryngectomy. Acta Otolaryngol 2004;124:117–20.
31. Hom DB, Adams G, Koreis M, et al. Choosing the optimal wound dressing for irradiated soft tissue wounds. Otolaryngol Head Neck Surg 1999;121:591–8.
32. Lambert PM, Patel M, Gutman E, et al. Dermal grafts to bony defects in irradiated and nonirradiated tissues. Arch Otolaryngol 1984;110:657–9.
33. Coleman JJ. Management of radiation-induced soft tissue injury to the head and neck. Clin Plast Surg 1993;20:491–505.
34. Hopewell JW, Calvo W, Reinhold HS. Radiation effects on blood vessels: role in late normal tissue damage. The biological basis of radiotherapy. 2nd edition. New York: Elsevier; 1989. p. 223–4.
35. Dormand EL, Banwell PE, Goodacre TE. Radiotherapy and wound healing. Int Wound J 2005;2:112–27.
36. Shi HP, Most D, Efron DT, et al. The role of iNOS in wound healing. Surgery 2001;130:225–9.
37. Schaffer M, Weimer W, Wider S, et al. Differential expression of inflammatory mediators in radiation-impaired wound healing. J Surg Res 2002;107:93–100.
38. Illsley MC, Peacock JH, McAnulty RJ, et al. Increased collagen production in fibroblasts cultured from irradiated skin and effect of TGF beta(1)—clinical study. Br J Cancer 2000;83:650–4.
39. Gu Q, Wang D, Gao Y, et al. Expression of MMP1 in surgical and radiation-impaired wound healing and its effects on the healing process. J Environ Pathol Toxicol Oncol 2002;21:71–8.
40. Medrado AP, Soares AP, Santos ET, et al. Influence of laser photobiomodulation upon connective tissue remodeling during wound healing. J Photochem Photobiol B 2008;92:144–52.
41. Johnson LB, Jorgensen LN, Adawi D, et al. The effect of preoperative radiotherapy on systemic collagen deposition and postoperative infective complications in rectal cancer patients. Dis Colon Rectum 2005;48:1573–80.
42. Hom DH, Lee C. Irradiated skin and its postsurgical management. In: Hom DB, Hebda PA, Gosain AK, Friedman CD, editors. Essential tissue healing of the face and the neck. Shelton (CT): PMPH and BC Decker; 2009. p. 224–38.
43. Banwell PE. Topical negative pressure therapy in wound care. J Wound Care 1999;8:79–84.
44. Dhir K, Reino AJ, Lipana J. Vacuum-assisted closure therapy in the management of head and neck wounds. Laryngoscope 2009;119:54–61.
45. Friedman HI, Fitzmaurice M, Lefaivre JF, et al. An evidence-based appraisal of the use of hyper-baric oxygen on flaps and grafts. Plast Reconstr Surg 2006;117:175S–90S.
46. Tibbles PM, Edelsberg JS. Hyperbaric-oxygen therapy. N Engl J Med 1996;334:1642–8.
47. Mounsey RA, Brown DH, O'Dwyer TP, et al. Role of hyperbaric oxygen therapy in the management of mandibular osteoradionecrosis. Laryngoscope 1993;103:605–8.
48. Goldman R. Growth factors and chronic wound healing: past, present, and future. Adv Skin Wound Care 2004;17:24–35.
49. Steed D. Clinical evaluation of recombinant human platelet-derived growth factor for the treatment of lower extremity diabetic ulcers. Diabetic Ulcer Study Group. J Vasc Surg 1995;21:71–81.
50. Hom DB, Manivel JC. Promoting healing with recombinant human platelet-derived growth factor in a previously irradiated problem wound. Laryngoscope 2003;113:1566–71.
51. Hom DB. New developments in wound healing relevant to facial plastic surgery. Arch Facial Plast Surg 2008;10(6):402–6.
52. Pierce FG, Mustoe TA, Altrock BW, et al. Role of platelet-derived growth factor in wound healing. J Cell Biochem 1991;45:319–26.
53. Hom DB, Linzie BM, Huang TC. The healing effects of autologous platelet gel on acute human skin wounds. Arch Facial Plast Surg 2007;9:174–83.
54. Carter MJ, Fylling CP, Parnell LK. Use of platelet rich plasma gel on wound healing: a systematic review and meta-analysis. Eplasty 2011;11:e38.

Cutaneous Lasers

Fred G. Fedok, MD*, Frank Garritano, MD,
Antonio Portela, MD

KEYWORDS

• Laser • Cutaneous lesion • Vascular lesion • Facial resurfacing • Wrinkles • Lentigenes
• Hair removal • Scar

KEY POINTS

- The CO_2 and erbium lasers have been widely used for skin resurfacing for improvement of the aging skin. These technologies have been used to correct rhytids, dyschromias, lentigenes, elastosis, and other sign of photoaging. Recent fractionation of these laser wavelengths has resulted in more rapid healing, less downtime, and a reduced frequency of complications.
- Nonablative laser technology shows great promise and currently can produce significant improvements in fine lines and dyschromias.
- Laser therapy of hirsutism, vascular lesions, and tattoos is superior to most of the previously applied treatment modalities.
- A key to the safe and predicable use of lasers is in the selection of the optimal technology for the problem and patient being treated.

INTRODUCTION

Lasers are named for the medium that produces the wavelength of laser energy for a specific laser. The laser medium is contained within an optical cavity or resonator and may be a liquid, as in the case of a pulsed dye laser; a solid, as in the case of an erbium:yttrium-aluminum-garnet (YAG) laser; or a gas, as in the case of the carbon-dioxide (CO_2) laser. In a general design, photons from an energy source are made to move parallel to the axis of the optical cavity and are repeatedly reflected between opposing mirrors (**Fig. 1**). The summation of this repetitive interaction causes a stimulated emission to be generated.

Clinically, it is also helpful to describe the wavelengths of light at which particular lasers operate. These designations, such as "1064-nm neodymium (Nd):YAG," guide the clinician to the appropriate use and improve documentation and communication. Critical parameters of the laser emission include the wavelength, pulse characteristics, and fluence. Some lasers transmit their laser energy to the operator's handpiece by an articulated tube with mirrors, whereas other lasers transmit their energy by fiberoptic cable.

The following sections describe various lasers, along with their general physical characteristics and absorption spectra (**Table 1**).

LASERS FOR THE TREATMENT OF SKIN AGING

Ablative Resurfacing

The CO_2 10,600-nm laser

The CO_2 laser became popular for skin resurfacing in the early 1990s and has been the most widely used laser for ablative resurfacing.[1–6] In many ways, the dramatic results obtained by the full ablative CO_2 laser still represent the gold standard by which other resurfacing modalities are compared. However, its wide application has decreased because of the resulting prolonged healing time.

Disclosure: None.

Facial Plastic and Reconstructive Surgery, Otolaryngology/Head and Neck Surgery, Department of Surgery, Hershey Medical Center, The Pennsylvania State University, 500 University Drive, Hershey, PA 17033, USA
* Corresponding author.
E-mail addresses: drfredfedok@me.com; ffedok@hmc.psu.edu

Facial Plast Surg Clin N Am 21 (2013) 95–110
http://dx.doi.org/10.1016/j.fsc.2012.11.008
1064-7406/13/$ – see front matter

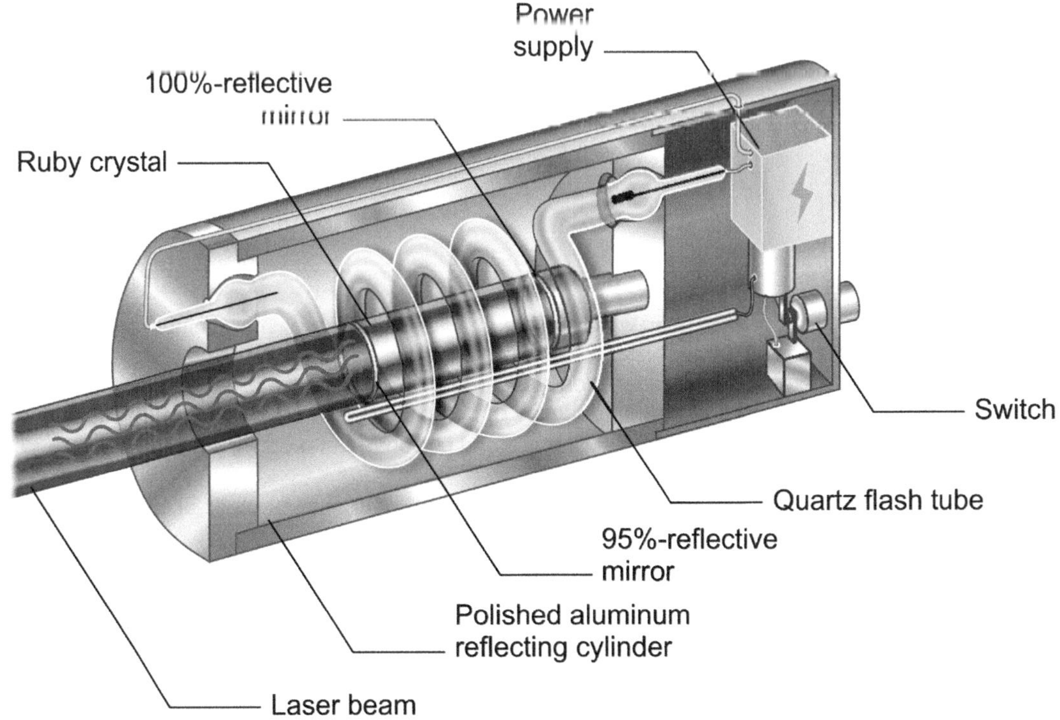

Fig. 1. Typical laser schematic.

Table 1
Table of commonly used clinical lasers

Energy Source	Wavelength	Targeted Chromaphore	Application
CO_2	10,600 nm	Water	Skin resurfacing
Erbium:yttrium-aluminum-garnet	2490 nm	Water	Skin resurfacing
Erbium:glass	1540–1550 nm	Water	Skin resurfacing
Erbium:yttrium-scandium-gallium-garnet	2790 nm	Water	Skin resurfacing
Neodynium:yttrium-aluminum-garnet	1440 nm/1064 nm	Water Red-green-brown pigment Blue-black pigment	Skin resurfacing Tattoo removal, hair removal (pigmented skin)
Q-switched potassium-titanyl-phosphate Frequency-doubled neodynium:yttrium-aluminum-garnet	532 nm	Hemoglobin Melanin Red pigment	Vascular lesions Pigmented lesions Tattoo removal
Q-switched ruby	694 nm	Melanin, dark blue-black pigment Green pigment	Tattoo removal
Q-switched alexandrite	755 nm	Melanin, black-blue pigment $\pm$ red-green pigment	Tattoo removal, hair removal
Pulsed dye laser	585–595 nm	Oxyhemoglobin	Vascular lesions
Pulsed diode	800–810 nm	Melanin	Tattoo removal, hair removal (fair skin)

The CO_2 laser emits invisible infrared radiation at a 10,600-nm wavelength. This wavelength is primarily absorbed by intracellular and extracellular water, resulting in several thermal effects, such as tissue necrosis, vaporization, carbonization, and coagulation. Clinically, CO_2 lasers have been applied in the treatment of a variety of cutaneous disorders including age-related photodamage, rhytids, and depressed scars (**Fig. 2**).

The use of fractionated CO_2 technologies was reported after 2007.[7–9] Similar to the fractionated erbium technologies that preceded, fractionated CO_2 technologies are based on the concept that cylinders of tissue are treated with laser energy while leaving interspersed areas of untreated tissue. As with the fractionated erbium technologies, this creates a productive balance between favorable tissue effects, such as correction of epithelial architecture and skin tightening, while reducing the propensity for prolonged healing, erythema, and scarring (**Figs. 3** and **4**).

The erbium:YAG 2940-nm laser

The erbium laser was introduced for clinical use in the latter part of the 1990s.[10–15] The second-generation erbium lasers possess favorable ablative and coagulation properties that make them favorable for skin resurfacing. Skin conditions that can be successfully treated with this laser include rhytids, solar elastosis, dyschromias, and actinic photodamage. The erbium:YAG laser has the highest absorption coefficient for water among ablative lasers. Given its particular tissue interaction characteristics, the erbium laser is touted to provide many of the benefits of CO_2 laser treatment with reduced unfavorable sequelae. This may be related to the favorable thermal relaxation times achievable with the erbium:YAG platforms compared with the CO_2 platforms.[16,17] The fractionated algorithm further improves its therapeutic margin (**Fig. 5**).[18]

Erbium:YAG versus CO_2 for photoaging

Rhytids, telangectasias, laxity, and actinic changes are characteristic signs of photoaging of the skin (**Table 2**). These findings can be improved with ablative and nonablative resurfacing technologies.[5,19–21] The erbium laser has been described to be more effective in the treatment of superficial dyschromias and other actinic changes in the superficial layers of the skin, whereas the CO_2 laser penetrates deeper and is more effective in the remodeling of the deeper layers of the dermis, causing the effacement of coarser rhytids. The major negative aspect of the use of CO_2 resurfacing is the prolonged healing time, prolonged erythema, and risk of hypopigmentation. Both lasers have been produced in fractionated platforms, allowing

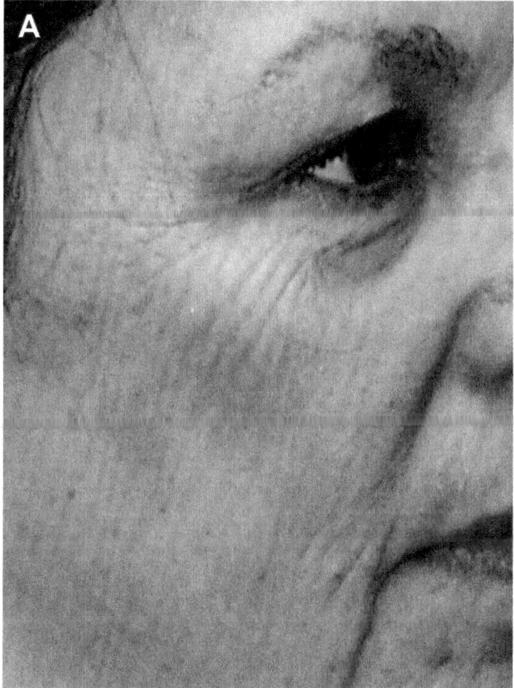

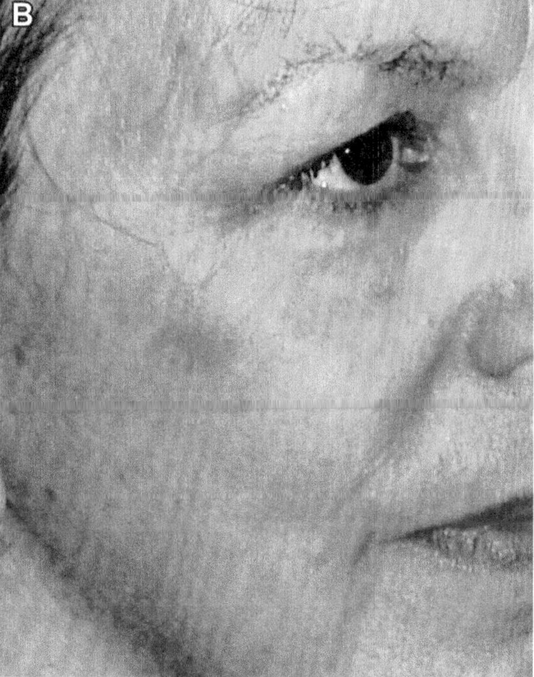

Fig. 2. Clinical photographs of patient after nonfractionated ablative CO_2 10,600-nm laser resurfacing. (*A*) Preoperative. (*B*) Postoperative.

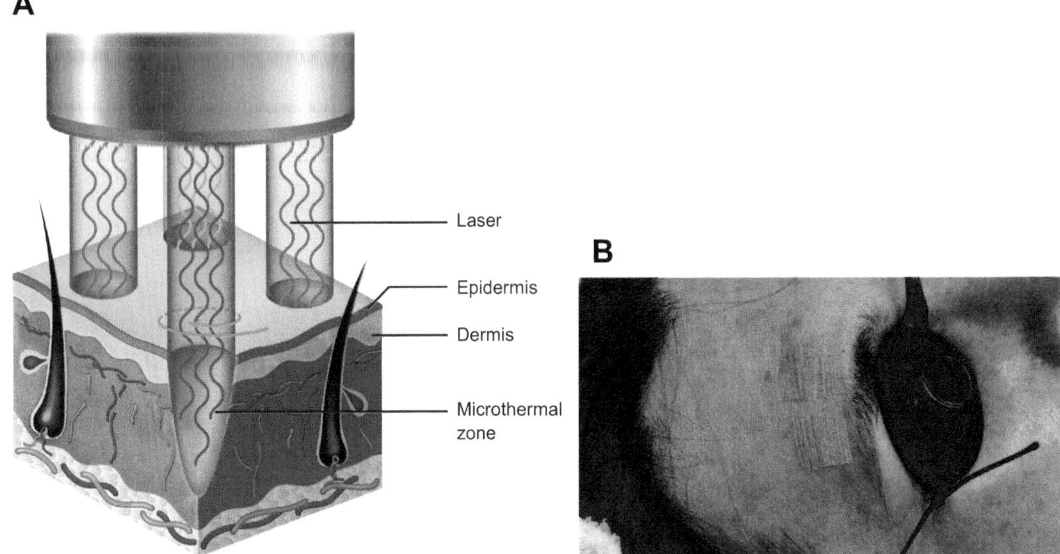

Fig. 3. The fractionated pattern. (*A*) Schematic. (*B*) Clinical intraoperative photograph showing fractionated pattern.

for an ability to adjust to a specific patient skin type and degree of photoaging. The result is a more measured effect, but a decreased downtime and healing time.

Other Superficial Ablative and Nonablative Lasers

The highly successful 1550-nm fractionated erbium laser expanded the use of erbium lasering for

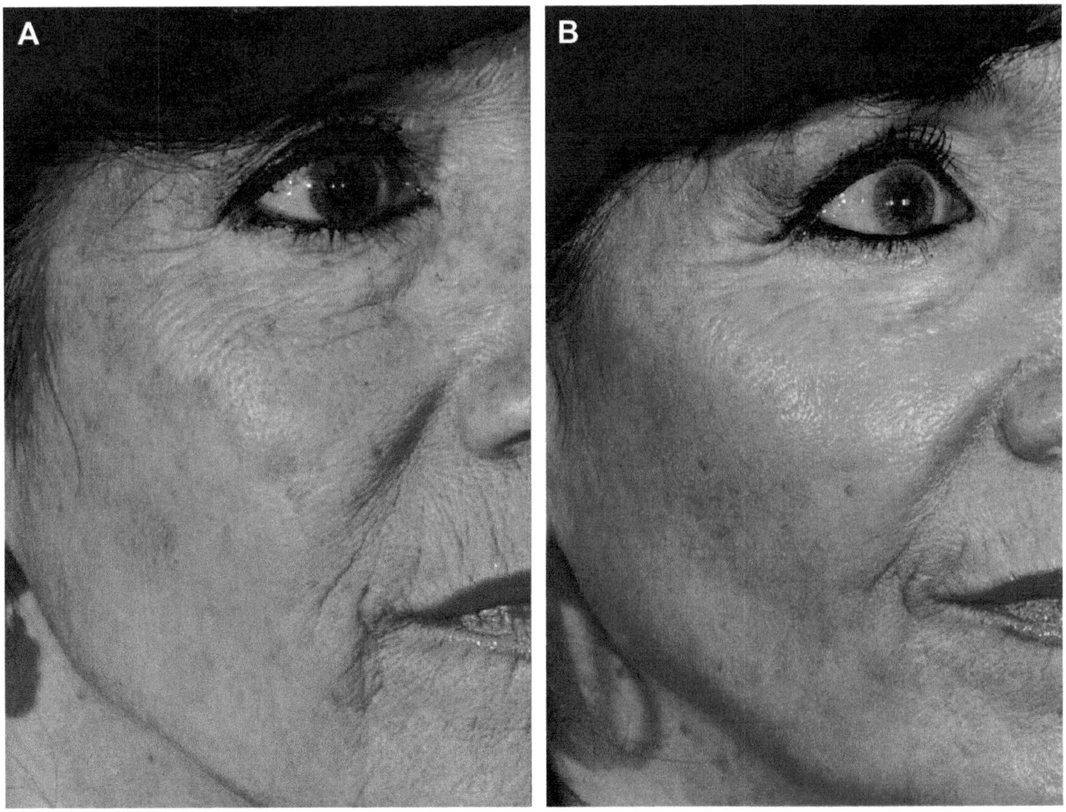

Fig. 4. Clinical photographs of patient after fractionated 10,600-nm CO_2 resurfacing for correction of rhytids and lentigenes. (*A*) Preoperative. (*B*) Postoperative.

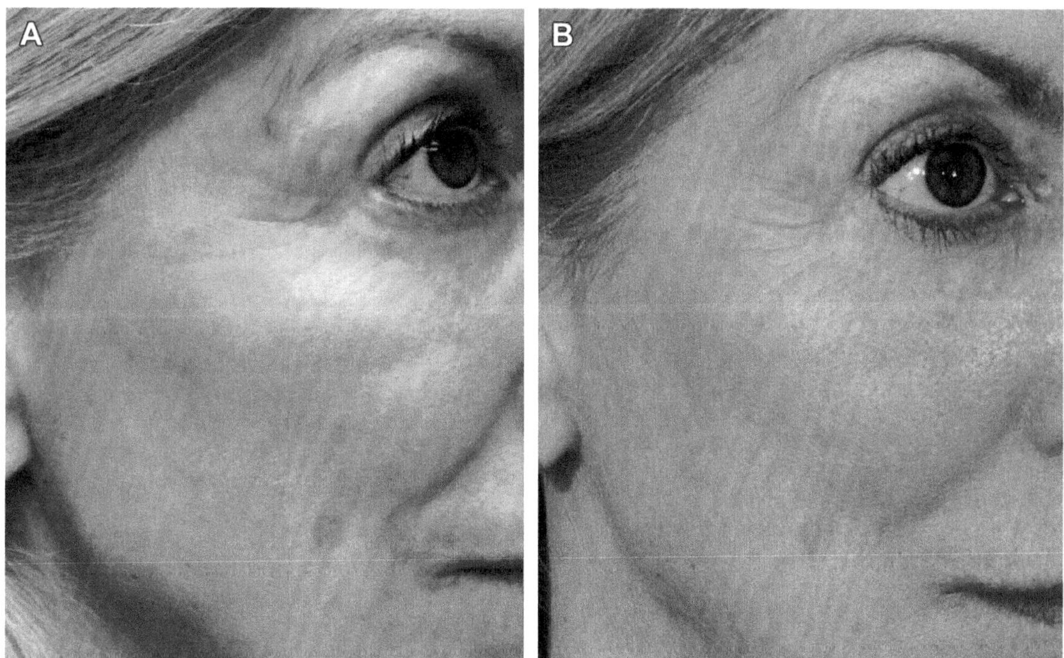

Fig. 5. Clinical photographs of patient after fractionated 2940-nm Er:YAG resurfacing for correction of rhytids and lentigenes. (*A*) Preoperative. (*B*) Postoperative.

cosmetic and reconstructive indications.[22–26] At this laser wavelength, patients could be offered a modest but significant improvement in texture, rhytids, and superficial lentigenes. The most significant benefit of this laser is the markedly reduced down time. However, because the results can be insufficient for several clinical conditions, the popularity of the fractionated CO_2 platforms continues.

Other superficial ablative and nonablative technologies are available for a spectrum of cutaneous applications. These lasers function at 2790 nm, 1440 nm, 1540 nm, 1550 nm, and 1064 nm, and other wavelengths.[27–32] The clinical effect of these lasers and technologies is frequently not as dramatic as with the ablative and fractionated technologies described previously, but the science continues to change, and more effective platforms are being developed.

There are many nonlaser skin improvement technologies available that include plasma, radiofrequency, and ultrasound technologies. A full discussion of these technologies is beyond the scope of this article, and the authors urge readers to investigate those reports further.

Table 2
The Glogou skin scale

Glogau Photodamage Classification		
Type 1	No wrinkles (age 20s to 30s)	Minimal to no discoloration or wrinkling, no keratoses, no need for makeup
Type 2	Wrinkles with motion (age 30s to 40s)	Wrinkling with movement, slight lines near eyes, no keratoses, need for some foundation or makeup
Type 3	Wrinkles at rest (age 50s to 60s)	Visible wrinkles all the time, noticeable discolorations, visible keratosis, need for heavy foundation or makeup
Type 4	Only wrinkles (age 60s to 70s)	Yellow or gray color to skin, wrinkles throughout, history of prior skin cancer, makeup unusable because of caking or cracking

Adapted from Glogau RG. Chemical peeling and skin aging. J Geriatr Dermatol 1994;2:5–10; with permission.

LASERS FOR THE TREATMENT OF BENIGN PIGMENTED LESIONS

The Nd:YAG laser produces laser energy at a wavelength of 1064 nm. It penetrates up to 2 to 3 mm into the dermis, making it useful in the removal of deeper dermal natural and artificial pigmentations. The 1064-nm wavelength of the Nd:YAG laser allows it to be helpful for the removal blue-black tattoos, but it is relatively poorly absorbed by green pigments.[33–35] When the laser beam is passed through a KTP crystal, the laser energy frequency is doubled and the resultant light wavelength is halved to 532 nm. This wavelength is absorbed more superficially in the skin, making it useful for the removal of benign superficial epidermal pigmentations.[36,37]

Lentigenes are frequently treated along with rhytids while doing ablative resurfacing. In the patient who does not need general ablative resurfacing, such as a younger patient, the lentigenes may be treated more directly. In cases where there is doubt about the diagnosis of the lesion, at least one area of the lesion should be biopsied. When one can be confident that the lesion is indeed benign, the Q-switched frequency-doubled Nd:YAG laser operating at 532 nm can produce good results (**Figs. 6** and **7**).[38–42]

LASERS FOR TATTOO REMOVAL

The removal of traumatic and cosmetic tattoo pigment can be effectively approached with lasers. Depending on the pigment, there are several lasers that are frequently used. **Table 3** depicts the lasers that are effective for various pigments. These include the Q-switched ruby 694-nm laser; the Q-switched Nd:YAG (532 and 1064) laser; and the Q-switched alexandrite (755 nm) laser.

The use of laser technology for the removal or lightening of artificially placed pigment in the skin, or tattoos, has some similarities to the treatment of naturally occurring pigment lesions. The wavelength of the laser to be used depends on the target pigment in the tattoo. There are several caveats to the treatment, and it is advisable that the practitioner (except for the most experienced) use test spots to assess the patient and pigment response before proceeding with treatment of the entire lesion. Various patient factors are important to assess before treatment including whether or not the patient has recently tanned, because this has an impact on resultant hypopigmentation and hyperpigmentation. It is also advisable to pretreat the patient with an antiviral agent if the perioral area is being treated.

The Q-switched alexandrite laser at 755 nm, the Q-switched ruby laser at 694 nm, and the Q-switched Nd:YAG laser at 1064 nm can be effective in the treatment of lighter-skinned individuals with a dark blue or black tattoo pigment. In darker-skinned individuals (ie, Fitzpatrick skin types IV–VI [**Table 4**]), the Q-switched Nd:YAG laser is preferred because the longer wavelength results in a greater

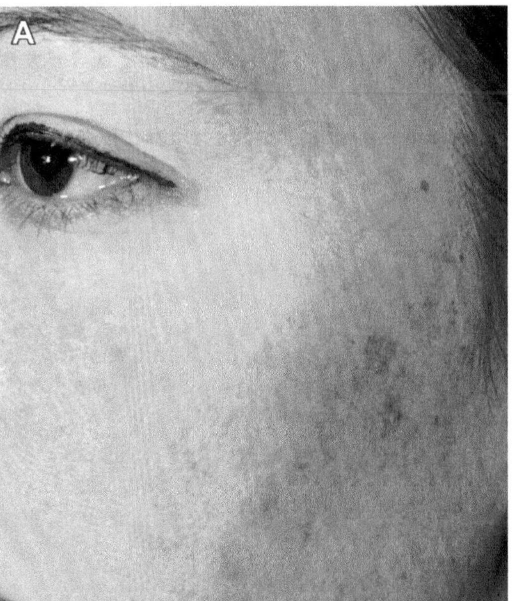

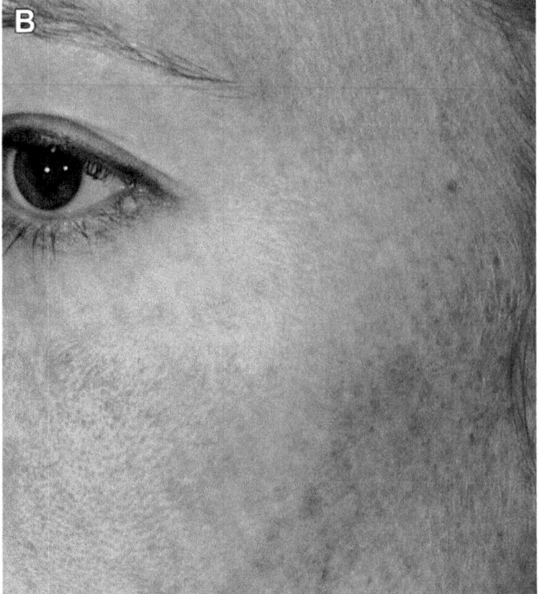

Fig. 6. Clinical photographs of patient after Q-switched 532-nm frequency-doubled Nd:YAG laser treatment of lentigenes. (*A*) Preoperative. (*B*) Postoperative.

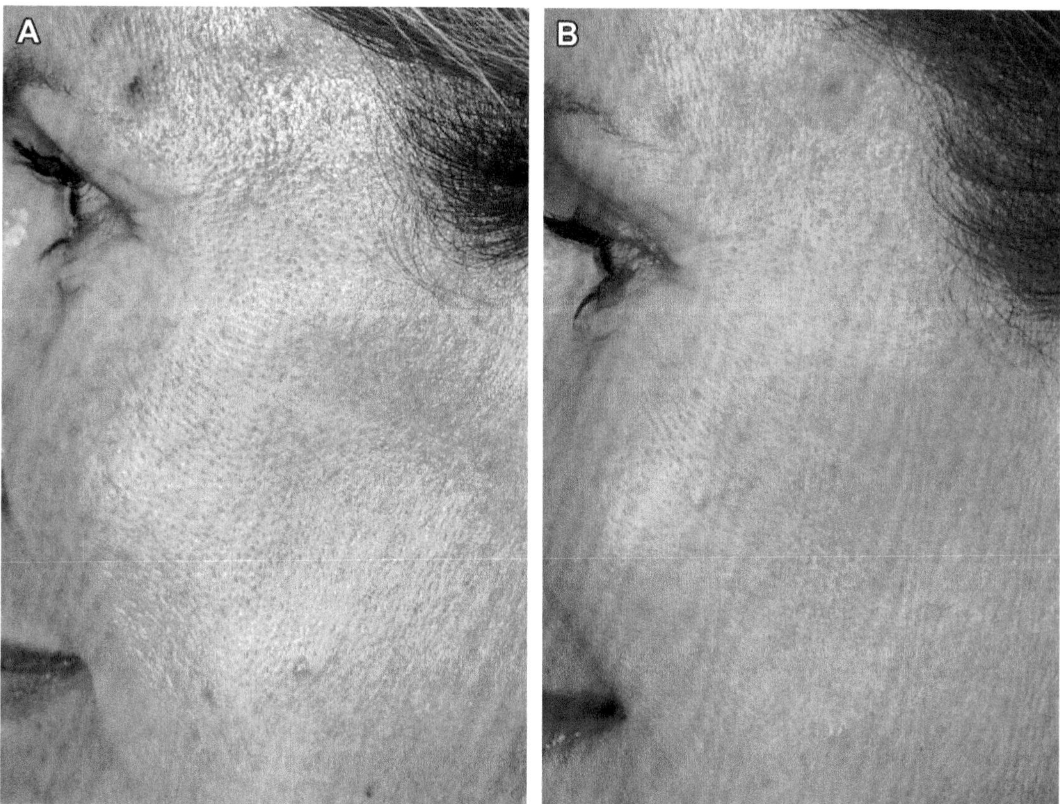

Fig. 7. Clinical photographs of second patient after Q-switched 532-nm frequency-doubled Nd:YAG laser treatment of upper eyelid and brow lentigenes and nevus, and 585-nm pulsed dye laser treatment of cheek telangectasias. (*A*) Preoperative. (*B*) Postoperative.

degree of epidermal sparing. For tattoos exhibiting red pigment, the Q-switched Nd:YAG laser operating at 532 nm can be used. Because of the risk of hyperpigmentation and hypopigmentation, treatment is usually limited to light-skinned individuals. Green pigment is frequently difficult to treat and best treated with the Q-switched ruby 694 nm laser (**Figs. 8** and **9**).[43–47]

Table 3
A clinical guide to the management of various tattoo pigments and effective lasers

Color of Tattoo Ink	Frequency-Doubled Nd:YAG (532 nm)	Ruby Laser (694 nm)	Alexandrite Laser (755 nm)	Nd:YAG Laser (1064 nm)
Red	++++	-	-	-
Orange	++	+	+	++
Yellow	-	-	-	-
Green	++	++++	+++	+
Blue	++	+++	++++	++
Blue-black	+++	++++	++++	++++
Violet	++	+	+	++
Tan	++	-	-	-
Brown	+	++	++	+
Black (amateur)	+++	++++	++++	++++
Black (professional)	+++	++++	++++	++++

Data from Parlette EC, Kaminer MS, Arndt KA. The art of tattoo removal. Plastic Surgery Practice Jan 18–20, 2008. Available at: http://www.plasticsurgerypractice.com/products/15374-the-art-of-tattoo-removal.

Table 4
The Fitzpatrick skin types

Fitzpatrick Phototyping Scale		
Fitzpatrick Type	**Description**	**Behavior in Sun**
Type I	Pale white, very fair, freckles	Burns easily, never tans
Type II	White, fair	Burns easily, tans with difficulty
Type III	Beige	Sometimes mild burn, gradually tans to a light brown
Type IV	Light brown	Rarely burns, tans easily to a moderate brown
Type V	Brown	Very rarely burns, tans easily
Type VI	Dark brown, black	Never burns, tans very easily

From Fitzpatrick TB. Soleil et peau. J Med Esthet 1975;2:33034.

LASERS FOR THE TREATMENT OF VASCULAR LESIONS

Vascular lesions are targeted by a variety of wavelength lasers including the KTP frequency-doubled Nd:YAG (532 nm), pulsed dye (585–595 nm), and Nd:YAG (1064 nm) laser systems.[48–55] The pulsed dye laser was introduced in 1989. The first version of these lasers emitted light at 577 nm, which corresponds with the oxyhemoglobin absorption spectrum. Current available pulsed dye lasers of emit a wavelength of 585 or 595 nm with longer pulse durations. The 585 nm wavelength gives it excellent specificity to hemoglobin with a minimal risk of hyperpigmentation, hypopigmentation, or skin breakdown. In general, the pulsed dye laser is considered to have a reliable safety margin, and for some authors has become the treatment of choice for vascular lesions, including port wine stains, telangectasias, and hemangiomas.[56–60] This laser can be used for vascular lesions of variable sizes ranging from small nasal telangectasias to large facial vascular malformations. The KTP frequency-doubled Nd:YAG (532 nm) laser is usually used for smaller lesions, such as spider-veins and telangectasias, and the Nd:YAG (1064 nm) laser has use in treating reticular veins (see **Fig. 7**; **Fig. 10**).[61–63]

LASERS FOR HAIR REMOVAL

Before the introduction of these laser technologies, such modalities as waxing and electrolysis had been used for hair removal. Laser technology has now become popular for the temporary and semipermanent removal of hair for women and men. Laser hair removal is performed for cosmetic purposes; for general grooming; or as part of the treatment or resolution of hirsutism associated with medical conditions, such as polycystic ovary disease. Laser hair removal was first noted to be available in the 1970s, with the first Food and Drug Administration approval coming in the mid-1990s.[64] The targeted chromaphore in these laser

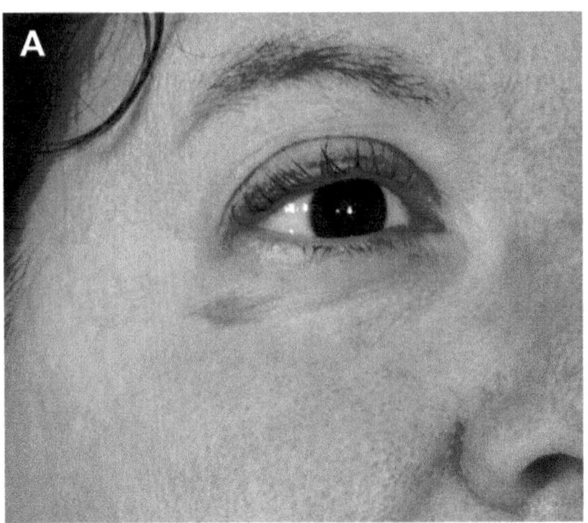

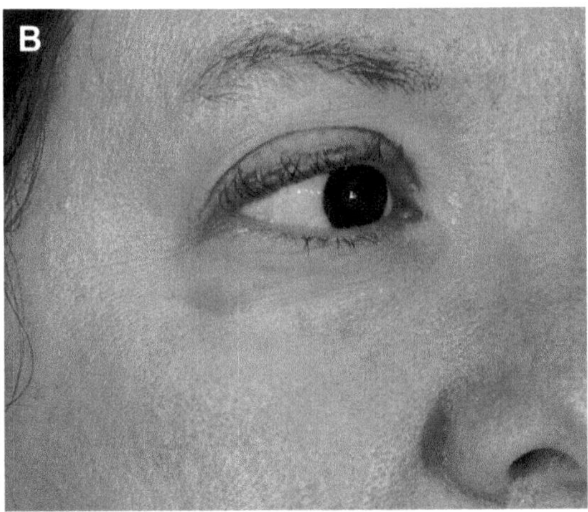

Fig. 8. Clinical photographs of second patient after Q-switched 1064-nm Nd:YAG laser treatment of traumatic tattoo. (*A*) Preoperative. (*B*) Postoperative.

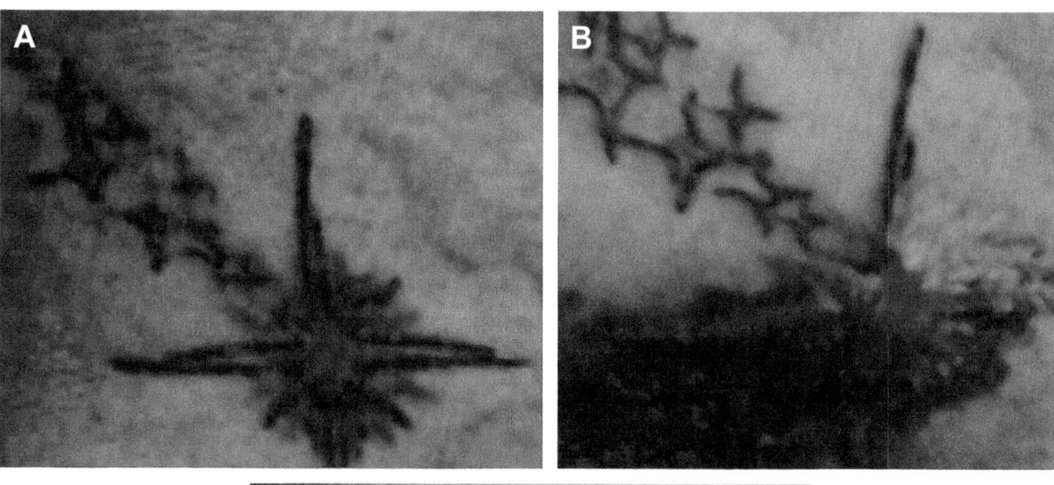

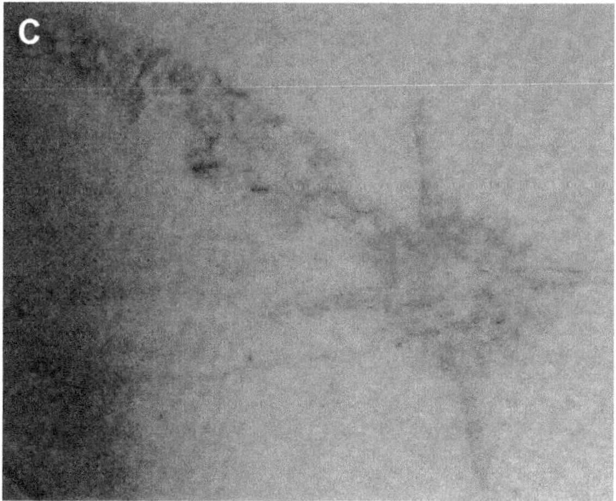

Fig. 9. Clinical photographs of patient after Q-switched 1064-nm Nd:YAG laser treatment of dark tattoo lines and treatment of red pigment with Q-switched 532-nm Nd:YAG laser. (*A*) Preoperative. (*B*) Intraoperative. (*C*) Postoperative intermediate result after two treatments.

systems is the melanin pigment. Because this is found in the hair shaft and hair follicle epithelium, these lasers are particularly effective.

Although laser hair removal was first introduced with the ruby laser in 1996, this laser has lost popularity with the development of other technologies that have improved specificity. Alexandrite lasers operating at 755 nm are among the most popular systems, touted to have improved penetration and the ability to treat Fitzpatrick skin types I to IV.[65] The 1064-nm Nd:YAG laser operating in the long pulse mode has reported success rates of 70% with five treatments and use for hair removal even in patients of higher Fitzpatrick skin types.[66]

Diode lasers are solid-state lasers that operate at 800 nm, reduce hair density through photothermal destruction of the melanin-containing portions of the hair follicle, can be used with Fitzpatrick skin types I to IV, and are among the most popular devices. These lasers are powerful devices that penetrate deeper into the dermis, necessitating epidermal cooling to minimize epidermal and superficial dermal damage, and to provide patient comfort. The diode lasers have shown efficacy rates up to 90%.[67,68] Patients with dark, coarse hair achieve the most successful outcomes (**Figs. 11** and **12**).[69]

Although it does not represent the laser technologies, intense pulsed light (IPL) has become increasingly popular for hair removal. IPL has shown effectiveness comparable with the ruby laser in several studies and statistical equivalence to other devices, such as the diode laser and the alexandrite laser.[69–83]

LASERS FOR THE TREATMENT OF SCARS

Red hypertrophic scars can be treated effectively with the pulsed dye laser; the results have been reliable and comparable with the use of intralesional

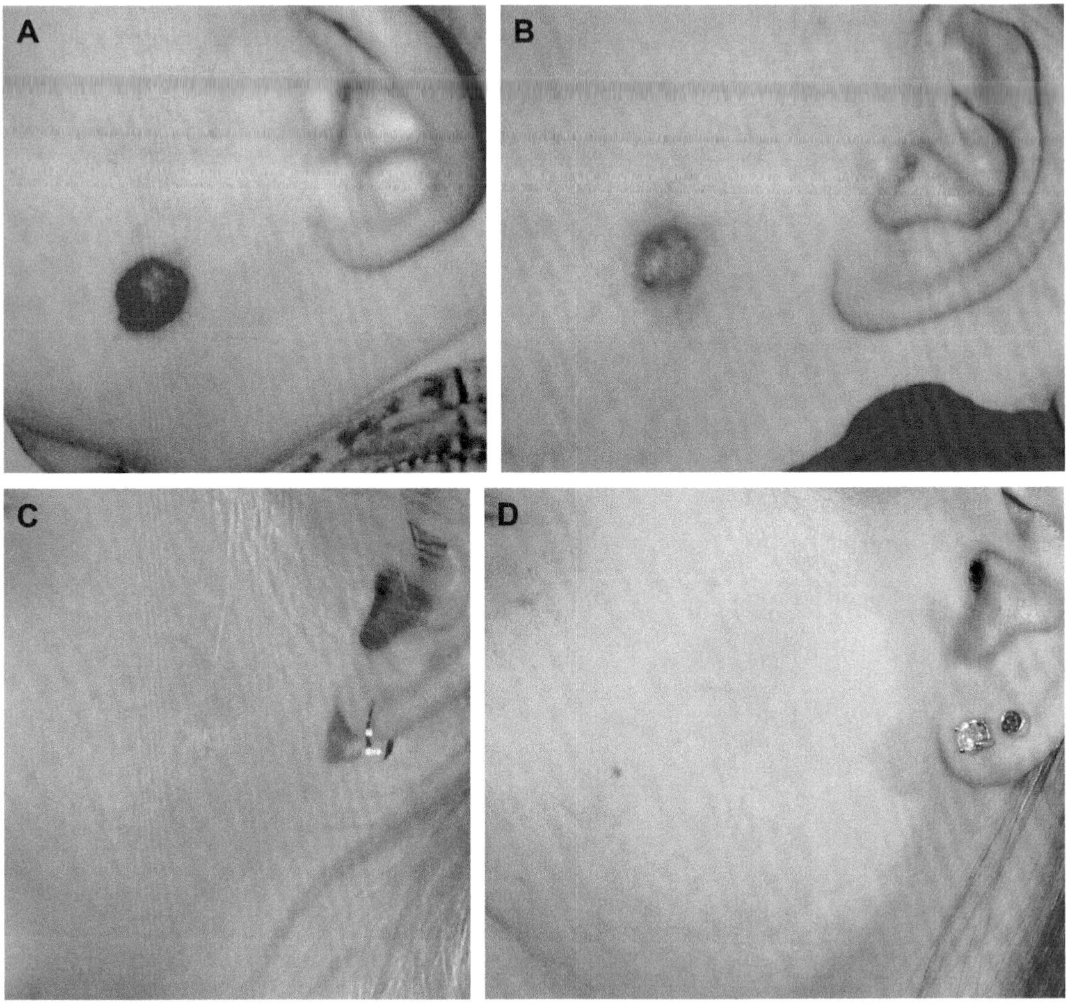

Fig. 10. Clinical photographs of patient after 585-nm pulse dye laser treatment of vascular lesion. (*A*) Preoperative. (*B*) Immediate postoperative. (*C*) Long-term postoperative - 5 years (*D*) Long-Term postoperative - 10 years.

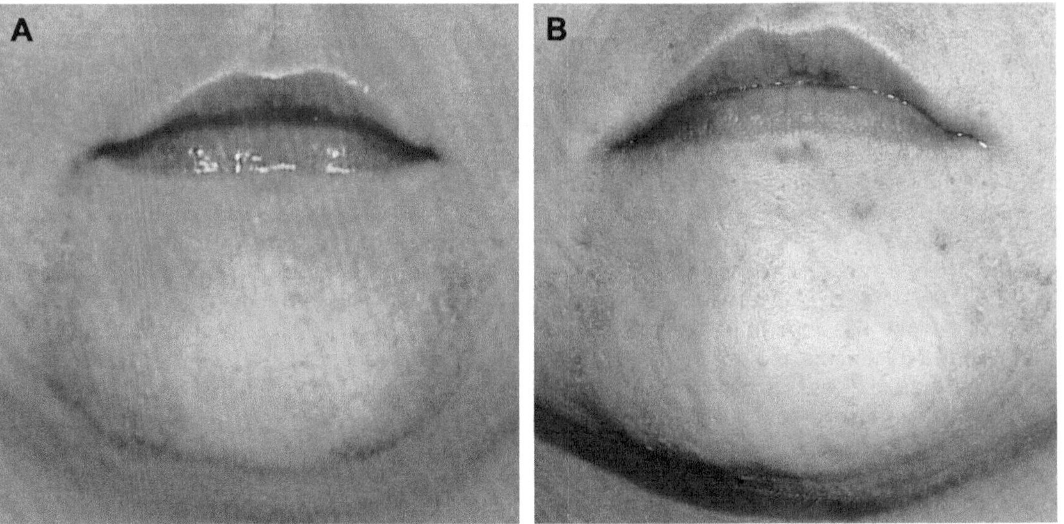

Fig. 11. Clinical photographs of patient after 800-nm pulsed diode laser treatment of hair excess. (*A*) Preoperative. (*B*) Postoperative.

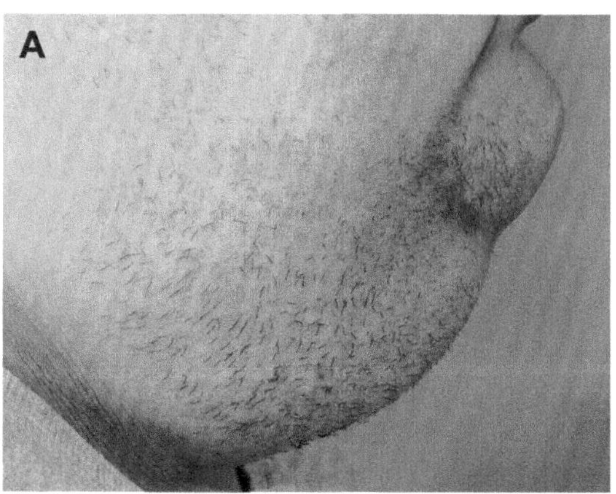

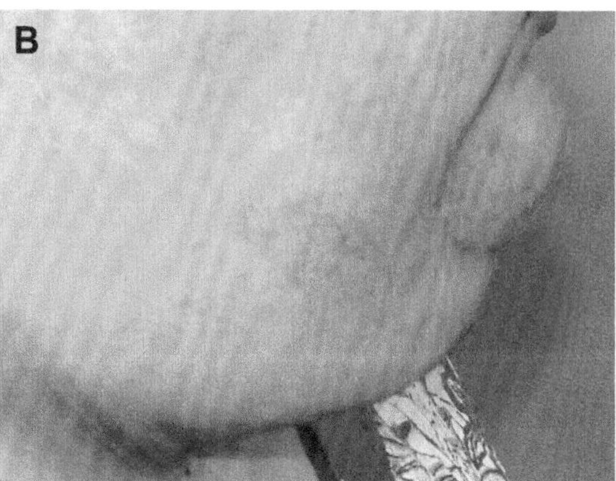

Fig. 12. Clinical photographs of patient with polycystic ovary disease and hirsutism after 800-nm pulsed diode laser treatment of hair excess. (*A*) Preoperative. (*B*) Postoperative.

steroid injections.[84] Depressed scars respond quite well to laser resurfacing with CO_2 and erbium lasers. Acne scars, in particular, can be treated with a combination of subcision and laser resurfacing (**Figs. 13–15**).[6,85,86]

LIGHT TECHNOLOGIES

IPL technologies, although not lasers, are frequently used by clinicians alongside available laser technologies. The IPL systems can be used with or without photosensitizers, such as 5-aminolevulinic acid, and are used to treat such disorders as acne, lentigenes, telangectasias and other smaller vascular lesions, actinic changes, and nonmelanoma skin cancers.[87,88]

GENERAL CLINICAL ISSUES

Preoperative Considerations

There are several general preoperative considerations for all patients undergoing laser therapy. Among the most common complications of laser therapy are pigmentary issues, such as hypopigmentation and hyperpigmentation.[89] It is therefore recommended that patient's skin type be considered with any laser use. In the more advanced Fitzpatrick skin types, there is a greater risk of permanent hypopigmentation with ablative resurfacing. Similar pigmentation concerns can arise with the use of lasers that target melanin and any other dark chromaphores, such as those used in hair and tattoo removal. Patients with darker skin types are also at greater risk of prolonged

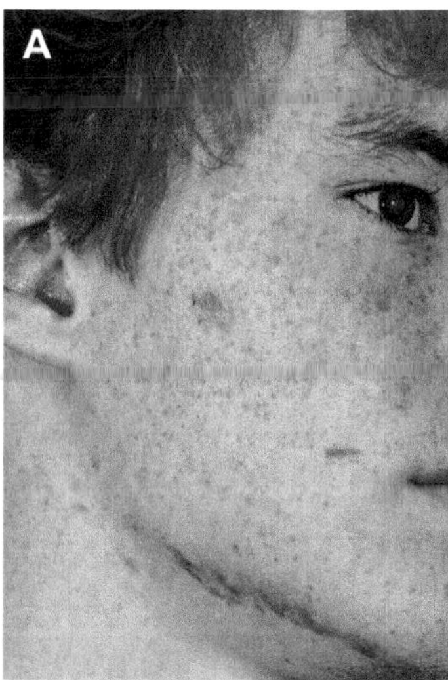

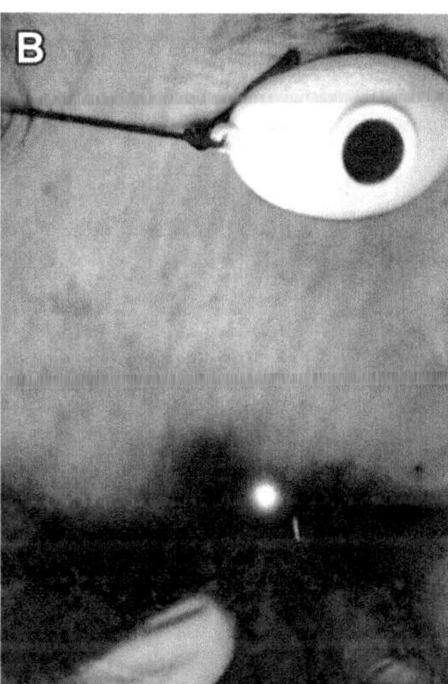

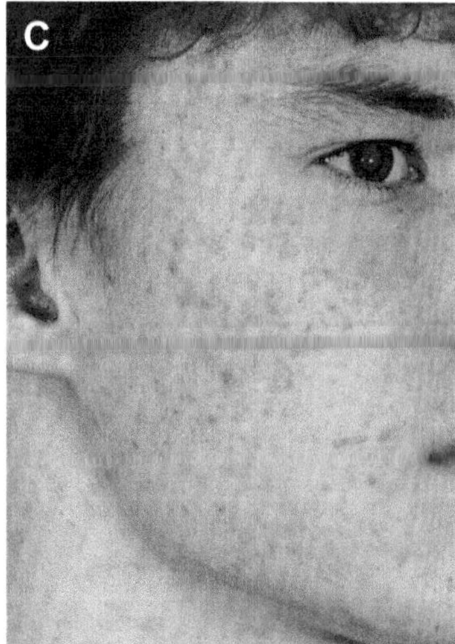

Fig. 13. Clinical photographs of patient after Q-switched 1064-nm Nd:YAG laser treatment of traumatic tattoos and treatment of hypertrophic scars with 585-nm pulsed dye laser. (*A*) Preoperative. (*B*) Intraoperative. (*C*) Postoperative.

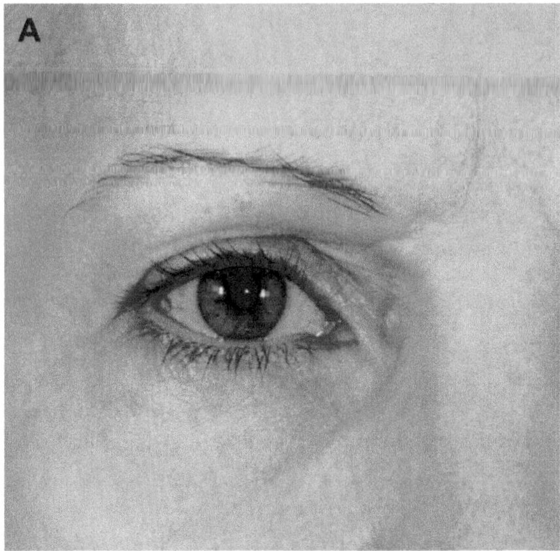

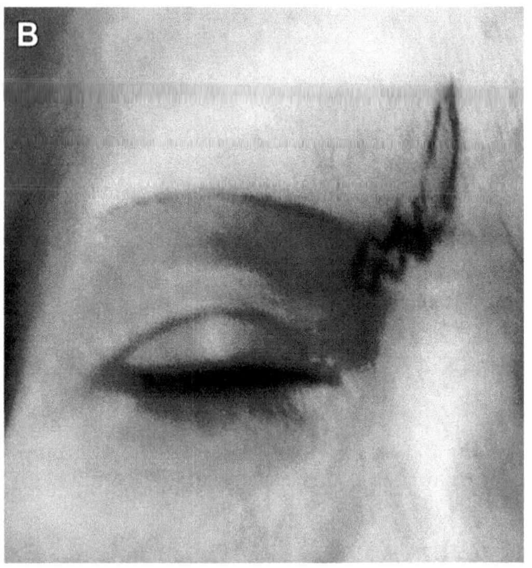

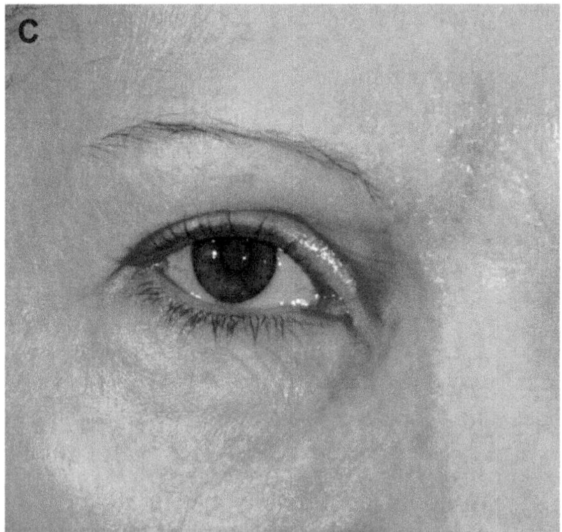

Fig. 14. Clinical photographs of patient after scar revision and fractionated 10,600-nm CO_2 laser treatment of depressed scar. (*A*) Preoperative. (*B*) Scar revision plan. (*C*) Postoperative after laser.

postinflammatory hyperpigmentation. To further reduce pigment-related problems, patients should be counseled that they should not tan before or for several weeks after laser therapy.

There is a variety of skin preparation or skin-conditioning regimens that clinicians use preoperatively. These generally include the use of bleaching agents containing 4% hydroquinone and retinoic

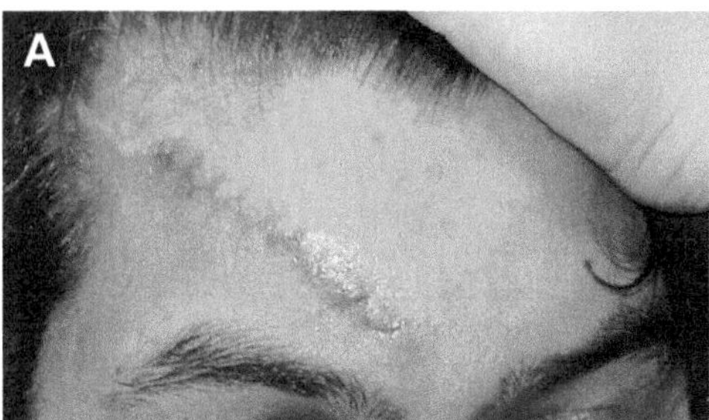

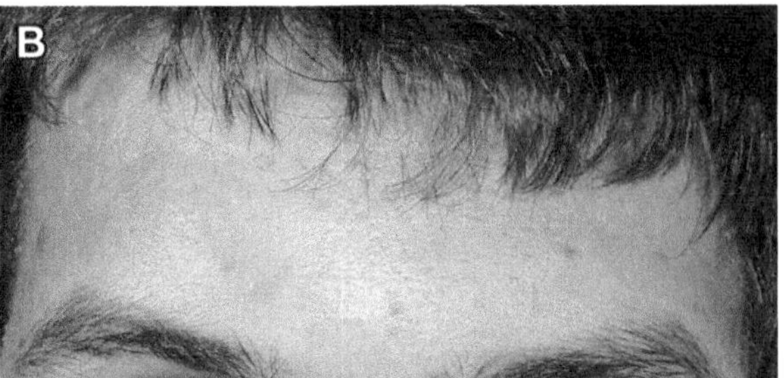

Fig. 15. Clinical photographs of patient after full ablative 10,600-nm CO_2 laser treatment of depressed scar after w-plasty. (*A*) Preoperative. (*B*) Postoperative.

creams. It is generally recommended that patients use these products for 2 weeks or more before the laser therapy.[90]

Another area of concern is the risk of infection. Although bacterial, viral, and fungal infections can occur, it is usually the consideration and prophylaxis for herpetic outbreaks that warrant most preprocedure attention. In all cases where the treatment area includes the perioral area or when the patient has had herpetic infections, it should be considered whether the patient should be treated with an antiviral agent preoperatively that is continued postoperatively. However, clinicians vary in their practices regarding the duration of preoperative and postoperative treatment, if prophylaxis is used in the patient without a history of herpetic infection, and what antiviral agent is used. Valacyclovir and acyclovir are commonly used.[91]

Procedural Anesthesia

In the adult patient, most laser procedures in the face and neck region can be performed in an awake patient. Frequently, an oral sedative is given. Anesthesia of the skin is obtained with the use of topical anesthetic creams and, at times, local infiltration of anesthesia into the skin area that is to be treated or with nerve blocks. When the procedure is being performed on a child, it is common for general anesthesia to be used.

Postoperative Care

There are some commonalities in the postoperative care of patients who have undergone laser therapy. The need for pain control after laser procedures is generally limited in intensity and duration. The lasered site should be monitored for infection, adverse healing issues, and pigmentation changes. The relevance of these issues is highly dependent on the type of laser being used, the condition being treated, the patient skin type, and other clinical issues.

The skin should be kept clean with the use of bland cleansers, and the patient should be cautioned about sun exposure and avoiding any trauma to the newly treated skin surface. Direct sunlight should be avoided. When the skin has been de-epithelialized, as in resurfacing, there should be instructions for the use of moist, bland occlusive dressings until the skin re-epithelialized.[92] In these cases, dilute acetic acid rinses can be helpful in freeing peeling skin and lowering the pH of the skin. This can reduce itching and prevent bacterial and yeast colonization of the healing, de-epithelialized area.

Complications and Concerns

Prolonged erythema after laser skin therapy, especially resurfacing procedures, is common. This is usually self-limited and of short duration. When deemed necessary, topical steroid cream or a silicone-based product can be used. If early scarring is detected, it may be improved with the use of topical steroids, intralesional steroid injection, and the use of pulse dye laser therapy.

Postinflammatory hyperpigmentation is also common after many laser procedures. The incidence is reduced by the selection of patients with lighter Fitzpatrick skin types I to III. When it occurs, hydroquinone creams are commonly used early in the course. Kojic and azeliac containing products are also advocated.[93–95] Hypopigmentation after resurfacing is difficult to reverse and can often be permanent. Hypersensitivity reactions can occur from exposure to topical preparations used after the laser treatment.

Infections are uncommon, but not rare. In the patient who has undergone resurfacing, the clinical appearance of skin infections may not have the same appearance as seen with untreated skin. The clinician should therefore exercise a high degree of suspicion when anything arises that might suggest infection. The recurrence of pain several days after the procedure can be a hint that an infection is present, because in most patients, pain dissipates within 24 hours even after a resurfacing procedure. Viral, bacterial, and fungal infection treatment should be guided by the results of clinical and laboratory study.

SUMMARY

Patients seek the advice of the facial plastic surgeon for a spectrum of skin problems, such as age-related concerns, pigmentation issues, lesions, and scars. Some of these problems are remedied with the prescription of medicated creams, some are treated with surgery, and some can be treated with laser therapy. Given the varied physical characteristics of many of these clinical issues and "lesions," it is necessary to use the laser technology that best targets the problem presented. A compendium of laser technologies for clinical use now exists, each laser with a spectrum of activity depending on the biologic chromaphore that is targeted. The surgeon's toolbox should therefore contain several lasers and knowledge of their best applications.

ACKNOWLEDGMENTS

The authors thank Beth Shultz and Cindy Wampler for their assistance in compiling the materials for this manuscript. The authors also thank Kim Gordon, MA, who did an ultimate bang-up job of editing!

REFERENCES

1. Fitzpatrick RE. Laser resurfacing of rhytides. Dermatol Clin 1997;15(3):431–47.
2. Fitzpatrick RE. CO2 laser resurfacing. Dermatol Clin 2001;19(3):443–51, viii.
3. David LM, Sarne AJ, Unger WP. Rapid laser scanning for facial resurfacing. Dermatol Surg 1995;21(12):1031–3.
4. Lowe NJ, Lask G, Griffin ME, et al. Skin resurfacing with the Ultrapulse carbon dioxide laser. Observations on 100 patients. Dermatol Surg 1995;21(12):1025–9.
5. Alster TS, Kauvar AN, Geronemus RG. Histology of high-energy pulsed CO2 laser resurfacing. Semin Cutan Med Surg 1996;15(3):189–93.
6. Alster TS, West TB. Resurfacing of atrophic facial acne scars with a high-energy, pulsed carbon dioxide laser. Dermatol Surg 1996;22(2):151–4 [discussion: 154–5].
7. Goldman MP. Observations on the use of fractionated CO2 laser resurfacing. J Drugs Dermatol 2009;8(1):82–6.
8. Hunzeker CM, Weiss ET, Geronemus RG. Fractionated CO2 laser resurfacing: our experience with more than 2000 treatments. Aesthet Surg J 2009;29(4):317–22.
9. Tierney EP, Eisen RF, Hanke CW. Fractionated CO2 laser skin rejuvenation. Dermatol Ther 2011;24(1):41–53.
10. Alster TS, Lupton JR. Erbium:YAG cutaneous laser resurfacing. Dermatol Clin 2001;19(3):453–66.
11. Bass LS. Erbium:YAG laser skin resurfacing: preliminary clinical evaluation. Ann Plast Surg 1998;40(4):328–34.
12. David LM. Erbium vs CO2 in laser resurfacing: the debate continues. J Cutan Laser Ther 1999;1(3):185–9.
13. Goldberg DJ. Erbium: YAG laser resurfacing: what is its role? Aesthet Surg J 1998;18(4):255–60.
14. Goldman MP. Techniques for erbium:YAG laser skin resurfacing: initial pearls from the first 100 patients. Dermatol Surg 1997;23(12):1219–21.
15. Weiss RA, Harrington AC, Pfau RC, et al. Periorbital skin resurfacing using high energy erbium:YAG laser: results in 50 patients. Lasers Surg Med 1999;24(2):81–6.
16. Ross EV, Naseef GS, McKinlay JR, et al. Comparison of carbon dioxide laser, erbium:YAG laser, dermabrasion, and dermatome: a study of thermal damage, wound contraction, and wound healing in a live pig model: implications for skin resurfacing. J Am Acad Dermatol 2000;42(1 Pt 1):92–105.
17. Shori RK, Walston AA, Stafsudd OM, et al. Quantification and modeling of the dynamic changes in the absorption coefficient of water at 2.94 um. IEEE 2001;7(6):955–70.
18. Cohen JL, Babcock MJ. Ablative fractionated erbium:YAG laser for the treatment of ice pick alar scars due to neodymium:YAG laser burns. J Drugs Dermatol 2009;8(1):65–7.
19. Alster T, Hirsch R. Single-pass CO2 laser skin resurfacing of light and dark skin: extended experience with 52 patients. J Cosmet Laser Ther 2003;5(1):39–42.
20. Fitzpatrick RE, Goldman MP, Satur NM, et al. Pulsed carbon dioxide laser resurfacing of photo-aged facial skin. Arch Dermatol 1996;132(4):395–402.
21. Goldman MP. CO2 laser resurfacing of the face and neck. Facial Plast Surg Clin North Am 2001;9(2):283–90, ix.
22. Tanzi EL, Wanitphakdeedecha R, Alster TS. Fraxel laser indications and long-term follow-up. Aesthet Surg J 2008;28(6):675–8 [discussion: 679–80].
23. Collawn SS. Fraxel skin resurfacing. Ann Plast Surg 2007;58(3):237–40.
24. Bass LS. Rejuvenation of the aging face using Fraxel laser treatment. Aesthet Surg J 2005;25(3):307–9.
25. Chiu RJ, Kridel RW. Fractionated photothermolysis: the Fraxel 1550-nm glass fiber laser treatment. Facial Plast Surg Clin North Am 2007;15(2):229–37, vii.
26. Pham AM, Greene RM, Woolery-Lloyd H, et al. 1550-nm nonablative laser resurfacing for facial surgical scars. Arch Facial Plast Surg 2011;13(3):203–10.
27. Alam M, Dover JS. Nonablative laser and light therapy: an approach to patient and device selection. Skin Therapy Lett 2003;8(4):4–7.
28. Ang P, Barlow RJ. Nonablative laser resurfacing: a systematic review of the literature. Clin Exp Dermatol 2002;27(8):630–5.
29. Carniol PJ, Farley S, Friedman A. Long-pulse 532-nm diode laser for nonablative facial skin rejuvenation. Arch Facial Plast Surg 2003;5(6):511–3.
30. Chua SH, Ang P, Khoo LS, et al. Nonablative 1450-nm diode laser in the treatment of facial atrophic acne scars in type IV to V Asian skin: a prospective clinical study. Dermatol Surg 2004;30(10):1287–91.
31. Doshi SN, Alster TS. 1,450 nm long-pulsed diode laser for nonablative skin rejuvenation. Dermatol Surg 2005;31(9 Pt 2):1223–6 [discussion: 1226].
32. Fulchiero GJ Jr, Parham-Vetter PC, Obagi S. Subcision and 1320-nm Nd:YAG nonablative laser resurfacing for the treatment of acne scars: a simultaneous split-face single patient trial. Dermatol Surg 2004;30(10):1356–9 [discussion: 1360].
33. Bernstein EF. Laser tattoo removal. Semin Plast Surg 2007;21(3):175–92.
34. Wenzel SM. Current concepts in laser tattoo removal. Skin Therapy Lett 2010;15(3):3–5.
35. Kent KM, Graber EM. Laser tattoo removal: a review. Dermatol Surg 2012;38(1):1–13.

36. Anderson RR, Margolis RJ, Watenabe S, et al. Selective photothermolysis of cutaneous pigmentation by Q-switched Nd:YAG laser pulses at 1064, 532, and 355 nm. J Invest Dermatol 1989;93(1):28–32.
37. Kim YJ, Whang KU, Choi WB, et al. Efficacy and safety of 1,064 nm Q-switched Nd:YAG laser treatment for removing melanocytic nevi. Ann Dermatol 2012;24(2):162–7.
38. DePadova-Elder SM, Milgraum SS. Q-switched ruby laser treatment of labial lentigines in Peutz-Jeghers syndrome. J Dermatol Surg Oncol 1994;20(12):830–2.
39. Kono T, Chan HH, Groff WF, et al. Long-pulse pulsed dye laser delivered with compression for treatment of facial lentigines. Dermatol Surg 2007; 33(8):945–50.
40. Bassichis BA, Swamy R, Dayan SH. Use of the KTP laser in the treatment of rosacea and solar lentigines. Facial Plast Surg 2004;20(1):77–83.
41. Li YT, Yang KC. Comparison of the frequency-doubled Q-switched Nd:YAG laser and 35% trichloroacetic acid for the treatment of face lentigines. Dermatol Surg 1999;25(3):202–4.
42. Fitzpatrick RE, Goldman MP, Ruiz-Esparza J. Clinical advantage of the CO2 laser superpulsed mode. Treatment of verruca vulgaris, seborrheic keratoses, lentigines, and actinic cheilitis. J Dermatol Surg Oncol 1994;20(7):449–56.
43. Pfeiffer N. Q-switched ruby laser brings scarless tattoo removal. J Clin Laser Med Surg 1990;8(6):10–3.
44. Watts MT, Downes RN, Collin JR, et al. The use of Q-switched Nd:Yag laser for removal of permanent eyeliner tattoo. Ophthal Plast Reconstr Surg 1992; 8(4):292–4.
45. Wheeland RG. Tattoo removal using the ruby laser. West J Med 1992;156(2):190.
46. Fitzpatrick RE, Goldman MP, Ruiz-Esparza J. Use of the alexandrite laser (755 nm, 100 nsec) for tattoo pigment removal in an animal model. J Am Acad Dermatol 1993;28(5 Pt 1):745–50.
47. Adrian RM, Griffin L. Laser tattoo removal. Clin Plast Surg 2000;27(2):181–92.
48. Barcot Z, Zupancic B. Pulsed dye laser treatment of vascular lesions in childhood. Acta Dermatovenerol Croat 2010;18(3):201–8.
49. Dias Coelho J, Serrao V. Treatment of vascular lesions of the tongue with Nd:YAG laser. Case Report Med 2009;2009:795363.
50. Cole PD, Sonabend ML, Levy ML. Laser treatment of pediatric vascular lesions. Semin Plast Surg 2007; 21(3):159–66.
51. Railan D, Parlette EC, Uebelhoer NS, et al. Laser treatment of vascular lesions. Clin Dermatol 2006; 24(1):8–15.
52. Rothfleisch JE, Kosann MK, Levine VJ, et al. Laser treatment of congenital and acquired vascular lesions. A review. Dermatol Clin 2002;20(1):1–18.
53. Goldberg DJ. Laser treatment of vascular lesions. Clin Plast Surg 2000;27(2):173–80, ix.
54. Ross BS, Levine VJ, Ashinoff R. Laser treatment of acquired vascular lesions. Dermatol Clin 1997; 15(3):385–96.
55. McKeown A. Pulsed-dye laser treatment of vascular lesions. Dermatol Nurs 1991;3(5):330–4.
56. Bernstein EF, Kligman A. Rosacea treatment using the new-generation, high-energy, 595 nm, long pulse-duration pulsed-dye laser. Lasers Surg Med 2008;40(4):233–9.
57. Bernstein EF, Kornbluth S, Brown DB, et al. Treatment of spider veins using a 10 millisecond pulse-duration frequency-doubled neodymium YAG laser. Dermatol Surg 1999;25(4):316–20.
58. Bernstein EF, Lee J, Lowery J, et al. Treatment of spider veins with the 595 nm pulsed-dye laser. J Am Acad Dermatol 1998;39(5 Pt 1):746–50.
59. Choi YS, Suh HS, Yoon MY, et al. Intense pulsed light vs pulsed-dye laser in the treatment of facial acne: a randomized split-face trial. J Eur Acad Dermatol Venereol 2010;24(7):773–80.
60. Cordoro KM, Frieden IJ. Pulsed dye laser for port wine stains. J Am Acad Dermatol 2010;62(6): 1065–6.
61. Eremia S, Li CY. Treatment of leg and face veins with a cryogen spray variable pulse width 1064-nm Nd:YAG laser: a prospective study of 47 patients. J Cosmet Laser Ther 2001;3(3):147–53.
62. Rogachefsky AS, Silapunt S, Goldberg DJ. Nd:YAG laser (1064 nm) irradiation for lower extremity telangiectases and small reticular veins: efficacy as measured by vessel color and size. Dermatol Surg 2002;28(3):220–3.
63. Omura NE, Dover JS, Arndt KA, et al. Treatment of reticular leg veins with a 1064 nm long-pulsed Nd:YAG laser. J Am Acad Dermatol 2003;48(1): 76–81.
64. Dierickx CC, Grossman MC, Farinelli WA, et al. Permanent hair removal by normal-mode ruby laser. Arch Dermatol 1998;134(7):837–42.
65. McDaniel DH, Lord J, Ash K, et al. Laser hair removal: a review and report on the use of the long-pulsed alexandrite laser for hair reduction of the upper lip, leg, back, and bikini region. Dermatol Surg 1999;25(6):425–30.
66. Lorenz S, Brunnberg S, Landthaler M, et al. Hair removal with the long pulsed Nd:YAG laser: a prospective study with one year follow-up. Lasers Surg Med 2002;30(2):127–34.
67. Dierickx CC. Hair removal by lasers and intense pulsed light sources. Dermatol Clin 2002;20(1): 135–46.
68. Handrick C, Alster TS. Comparison of long-pulsed diode and long-pulsed alexandrite lasers for hair removal: a long-term clinical and histologic study. Dermatol Surg 2001;27(7):622–6.

69. Campos VB, Dierickx CC, Farinelli WA, et al. Hair removal with an 800-nm pulsed diode laser. J Am Acad Dermatol 2000;43(3):442–7.
70. Vachiramon V, McMichael AJ. Laser hair removal in ethnic skin: principles and practical aspects. J Drugs Dermatol 2011;10(Suppl 12):s17–9.
71. Battle EF Jr. Advances in laser hair removal in skin of color. J Drugs Dermatol 2011;10(11):1235–9.
72. Lapidoth M, Dierickx C, Lanigan S, et al. Best practice options for hair removal in patients with unwanted facial hair using combination therapy with laser: guidelines drawn up by an expert working group. Dermatology 2010;221(1):34–42.
73. Eremia S, Li C, Newman N. Laser hair removal with alexandrite versus diode laser using four treatment sessions: 1-year results. Dermatol Surg 2001; 27(11):925–9 [discussion: 929–30].
74. Goldberg DJ, Silapunt S. Hair removal using a long-pulsed Nd:YAG laser: comparison at fluences of 50, 80, and 100 J/cm. Dermatol Surg 2001;27(5):434–6.
75. DiBernardo BE, Perez J, Usal H, et al. Laser hair removal. Clin Plast Surg 2000;27(2):199–211.
76. Goldberg DJ, Samady JA. Evaluation of a long-pulse Q-switched Nd:YAG laser for hair removal. Dermatol Surg 2000;26(2):109–13.
77. DiBernardo BE, Perez J, Usal H, et al. Laser hair removal: where are we now? Plast Reconstr Surg 1999;104(1):247–57 [discussion: 258].
78. Solomon MP. Hair removal using the long-pulsed ruby laser. Ann Plast Surg 1998;41(1):1–6.
79. Goldberg DJ, Littler CM, Wheeland RG. Topical suspension-assisted Q-switched Nd:YAG laser hair removal. Dermatol Surg 1997;23(9):741–5.
80. Wheeland RG. Laser-assisted hair removal. Dermatol Clin 1997;15(3):469–77.
81. Finkel B, Eliezri YD, Waldman A, et al. Pulsed alexandrite laser technology for noninvasive hair removal. J Clin Laser Med Surg 1997;15(5):225–9.
82. Bjerring P, Cramers M, Egekvist H, et al. Hair reduction using a new intense pulsed light irradiator and a normal mode ruby laser. J Cutan Laser Ther 2000;2(2):63–71.
83. Hovenic W, DeSpain J. Laser hair reduction and removal. Facial Plast Surg Clin North Am 2011; 19(2):325–33.
84. Alster T. Laser scar revision: comparison study of 585-nm pulsed dye laser with and without intralesional corticosteroids. Dermatol Surg 2003;29(1): 25–9.
85. Alexiades-Armenakas MR, Dover JS, Arndt KA. The spectrum of laser skin resurfacing: nonablative, fractional, and ablative laser resurfacing. J Am Acad Dermatol 2008;58(5):719–37 [quiz: 738–40].
86. Alster T, Zaulyanov L. Laser scar revision: a review. Dermatol Surg 2007;33(2):131–40.
87. Ciocon DH, Boker A, Goldberg DJ. Intense pulsed light: what works, what's new, what's next. Facial Plast Surg 2009;25(5):290–300.
88. Babilas P, Schreml S, Szeimies RM, et al. Intense pulsed light (IPL): a review. Lasers Surg Med 2010;42(2):93–104.
89. Duke D, Grevelink JM. Care before and after laser skin resurfacing. A survey and review of the literature. Dermatol Surg 1998;24(2):201–6.
90. Horton S, Alster TS. Preoperative and postoperative considerations for carbon dioxide laser resurfacing. Cutis 1999;64(6):399–406.
91. Beeson WH, Rachel JD. Valacyclovir prophylaxis for herpes simplex virus infection or infection recurrence following laser skin resurfacing. Dermatol Surg 2002;28(4):331–6.
92. Fitzpatrick RE, Williams B, Goldman MP. Preoperative anesthesia and postoperative considerations in laser resurfacing. Semin Cutan Med Surg 1996; 15(3):170–6.
93. Alster TS, Lupton JR. Treatment of complications of laser skin resurfacing. Arch Facial Plast Surg 2000; 2(4):279–84.
94. Apfelberg DB. Side effects, sequelae, and complications of carbon dioxide laser resurfacing. Aesthet Surg J 1997;17(6):365–72.
95. Goldman MP. The use of hydroquinone with facial laser resurfacing. J Cutan Laser Ther 2000;2(2): 73–7.

Cutaneous Vascular Lesions

Ravindhra G. Elluru, MD, PhD[a,b,*]

KEYWORDS

• Vascular anomalies • Vascular malformations • Hemangiomas • Capillary malformations • Venous malformations • Lymphatic malformations • Arteriovenous malformations

KEY POINTS

- All cutaneous vascular lesions (more appropriately called vascular anomalies) can be divided into vascular tumors and vascular malformations.
- The most common vascular tumors are infantile hemangiomas, which present shortly after birth, grow for 6 to 9 months, and then undergo programmed cell death, leading to involution.
- Vascular malformations are present at birth and are composed of dysmorphic blood vessels, which grow proportionate with the size of the child and do not involute as the child gets older.
- Kasabach-Merritt phenomenon is associated with kaposiform hemangioendotheliomas and tufted angiomas, and not infantile hemangiomas.
- Infantile hemangiomas that have the potential of causing long-term functional or aesthetic issues should be treated with medicine or surgery.
- Management of vascular malformations is limited mostly to laser, sclerotherapy, or surgical treatment.

VASCULAR TUMORS

Infantile Hemangioma

The most commonly occurring vascular tumor is the infantile hemangioma, affecting 1 in 10 white infants in North America, although it is less common in children of African or Asian descent (**Fig. 1**).[1,2] These tumors are more common in females (3:1) and in infants with low birth weight.[3] They are typically observed at birth or during the first several weeks of life. Lesions generally present cutaneously in the head and neck (60%), but can involve any anatomic site, including the extremities (15%), visceral organs, and brain.[3]

Infantile hemangiomas are clinically characterized as superficial, deep, or combined, depending on their anatomic depth. Superficial lesions are typically soft, red, and raised, whereas deep lesions show a spectrum of appearance and consistency, ranging from soft and supple to raised and firmer warm masses with a bluish hue. Combined lesions have both a red epidermal coloration and a subcutaneous mass that is either blue or flesh-colored.

Although most tumors present singularly, up to 20% of affected infants have multiple cutaneous lesions. When a patient has 6 or more cutaneous hemangiomas, there is an increased risk of having visceral hemangiomas, which in turn can give rise to serious or life-threatening conditions such as hepatomegaly, gastrointestinal bleeding, profound hypothyroidism, anemia, or congestive heart failure.[4,5]

Hemangiomas of infancy generally follow a predetermined clinical course of active growth (proliferation) and later tumor regression (involution); however, there is wide variation in the rate,

Disclosures: None.

[a] Division of Pediatric Otolaryngology-Head and Neck Surgery, Cincinnati Children's Hospital Medical Center, 3333 Burnet Avenue, MLC 2018, Cincinnati, OH 45229-3039, USA; [b] Department of Otolaryngology-Head and Neck Surgery, University of Cincinnati College of Medicine, Medical Sciences Building, Room 6507, 231 Albert Sabin Way, Cincinnati, OH 45267-0528, USA

* Division of Pediatric Otolaryngology-Head and Neck Surgery, Cincinnati Children's Hospital Medical Center, 3333 Burnet Avenue; MLC 2018, Cincinnati, OH 45229-3039.

E-mail address: ravi.elluru@cchmc.org

Facial Plast Surg Clin N Am 21 (2013) 111–126
http://dx.doi.org/10.1016/j.fsc.2012.11.001
1064-7406/13/$ – see front matter

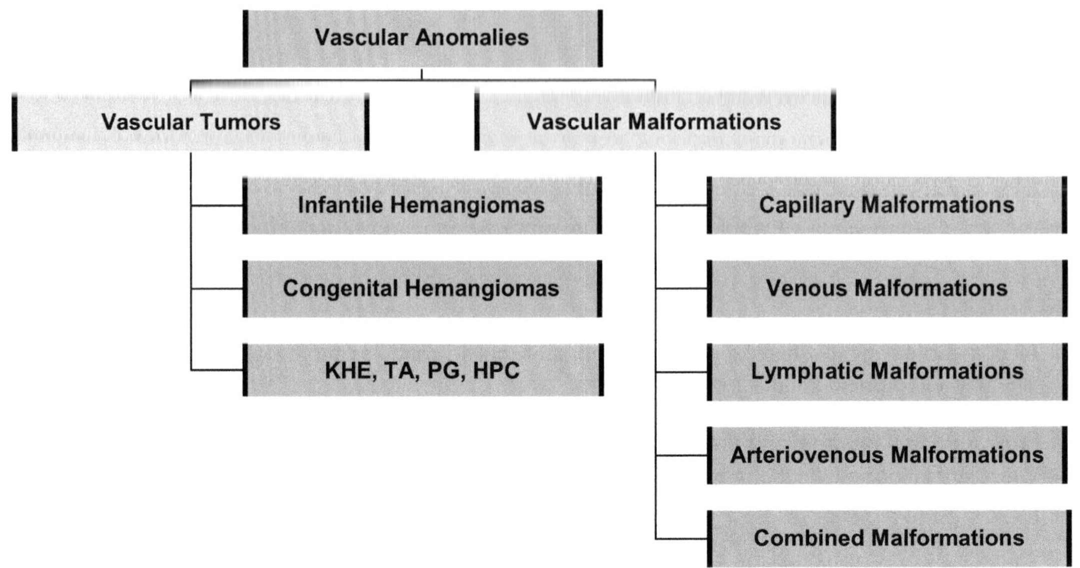

Fig. 1. The 1996 International Society for the Study of Vascular Anomalies classification of vascular anomalies. HPC, hemangiopericytoma; KHE, kaposiform hemangioendothelioma; PG, pyogenic granuloma; TA, tufted angioma.

duration, and degree of growth and spontaneous tumor regression. Proliferation begins during the first few weeks of life and generally continues for 4 to 10 months, although deep lesions may proliferate until age 2 years. The proliferative phase is followed by a period of quiescence, during which the growth rate of the lesion stabilizes. Involution occurs at 12 to 18 months and can last up to 5 to 6 years. During this time, the color of the lesion fades, becoming grayish or dull purple (**Fig. 2**). Clinical studies show that maximum involution occurs in 50% of children by age 5 years and in 90% by age 9 years.[6–12]

The cosmetic outcome after involution varies considerably and is generally unpredictable. In many patients, involution results in the restoration of normal skin. In others (20%–40%), residual changes of the skin such as laxity, discoloration, telangiectasia, fibrofatty masses, or scarring are seen in the affected area. Given this unpredictability, for patients who are not at risk, clinical monitoring, parental education, and ongoing support are preferable to early intervention.

There is sound evidence that hemangiomas of infancy are related to placental endothelial cells. Four markers of hemangioma cells that are coexpressed in placental vessels have been identified[13]:

1. GLUT1 (a glucose transporter enzyme)
2. Merosin
3. Lewis Y antigen
4. Fcγ-RIIb

GLUT1 is strongly expressed in infantile hemangiomas, placentas, and the blood-brain barrier; however, it is not expressed in normal surrounding vascular endothelium or in vascular malformations, nor is it generally expressed in congenital hemangiomas (see later discussion). Because the positive expression of GLUT1 persists throughout all phases of the hemangioma life cycle, this histochemical marker is particularly useful in distinguishing hemangiomas of infancy from other vascular tumors and from vascular malformations.

Congenital Hemangiomas

Congenital hemangiomas are an uncommon variant of infantile hemangiomas. They differ from infantile hemangiomas in clinical behavior, appearance, and histopathology, and are occasionally diagnosed in utero. Unlike infantile hemangiomas, congenital hemangiomas present at birth as fully grown lesions and do not undergo additional postnatal growth. Congenital hemangiomas fall into distinct subgroups: rapidly involuting congenital hemangiomas (RICHs) and noninvoluting congenital hemangiomas (NICHs).[14] RICHs typically involute by age 12 to 14 months, leaving a residual patch of thin skin with prominent veins and little, if any, subcutaneous fat. NICHs do not undergo involution. Both tumor types have a predilection for the head or limbs. Both tumor types generally present as solitary violaceous lesions at birth and rarely coexist in a patient with a typical infantile hemangioma. Both are high-flow lesions

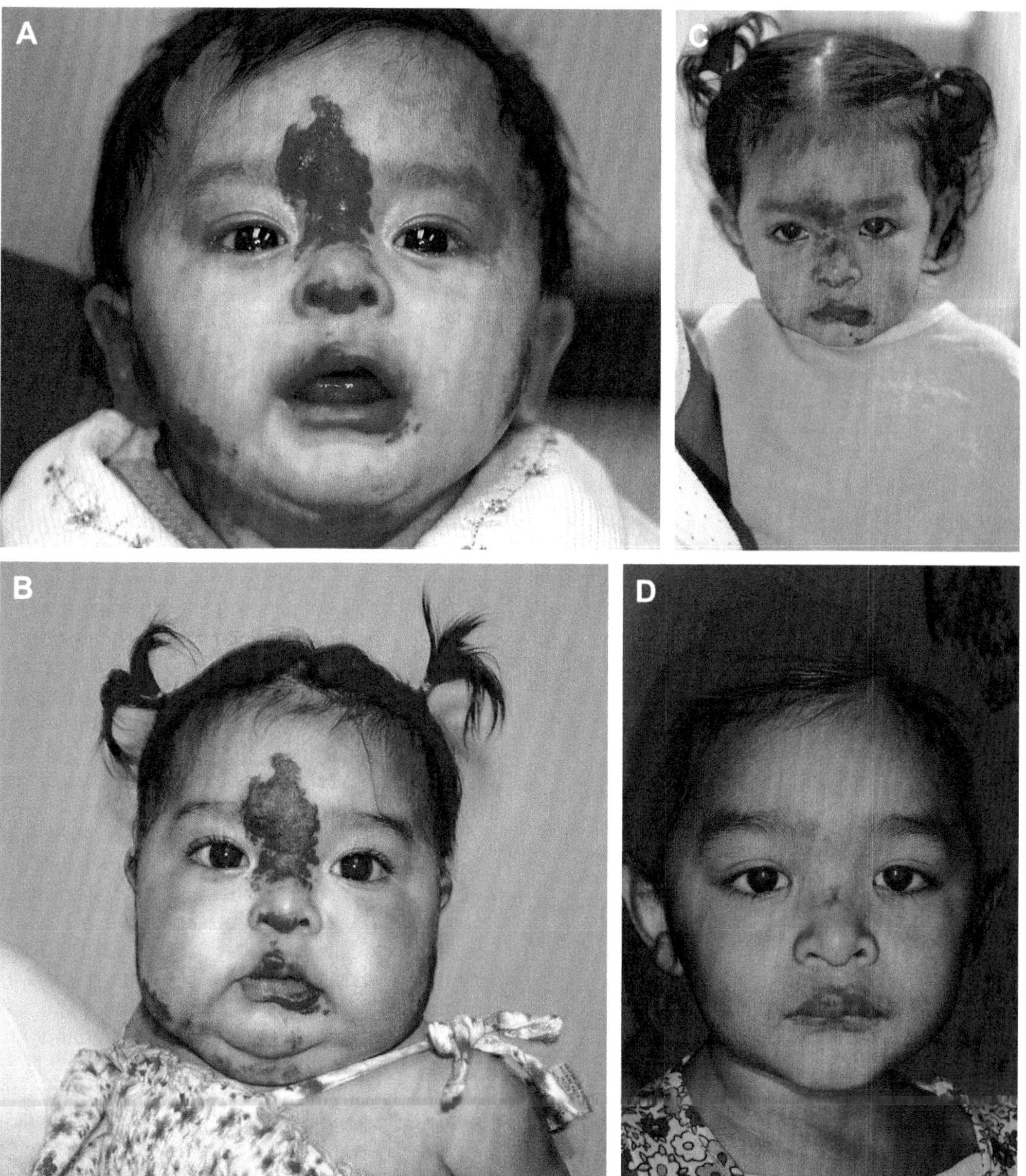

Fig. 2. Infantile hemangiomas undergo a process of natural regression. (*A*) A young girl at 2 months, (*B*) 6 months, (*C*) 18 months, and (*D*) 36 months of age. As the child grows older, the hemangioma changes from bright red to a grayish red, and finally to the natural skin color. The mass of the lesion also decreases, leaving little evidence of the hemangioma over time.

that can be misdiagnosed as arteriovenous malformations (AVMs). In contrast to infantile hemangiomas, congenital hemangiomas are GLUT1 negative and comprise less than 3% of all hemangiomas seen in infancy.[15]

Problematic Head and Neck Hemangiomas

Hemangiomas can occur anywhere in the head and neck region. Hemangiomas can occur singularly on the neck, cheek, nose, ears, forehead, or scalp, or multifocally at several of these sites. The head and neck can also be the site of segmental hemangiomas that occupy an entire developmental subunit (**Fig. 3**).

PHACES

Hemangiomas that present in developmental segments are referred to as segmental lesions. These lesions are less common than focal lesions

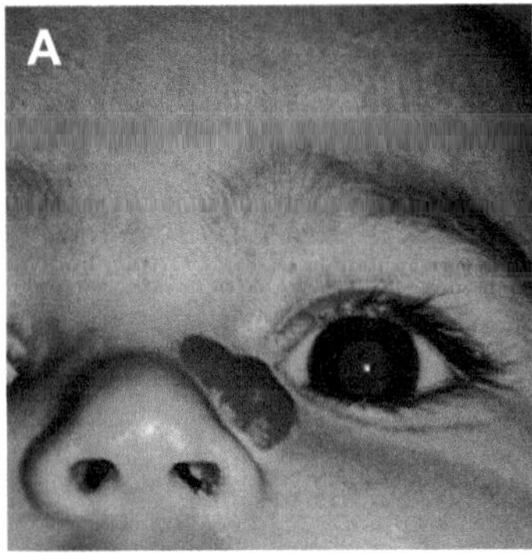

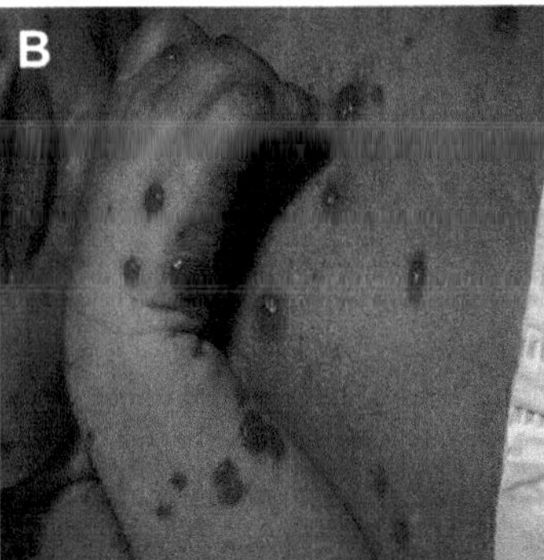

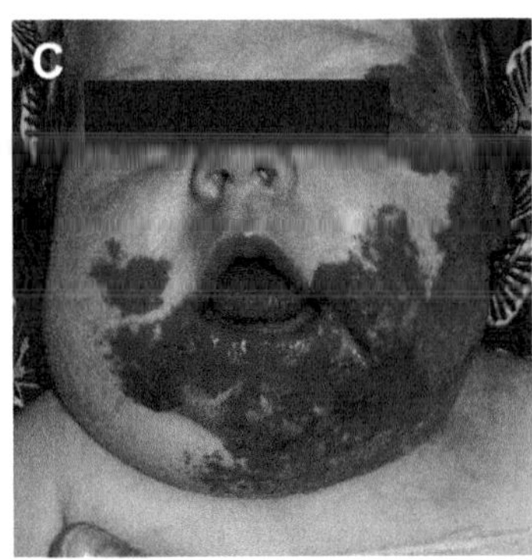

Fig. 3. Children with hemangiomas demonstrating variations in morphology. (*A*) A child with an isolated focal hemangioma. (*B*) A child with multiple cutaneous hemangiomas. (*C*) A child with a facial segmental hemangioma occupying the periorbital, temporal, cheek, and chin areas of the face. Segmental hemangiomas are prone to ulceration as can be seen in this child around the left nasolabial crease.

and have a higher risk of being life-threatening or function-threatening and of having associated structural anomalies. Large cervicofacial segmental hemangiomas, particularly those on the forehead, temple, upper cheek, and around the periorbital area can be accompanied by a constellation of anomalies referred to as PHACES association.[16] This association is more common in females. Accompanying anomalies include:

- Posterior fossa brain malformations (eg, Dandy-Walker malformation)
- Hemangiomas
- Arterial abnormalities
- Cardiac and aortic arch defects (eg, aneurysms, and congenital valvular aortic stenosis)
- Eye abnormalities (eg, congenital cataract, microphthalmia, and abnormal retinal vessels)
- Sternal clefts or supraumbilical raphes

More than 50% of patients are affected by neurologic sequelae, including seizures, stroke, developmental delay, and migraines.[17]

Segmental hemangiomas are plaquelike in contour, typically undergo an extended proliferative period of 18 months, and unlike most hemangiomas of infancy, they do not completely regress. Furthermore, segmental hemangiomas are at a higher risk of ulceration and residual scarring.[16] When there is an index of suspicion for PHACES association, referral should be made for an ophthalmologic and neurologic examination, screening echocardiogram, and possibly magnetic resonance imaging (MRI) or magnetic resonance angiography (MRA) of the head, neck, and chest. Patients in whom imaging reveals a central nervous system abnormality should be closely monitored. The frequency of repeated imaging depends on symptom presentation and disease progression.

Hemangiomas in a beard distribution

Sixty-five percent of patients with hemangiomas that occur in a beard distribution (ie, the chin, jawline, and preauricular areas) have associated airway involvement,[18] and most airway hemangiomas are localized in the supraglottic or subglottic region. Patients must be closely followed and treatment should be initiated when airway involvement is suspected. Localized lesions are managed with laser ablation, intralesional steroids, surgical resection, or medical therapy (see later discussion). Tracheotomy placement is used only in refractory cases or in cases in which the airway hemangioma is extensive. Hemangiomas that occur in the beard distribution often involve the parotid glands. Parotid gland hemangiomas typically occupy the entire gland and adjacent parapharyngeal space. They grow rapidly, causing extrinsic compression of the upper pharyngeal airway. These lesions frequently have a prolonged proliferative phase (12–16 months) and may require systemic therapy if the airway is compromised.[19] Children with extensive hemangioma of the parotid region and pharyngeal area often have chronic recurrent otitis media, likely secondary to extrinsic compression of the eustachian tube.

Periocular hemangiomas

Periocular hemangiomas can involve the upper lid, lower lid, or the retrobulbar space (**Fig. 4**). Pressure from the hemangioma on the globe may lead to astigmatism and amblyopia. Early ophthalmologic evaluation and treatment are indicated for all cases of periocular hemangiomas to avoid deprivation amblyopia, which can occur with as little as

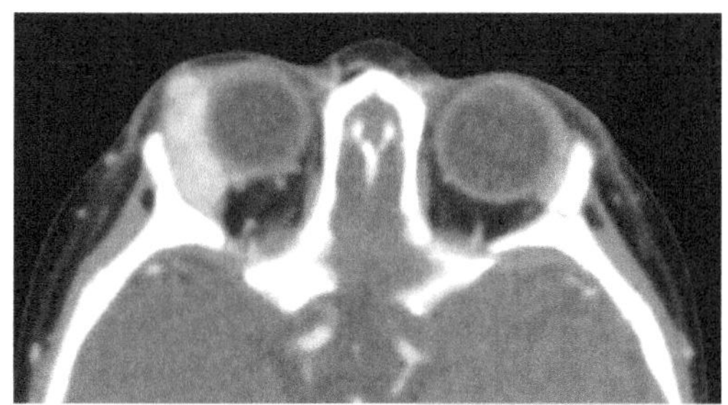

Fig. 4. An axial cut through the orbit of a child with a right preseptal and postseptal orbital hemangioma.

1 week of deprivation during key developmental periods. Treatment options for vision obstructing periocular hemangiomas include either medical therapy or surgical excision. Children older than 1 year who have gone untreated have rates of deprivation amblyopia as high as 75%.

Nose, lip, and ear hemangiomas

Hemangiomas involving the nose occur in close to 16% of facial hemangiomas.[20,21] Proliferation of lesions on the nasal tip often distort the anatomy of the nose, causing misalignment of the nasal cartilages and mild to severe nasal volume increase. Management approaches must consider the depth, location, rate of involution, and functional and cosmetic disturbance caused by the lesion. In view of possible complications such as severe cutaneous infiltration, the consequences on nasal growth, and the psychological impact of nasal distortion, surgical excision before school age is recommended. Various surgical techniques have been reported.[22]

Lesions of the pinna of the ear can deform normal anatomic structures and result in ulceration, with focal destruction of the auricle. Lesions obstructing the auditory canal can cause temporary conductive hearing loss. Lip lesions frequently involute slowly, sometimes leaving residual skin changes. In addition, lip ulcerations can result in feeding difficulties, secondary infection, and significant scarring.

Subglottic hemangiomas

Hemangiomas can occur anywhere within the tracheobronchial tree; however, they are most commonly seen in the subglottis (**Fig. 5**). As mentioned earlier, there is a close association of hemangiomas in a beard distribution with airway hemangiomas. However, airway hemangiomas can occur without associated cutaneous hemangiomas. Only 50% of patients with airway hemangiomas have cutaneous hemangiomas.[23] Presentation usually occurs within the first 6 months of life, and the earlier the presentation, the greater the likelihood that patients will require surgical intervention. Symptoms typically include progressive stridor and retractions. The diagnosis is made on rigid bronchoscopy, and although radiologic evaluation (MRI with contrast enhancement) is indicated, it rarely shows extension of the lesion beyond the confines of the subglottis. Lesions are typically asymmetric and usually covered by a normal smooth mucosa. Treatment options range from medical management to laser ablation and surgical excision.

Kasabach-Merritt phenomenon

Kasabach-Merritt phenomenon is a rare, life-threatening condition associated with 2 specific subtypes of vascular tumors: tufted angioma or kaposiform hemangioendothelioma. Kasabach-Merritt phenomenon is included in this section only to highlight the fact that it is not associated with infantile hemangiomas, as sometimes construed. In Kasabach-Merritt phenomenon, the tumor traps and destroys platelets. In addition to platelet trapping, there are other associated coagulopathies. As the tumor grows, it causes more platelet trapping. No single treatment approach is effective, and responses to various treatments are inconsistent.

Diagnostic Evaluation of Infantile Hemangiomas

The diagnosis of infantile hemangiomas is generally established by clinical presentation, history, and physical examination. In patients with complex lesions that require surgical intervention, additional investigations can be helpful in determining the extent of involvement. Ultrasonography (US) with color flow Doppler can be useful in differentiating hemangiomas from vascular malformations that may have a similar appearance. On US, an infantile hemangioma appears hypoechoic, well-defined, and heterogeneous in texture, with small cystic and sinusoidal spaces. In most proliferating hemangiomas, a characteristic fast-flow pattern and blood vessel density (>5 blood vessels/cm^2) is visualized by Doppler US (**Fig. 6**).

MRI and computed tomography (CT) scans can delineate the extent and involvement of the hemangioma and can also be helpful in distinguishing hemangiomas from other malformations (**Table 1**).[24] In the proliferative phase, a hemangioma appears as a well-circumscribed tumor with homogeneous parenchymatous density and intense enhancement. In the involutive phase, it appears heterogeneous, with distinct lobular architecture and large draining veins in the center and the periphery. Biopsy is indicated when the

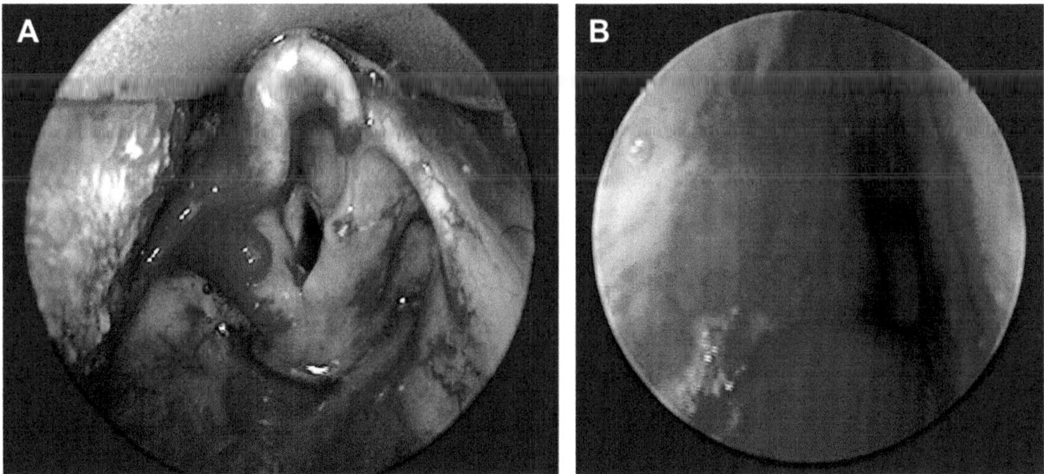

Fig. 5. Endoscopic photographs of (*A*) a child with flat supraglottic hemangiomas occupying the left epiglottis and aryepiglottic fold and (*B*) a child with a large left subglottic hemangioma that severely narrows the subglottic lumen.

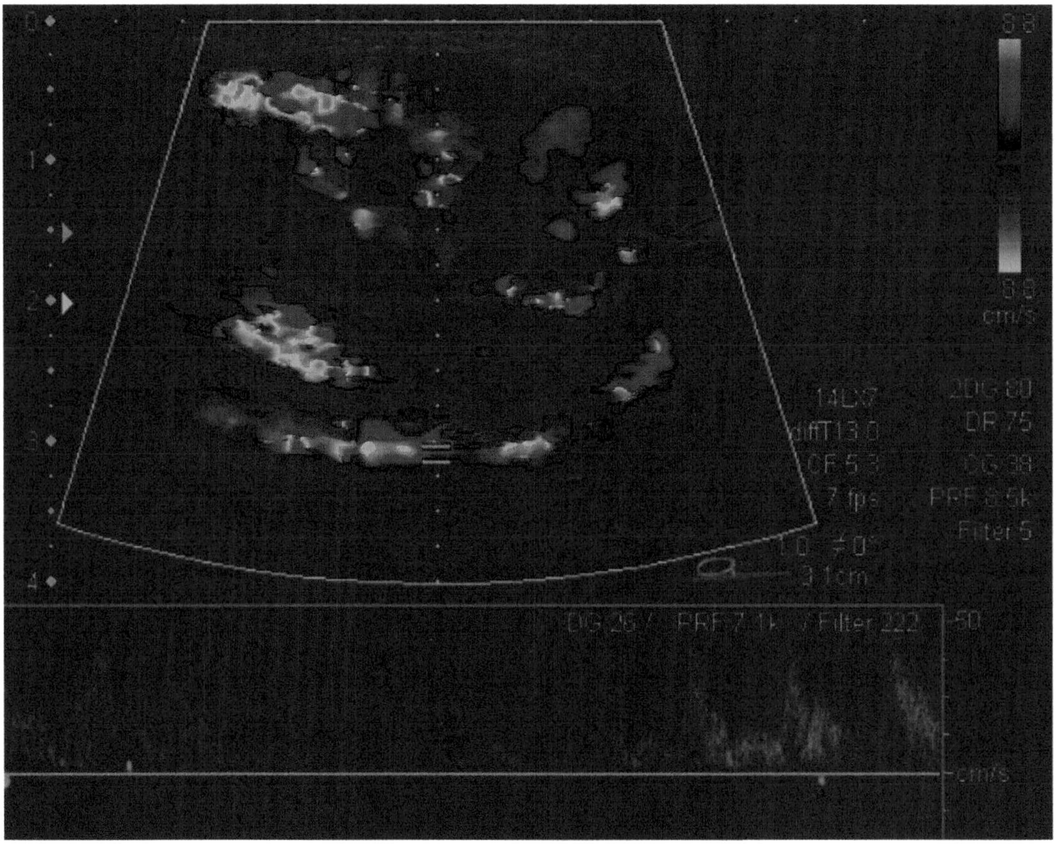

Fig. 6. Color US Doppler image of an infantile hemangioma. Infantile hemangiomas are composed of small blood vessels conducting blood at high flow rates (*top panel*). Doppler shows that the blood flow in these small blood vessels is pulsatile, characterized by a rapid upstroke and a gradual down stroke in flow rates (*bottom panel*).

Table 1
MRI characteristics of vascular anomalies

Anomaly Type	T1-Weighted	T2-Weighted	Contrast	Gradient
Hemangioma	Soft-tissue mass, isointense or hypointense, flow voids	Lobulated soft-tissue mass, increased signal, flow voids	Uniform intense enhancement	High-flow vessels within and around soft-tissue mass
Venous malformation	Isointense to muscle, possible high signal thrombi	Septated soft-tissue mass, high signal, signal voids (phleboliths)	Diffuse or inhomogeneous enhancement	No high-flow vessels
Lymphatic malformation	Septated soft-tissue mass, low signal	Soft tissue mass, high signal, fluid levels	Rim enhancement or no enhancement	No high-flow vessels
Arteriovenous malformation	Soft tissue thickening, flow voids	Variable increased flow voids	Diffuse enhancement	High-flow vessels throughout abnormal tissue

Data from Dubois J, Garel L. Imaging and therapeutic approach of hemangiomas and vascular malformations in the pediatric age group. Pediatr Radiol 1999;29(12):879–93.

diagnosis is uncertain or when the possibility of malignancy must be ruled out.

Treatment of Infantile Hemangiomas

Most uncomplicated focal hemangiomas involute spontaneously and do not require intervention. Nevertheless, rapidly proliferating lesions are sometimes problematic and can cause a wide array of complications, including ulceration, infection, hemorrhage, necrosis, airway obstruction, loss of vision, and cardiac failure. To ensure timely intervention should any of these complications occur, patients should be closely monitored during the proliferative phase. Optimally, management strategies for complex lesions should be planned by a multidisciplinary team of clinicians with expertise in treating vascular anomalies. Management decisions should consider the size and location of the lesion, the presence of complications at diagnosis, the age of the patient, and the rate of tumor growth. Large segmental hemangiomas and life-threatening or function-threatening hemangiomas are likely to require immediate treatment. Immediate treatment is also essential in the presence of ulceration or secondary infection. Serious aesthetic concerns such as the possibility of permanent disfigurement or scarring warrant early intervention.

These patients almost always require multimodal therapy. Major therapies include pharmacotherapy, chemotherapy, laser therapy, and surgical excision. Recently, the dramatic effect of oral propranolol has been reported in several small case series,[25–27] and prospective studies are under way at several major centers. Although research regarding propranolol is in its infancy, this medication has replaced steroids as the first line in medical management. Propranolol is discussed further later.

Ulceration is the most common complication of hemangiomas, often occurring in lesions involving the nose, lips, and periorbital region.[28] Most ulcers develop during a phase of rapid growth. They are often painful and can lead to infection, anemia, scarring, and disfigurement. Treatment should focus on decreasing pain, preventing secondary infections, and promoting reepithelialization. Painful ulcerations may require oral medications such as acetaminophen or acetaminophen with codeine. Superficial ulcerations generally respond to supportive therapy such as gentle cleansing and the daily application of a topical antibiotic. Dressings that cover the ulceration such as DuoDERM (Convatec, Skillman, New Jersey) or Mepilex (Molnlycke Health Care US, LLC, Norcross, Georgia) can provide pain relief and promote healing. When an associated cellulitis occurs, oral systemic antibiotics are given. Ulcerations on localized cervicofacial lesions are amenable to surgical resection, which generally results in excellent cosmetic outcomes. When resection is not feasible or desirable, Pulse Dye Laser (PDL) is used to promote reepithelialization and decrease pain. This approach is particularly helpful in anatomic areas that are not amenable to resection, such as extensive facial lesions. Products such as imiquimod, which stimulates endogenous interferon production, and becaplermin gel, which seems to accelerate reepithelialization, have been used for treating refractory ulcerated hemangiomas, but require further study.

Until recently, corticosteroids have remained the first line of therapy for the treatment of complicated hemangiomas.[29,30] Currently, the 2 indications for the use of corticosteroids in the treatment of infantile hemangiomas is for those patients who fail propranolol treatment or for intralesional injection in small focal hemangiomas.[31] Local injection is especially effective in the periorbital region, nasal tip, and subglottic region. Some surgeons and ophthalmologists recommend using general anesthesia, whereas others perform the procedure on an outpatient basis using a topical anesthetic. A long-acting steroid (eg, triamcinolone acetonide) and a short-acting steroid (eg, betamethasone acetate) can be combined in a total volume that generally does not exceed 2.5 mL. The dose and volume are individualized according to the size of the lesion. A 25-gauge needle is used and injections are made directly into the hemangioma in different directions through the same needle hole. After this stage, direct pressure is applied for 2 to 10 minutes to stop bleeding. In subglottic lesions, it is important to avoid direct injection of the cricoid plate, because cartilage resorption may occur. Although this approach is associated with a 70% to 90% response rate in periorbital hemangiomas, a known complication is the risk of retinal artery embolization and thrombosis, with resulting blindness.[32–36] To lessen this risk, fundoscopic retinal examination should be performed as the lesion is slowly injected so as to recognize early signs of retinal arterial flow interruption. Adrenal suppression and failure to thrive have also been reported after local injection for periocular hemangioma.[31]

Propranolol, a nonselective β-blocker, has recently been introduced as a novel modality for the treatment of proliferating hemangiomas. The dramatic effect of propranolol therapy on hemangiomas was first described in 2008 by Leaute-Labreze and colleagues.[25] These investigators serendipitously discovered that propranolol induced early regression of infantile hemangiomas during their proliferative phase. Their reported findings in a small series of infants sparked the enthusiasm of clinicians eager to identify appropriate uses for propranolol. Buckmiller and colleagues[27] reported the successful management of tracheal hemangiomas in a young patient with otherwise treatment-resistant airway lesions. Within 6 weeks of beginning oral propranolol (2 mg/kg/d), airway compromise was eliminated and the patient had complete resolution of endoscopically visible disease. No side effects occurred. Denoyelle and colleagues[26] reported the successful management of 2 infants with subglottic hemangiomas that were resistant to established medical treatments. Both patients' subglottic hemangiomas responded dramatically to propranolol and no side effects were noted. The mechanisms of action are speculative, but may involve the downregulation of angiogenic factors and upregulation of apoptosis. Early research shows that propranolol may be a safe and effective therapeutic strategy for both cutaneous and airway lesions. There is controversy as to the diagnostic testing needed before drug administration and the appropriate venue (inpatient or outpatient) for the drug. **Box 1** shows an inpatient and outpatient algorithm developed by our vascular anomalies team. In general, we advocate inpatient protocol for infants younger than 2 years and children with comorbidities. The parents of all other children are given the choice of inpatient or outpatient treatment. Side effects that have been reported to date include hypoglycemic seizures and sleep disturbance.

Lasers have a limited role in the treatment of hemangiomas. The PDL is often used at the end of the involution phase to reduce any residual vascular markings. PDLs are also used as mentioned earlier to promote wound healing, reepithelialization, and pain control for ulcerated hemangiomas that are refractory to medical management. CO_2 and ND:YAG (neodymium-doped yttrium aluminum garnet) lasers have been used to ablate airway hemangiomas, although overaggressive use of these lasers can cause scar deposition and subglottic stenosis.

The indications for the surgical excision of hemangiomas are in evolution, especially given the natural regression of these lesions and the efficacy of medical management. Nonetheless, there are several clinical situations in which surgical excision is an attractive treatment option (**Box 2**). Large hemangiomas that are likely to leave large amounts of fibrofatty residuum or excess skin are often good candidates for surgical excision. Ulcerative hemangiomas that fail medical management and can be excised completely are another candidate for surgical excision (**Fig. 7**). Periorbital hemangiomas and airway hemangiomas that are causing significant signs and symptoms and are unlikely to respond quickly or do not respond to medical management are often best treated by surgical excision. Hemangiomas that are not completely resolved by school age and cause psychosocial distress can also be treated with surgical excision. The timing of surgery remains a controversial subject, particularly in regard to early surgery on hemangiomas that are disfiguring and in which the results of spontaneous involution are difficult to predict. Surgical intervention should be considered when surgery is believed to provide

Box 1
Algorithm or propranolol initiation

Inpatient Propranolol Algorithm

- Preadmission diagnostic testing: echocardiogram to rule out congenital anomalies in patients with a history of murmurs, failure to thrive, or other significant medical comorbidities; electrocardiography (EKG) to rule out cardiac arrhythmia
- Admit to telemetry unit with continuous heart rate and blood pressure monitoring
- Initiate propranolol at 0.5 mg/kg by mouth twice a day for 2 doses; increase to 1 mg/kg by mouth twice a day for 2 doses; increase to 2 mg/kg by mouth twice a day
- Propranolol is increased in this manner if the patient shows no adverse response to the administration of the medication
- Check blood glucose 2 hours after each dose of propranolol
- Check EKG 24 hours after initiation of propranolol
- Discharge home after second dose of propranolol at 2 mg/kg, with contact information if questions or problems arise
- Parents are instructed to maintain a strict feeding regimen. If the child is younger than 6 months, feeds should be every 2 to 4 hours. Older children can be spaced to feeds every 6 to 8 hours
- Parents are instructed to hold medication if the child becomes ill or has decreased oral intake

Outpatient Propranolol Algorithm

- Diagnostic testing: same as for inpatient algorithm
- Monitor on telemetry unit for 6 hours with continuous blood pressure and heart rate monitoring
- Initiate propranolol at 0.5 mg/kg
- Check blood glucose 2 hours after each dose of propranolol
- Discharge instructions as for inpatient algorithm, with contact information if questions or problems arise
- Continue propranolol at 0.5 mg/kg by mouth twice a day or 1 week
- Return to hospital for 6-hour admission on telemetry unit, during which propranolol is increased to 1 mg/kg. An EKG is obtained before increasing the dose, and blood glucose is checked 2 hours after dose. Discharge home at this dose for a week, with discharge instructions as previously
- Return to hospital for 6-hour admission, during which propranolol is increased to 2 mg/kg. Blood glucose is again checked 2 hours after dose. Patient is discharged home, with discharge instructions as previously with follow-up in 4 weeks

a better overall outcome to the patient than natural regression or medical management.

VASCULAR MALFORMATIONS

Vascular malformations are the second major category of vascular anomalies (see **Fig. 1**). In contrast to vascular tumors, vascular malformations are present at birth and grow commensurately with size of the child. Although the molecular mechanisms underlying the formation of these lesions remain unclear, they are known to result from abnormal development and morphogenesis. Histologic examination of vascular malformations shows no evidence of cellular proliferation, but rather progressive dilation of abnormal channels. Vascular malformations are designated according to the predominant channel type present. They are classified as capillary, venous, lymphatic, arterial, or combined malformations. Malformations with an arterial component are rheologically fast-flow, whereas capillary, lymphatic, and venous malformations are slow-flow in nature. The morbidity of vascular malformations varies greatly both within and among the clinical subgroups cited earlier.

Diagnostic Modalities

Accurate and expeditious diagnosis is essential to the proper treatment of vascular malformations. A diagnosis is arrived at only after a thorough and complete history and physical examination. Key parts of the history include the age at which parents initially noticed the lesion; overall rate of growth of

Box 2
Relative indications for surgical management of hemangiomas

- Noninvoluting congenital hemangioma.
- Ulcerative hemangioma that will likely leave a large scar.
- A hemangioma that is causing significant functional compromise or signs and symptoms and is not responding expeditiously to medical management. Examples of functional compromise include obstruction of visual axis with changes in vision, or airway obstruction.
- A hemangioma that has a pedunculated appearance, and therefore will likely not involute completely.
- A hemangioma that causes significant psychosocial or appearance issues to the patient as they enter school and that can be removed with a satisfactory cosmetic outcome.

the lesion as well as recent changes in the size of the lesion; and acute changes in the size of the lesion concordant with upper respiratory tract infections, trauma, hormonal changes, body position, Valsalva maneuver, or high cardiac output states. In addition to the history, a complete review of systems is essential. Fundamental aspects of the physical examination include the extent and color of the lesion, the three-dimensional morphology of the lesion, temperature, presence of vascular marking, compressibility of the lesion, and whether the lesion is pulsatile.

Radiologic imaging is frequently the next step in the diagnostic algorithm, which is used not only to validate the clinical diagnosis but also to determine the extent of the lesion. Imaging modalities used include US, MRI, and, infrequently, arteriograms. Each subclass of vascular malformation has classic radiologic findings that are helpful in diagnosis (see **Table 1**). The success of using radiologic imaging as a tool in the diagnosis of vascular malformations depends on the expertise of the radiologist. In most institutions, the radiologist is a key member of the multidisciplinary team that delivers care to children with vascular anomalies.

Capillary Malformations

Capillary malformations are the most commonly occurring subgroup of vascular malformations. The 2 most common types of capillary malformations are salmon patches (naevus simplex) and port-wine stains (naevus flammeus) (**Fig. 8**). This malformation consists of a superficial collection of ectatic vessels that is located in the papillary and superficial reticular dermis, with a mean depth of 0.46 mm.[37] Salmon patches are common and manifest as macular capillary stains, colloquially referred to as angel kisses or stork bites. They generally appear as pink macules on the forehead, eyelids, nose, and nuchal region, and characteristically fade or disappear during childhood. Port-wine stains also present at birth as flat, light-pink, macular lesions. However, in contrast to angel kisses or stork bites, port-wine stains become raised, nodular, or darken to a deep red and persist throughout life. Port-wine stains occur in 0.3% of newborns and frequently appear within the distribution of the trigeminal nerve.[38]

Most isolated port-wine stains occur sporadically, although an autosomal-dominant inheritance pattern has been reported in some families. Port-wine stains may occur in conjunction with other vascular anomalies or congenital malformations. For example in Wyburn-Mason syndrome, port-wine facial stains are associated with a unilateral

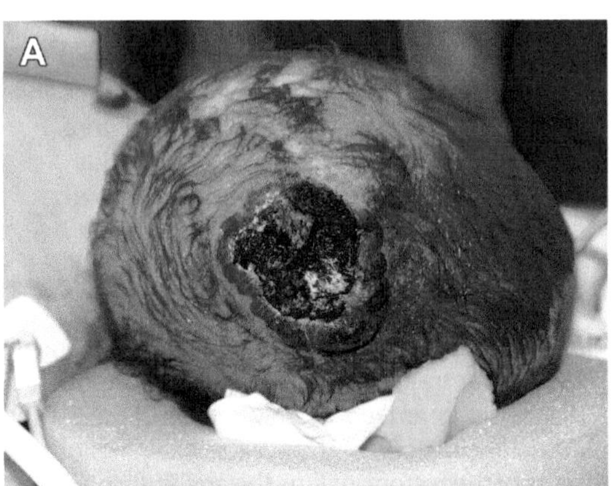

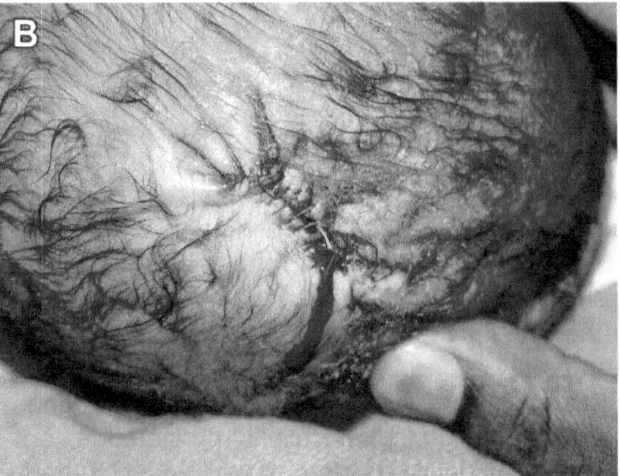

Fig. 7. A patient with a large ulcerative scalp hemangioma (*A*) that was surgically excised (*B*).

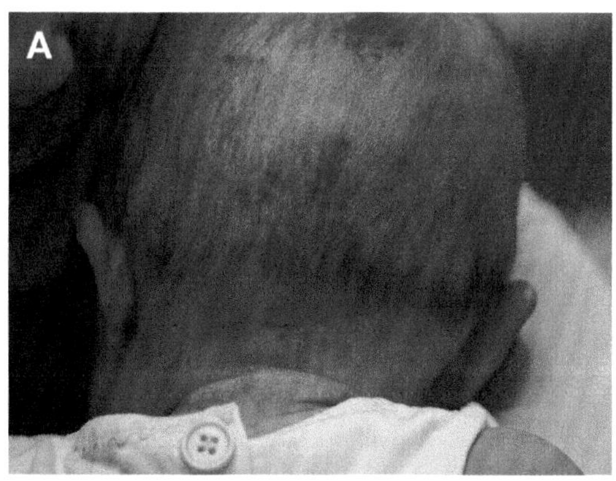

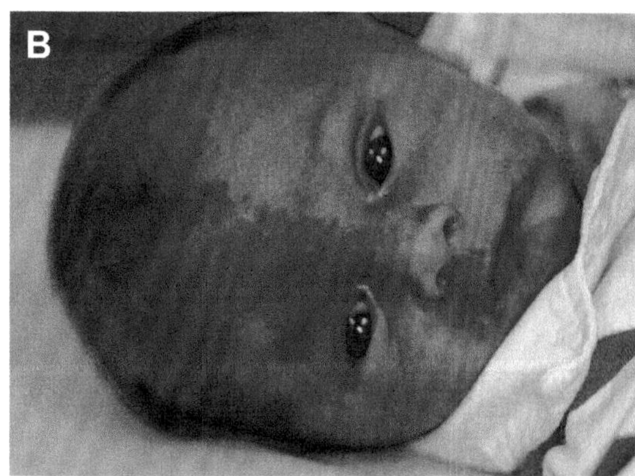

Fig. 8. (*A*) A salmon patch on the posterior neck of a patient. (*B*) A port-wine stain covering the upper right half of the face.

AVM of the retina and intracranial optic pathway.[38] When port-wine stains appear in the trigeminal nerve distribution, there may be associated structural and vascular abnormalities of the face and leptomeninges (Sturge-Weber syndrome) (see **Fig. 8**).[39] Glaucoma occurs in approximately 10% of patients with facial port-wine stains and can occur without leptomeningeal involvement. For these reasons, children with craniofacial involvement should undergo an MRI or CT scan to rule out central nervous system disease.

Sturge-Weber syndrome deserves additional attention, given its unique clinical manifestations. Sturge-Weber syndrome typically presents with a facial port-wine stain in the ophthalmic distribution of the trigeminal nerve, glaucoma and vascular eye abnormalities, and an ipsilateral intracranial vascular malformation. Children with Sturge-Weber syndrome often develop progressive neurologic problems, including seizures, migraines, strokelike episodes, learning difficulties or mental retardation, visual field impairment, or hemiparesis. Furthermore, overgrowth of the craniofacial skeleton can sometimes be noted on the side of the lesion, causing most notably a cross-bite deformity. The specific genetic and environmental factors that result in the disorder are unknown, but the localized abnormalities of blood vessel development and function affecting the facial skin, eye, and brain suggest that a developmental disruption occurs during the first trimester of pregnancy.[39]

Treatment with PDL is often used to mitigate the red coloration of port-wine stains and prevent the progression to more darkly colored and raised lesions. Based on the theory of selective photothermolysis,[40] PDL is able to preserve the epidermis by allowing hemoglobin to be more precisely targeted within lesions, resulting in less injury to adjacent nontargeted tissue. In capillary lesions that have thickened and become darker with age, the Nd:YAG laser has been used successfully, although patients are often left with some residual scarring. Other options, although of limited use, include surgical debulking of hypertrophied lip and eyelid tissue, and skin grafting of facial aesthetic units.[38] Medical management usually takes priority and consists of ameliorating associated health problems such as glaucoma and seizures.

Venous Malformations

Congenital venous malformations consist of either localized or diffuse ectatic veins with abnormal collections of irregular venous channels having flat, mitotically inactive endothelia and scant mural smooth muscle. These lesions may be superficial (ie, intradermal or subcutaneous) or deep (ie, intramuscular or intraosseous) (**Fig. 9**). For the most part, they are asymptomatic. Superficial venous malformations have a bluish compressible mass,

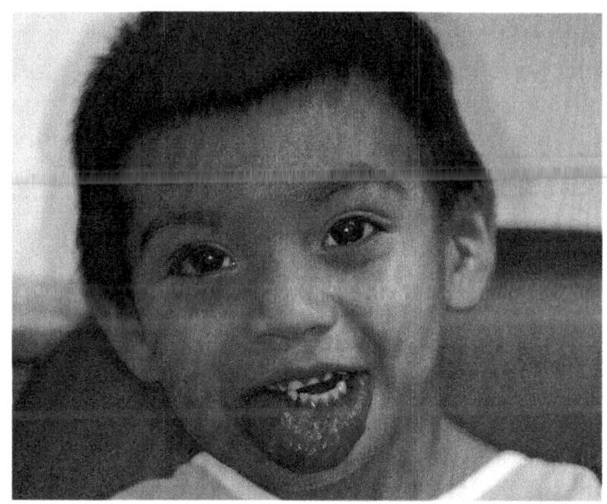

Fig. 9. A young boy with an extensive venous malformation of the right check and lower lip.

with no palpable thrill or audible bruit. These lesions often enlarge when the lesion is in a dependent position, with Valsalva maneuver, or high cardiac output states. Phleboliths can be seen on radiograph and are pathognomonic for venous malformations. Doppler echocardiography, MRI or MRA, and direct-puncture phlebography may be required to confirm the diagnosis and assess the extent of the lesion. When malformations are extensive, a blood coagulation profile should be performed. Because patients with extensive venous malformations are at risk for a pulmonary embolus after surgery, they require antithromboembolic prophylactic treatment.[29]

Treatment depends on the location, associated symptoms, and extent of the venous malformation. Phleboliths within the malformation often cause pain. Symptoms caused by phleboliths can be treated medically with aspirin, nonsteroidal antiinflammatory drugs, or low-molecular-weight heparin. When a lesion is localized and accessible, surgical excision results in excellent outcomes. More extensive lesions are often not amenable to resection or only partially resectable. To preserve function when vital structures are involved, a series of sclerotherapy procedures with one of a variety of sclerosing agents (see section on lymphatic malformations) is often performed.[41] Superficial lesions or the superficial component of deep lesions can be treated with the Nd:YAG laser.[42,43] Recurrent painful intramuscular or intra-articular bleeding or thrombosis and phlebolith formation can be ongoing problems.

Lymphatic Malformations

Lymphatic malformations are benign vascular lesions that arise from embryologic disturbances in the development of the lymphatic system. They encompass a wide spectrum of abnormalities, including cystic lymphatic lesions (formerly referred to as lymphangiomas), lymphangiectasis, and lymphedema. Given that lymphangiectasis and lymphedema usually involve sites other than the head and neck, these topics are not further discussed in this article.

Cystic lymphatic malformations can be seen in any anatomic region but are more commonly seen in rich lymphatic areas, such as the head and neck (45%–52%), axilla, mediastinum, groin, and retroperitoneum. These malformations are believed to be the result of maldevelopment of the embryonic lymphatics or lymphatic jugular sacs, with failure of these structures to connect or drain into the venous system. In some patients, a venous malformation can be seen in association with a cystic lymphatic lesion. There are 3 morphologic types of cystic lymphatic lesions: microcystic, macrocystic, and combined. Microcystic malformations present as clear, tiny vesicles that permeate the subcutaneous tissue and muscles. Microcystic lesions are commonly found above the level of the mylohyoid muscle and involve the oral cavity, oropharynx, tongue, parotid gland, submandibular gland, and pre-epiglottic space (**Fig. 10**). These vesicles are often firm and may give the impression of a brawny edema. Macrocystic lesions are large, compressible or noncompressible, smooth, translucent masses under normal or bluish skin. Most macrocystic lesions are multilocular structures consisting of numerous cysts that vary in size. Macrocystic lesions are often located below the level of the mylohyoid muscle and involve the anterior and posterior cervical triangles.[38]

Large cystic lymphatic lesions can be diagnosed in utero by US as early as the beginning of the second trimester, but lesions are more commonly noted at birth; most are evident by age 2 years. Although large cervical or axillary lesions identified in the perinatal period have been referred to as cystic hygromas, this term is incorrect, because it does not encompass the morphology and distribution of most cystic malformations. The prenatal diagnosis of anterior and posterior cervical lymphatic malformations has significant clinical implications. They may be associated with airway obstruction, and prenatal diagnosis can influence the mode, timing, and place of delivery. Specifically, the prenatal diagnosis of large cervicofacial lymphatic malformations can signal the need to prepare for possible interventions to control a precarious airway in the delivery room. These patients may require the presence of a skilled surgical team capable of performing an EXIT (ex utero intrapartum treatment) procedure as well as a spectrum of other techniques, including fiber-optic and rigid endoscopy and direct surgical airway access.

Postnatally, most cases are readily diagnosed by physical examination. Transillumination can be helpful in differentiating some cystic lesions from solid masses. All patients with cervical cystic lesions should have a chest radiograph to determine the presence or absence of mediastinal involvement. Although US is helpful in confirming the diagnosis in superficial lesions, it is less valuable for showing extension into deep structures of the neck, thoracic cavity, and retroperitoneum. CT or MRI can clearly show the anatomic extent of cystic lesions and their relationship to soft tissues, muscle, and vascular structures.

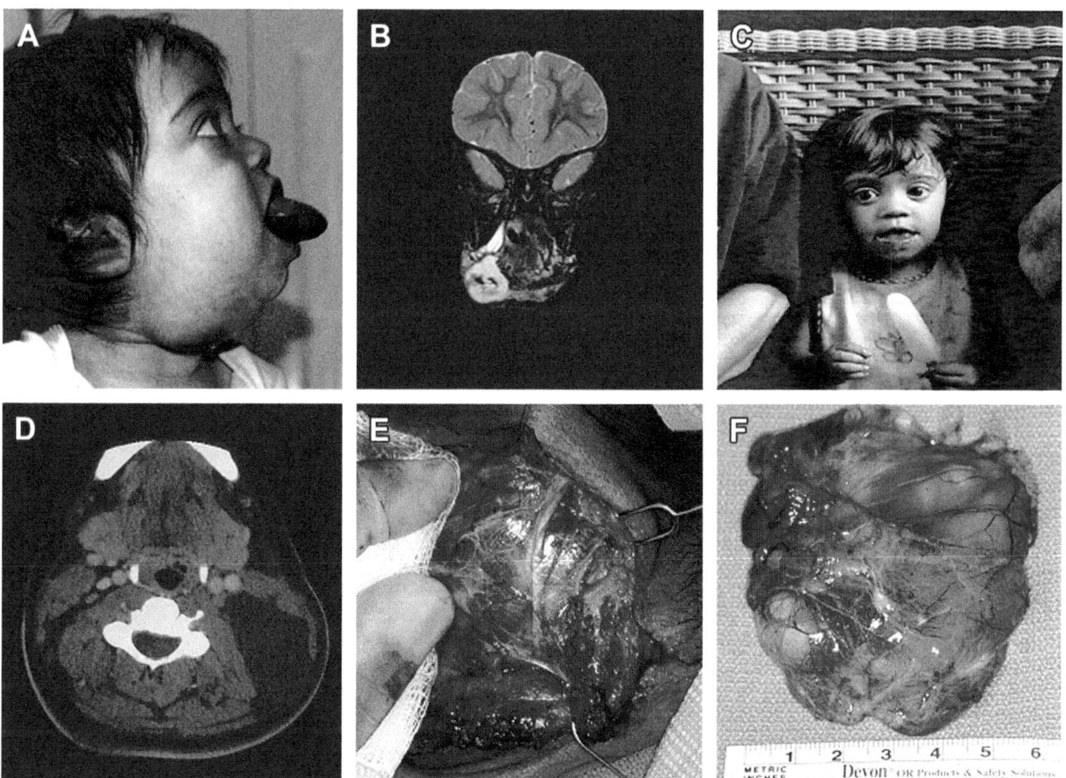

Fig. 10. (*A*) Combined microcystic and macrocystic malformation of the tongue, floor of mouth, and anterior neck. (*B*) MRI with gadolinium of the same patient. (*C*) Postoperative image after excision of cervical disease and tongue reduction. (*D*) CT scan of the neck showing macrocystic malformation of the lateral neck. (*E, F*) Intraoperative images demonstrating the appearance of a macrocystic lymphatic malformation.

Cystic lymphatic malformations are associated with numerous complications. Cutaneous involvement can be associated with spontaneous lymphatic leakage from pathologic vesicles. Bacteria can readily enter via these vesicles and quickly spread through tissues affected by the lymphatic lesion. The result is acute cellulitis or recurrent cellulitis, which in turn can lead to cosmetic disfigurement and life-threatening sepsis. Given the morbidity of such infections, aggressive antimicrobial therapy is mandatory.[38]

Another serious complication caused by large lymphatic malformations of the head and neck is respiratory obstruction of the larynx and trachea. Management is difficult and requires staged operative procedures, speech and physical therapy, and long-term follow-up, preferably by a multidisciplinary team. Less commonly, dysphagia is caused by the involvement of the hypopharynx and the esophagus. Other complications include localized hemorrhage into cysts and nerve compressions that can cause paresthesias and pain. Chylothorax and chylopericardium have been reported as rare complications of cervicomediastinal lesions.

Treatment depends on the clinical presentation, the size of the lesion, the anatomic location, and the complications. Although complete excision of the lesion is the treatment of choice, this is sometimes impossible. Whereas small lesions are generally amenable to excision with excellent results, large lesions that involve deep structures of the neck, tongue, and mediastinum entail the risk of multiple complications, including fistula formation, infection, damage to vascular structures, damage to nerves, and cosmetic deformity. Past reported mortality of such complex lesions varies from 2% to 6%. Persistent disease manifests in about 30% of patients who have undergone gross excisions. In the absence of signs and symptoms, it is reasonable and appropriate to manage lymphatic lesions nonoperatively. Surgical excision cannot be performed without scarring, and undesirable scars can develop after excision of large intradermal and subcutaneous microcystic and vesicular lymphatic lesions. In some patients with extensive microcystic disease, lymphatic vesicles may become apparent in or around the scar, years after excision.[44–47]

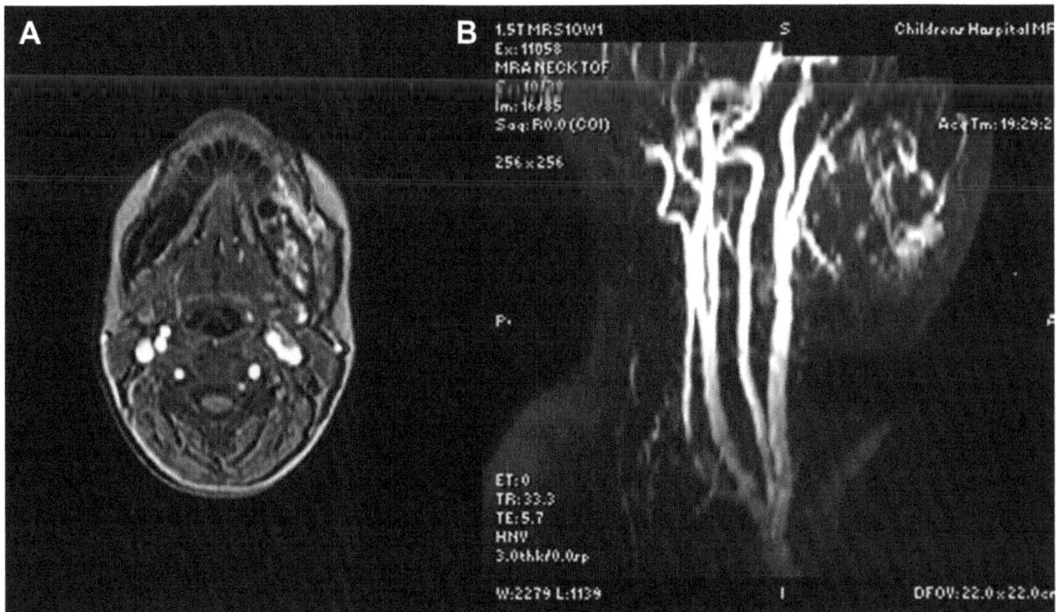

Fig. 11. (*A*) MRI and (*B*) MRA of the neck showing an AVM of the left mandible.

Sclerotherapy is frequently used as an alternative to surgery for patients with macrocystic disease, and although it is not generally curative, approximately 40% of patients have amelioration of their symptoms.[38] Several sclerosing agents have been used, including ethanol, bleomycin, OK-432 (known as picibanil), doxycycline, and sodium tetradecyl sulfate.

AVMs

AVMs are congenital vascular lesions associated with a variable degree of arteriovenous shunting.[38] Some of these lesions are believed to originate from arteriovenous channels that have failed to regress during development. These high-flow communications between arteries and veins are among the most dangerous vascular anomalies. They are always multiple and vary in diameter from several millimeters to the size of the normal precapillary anastomosis. The length of the channels between the arteries and the veins can vary from millimeters to centimeters, and convoluted or cavernous abnormal vascular structures may be intercalated between the arterial and venous ends of the malformation. The fast-flow character of AVMs usually becomes evident in childhood or during puberty. Rapid expansion has been reported after pregnancy, trauma, or inadequate surgical intervention. Complications associated with AVMs include cardiac hypertrophy, cardiac failure, and cardiac instability, as well as hemorrhage and stroke.

It is clinically useful to identify 3 major groups of AVMs, based on structural criteria: truncal, diffuse, and localized. Truncal fistulae arise from major arterial branches and commonly occur in the head and neck; however, trunk and extremity involvement is also seen. Diffuse AVMs are encountered particularly in the limbs and more frequently in lower than in upper limbs. Localized malformations are composed of a mass of abnormal intercalated tissues and can occur in any organ.[38]

Because of variations in position, size, length, and number, there is a wide pattern of clinical appearance. Nevertheless, these malformations are recognizable by warmth, a palpable thrill, and an audible bruit. Traditional angiography or MRA to show their vascular anatomy is essential for confirming the diagnosis and developing a treatment plan (**Fig. 11**).[48]

When a lesion is small and asymptomatic, a period of observation is often the most prudent initial strategy. However, pain, expansion, ulceration, bleeding, and cardiac decompensation can occur after a quiescent period. If so, more aggressive treatment is indicated. Intra-arterial embolization combined with surgical excision offers the best chance for cure, but complete excision may be impossible because of location and extent of the malformation. Complex lesions require creative operations tailored to individual disease and anatomy. When lesions cannot be excised, palliative embolization may be appropriate to control symptoms. Embolization techniques include the use of metal coils, particles, and glue (eg, *N*-butyl cyanoacrylate). In extremity lesions, amputation may eventually be required. The long- term outcomes of early versus late treatment and the different modalities of treatment are unknown.

SUMMARY

An understanding of cutaneous vascular lesions or vascular anomalies is essential for the practicing clinician, because these lesions can be common. The 2 key elements when treating cutaneous vascular lesions are to determine the effect of the lesion on function and cosmesis both for the short-term and long-term. Some vascular anomalies can have associated anomalies in other organ systems. For this reason, and because vascular anomalies are often managed with a combination of medicine and surgery, a multidisciplinary team approach is most efficacious in the treatment of these diseases.

REFERENCES

1. Mulliken JB, Glowacki J. Classification of pediatric vascular lesions. Plast Reconstr Surg 1982;70(1): 120–1.
2. Mulliken JB, Fishman SJ, Burrows PE. Vascular anomalies. Curr Probl Surg 2000;37(8):517–84.
3. Drolet BA, Swanson EA, Frieden IJ, Hemangioma Investigator Group. Infantile hemangiomas: an emerging health issue linked to an increased rate of low birth weight infants. J Pediatr 2008;153(5): 712–5, 715.e1.
4. Enjolras O, Riche MC, Merland JJ, et al. Management of alarming hemangiomas in infancy: a review of 25 cases. Pediatrics 1990;85(4):491–8.
5. Huang SA, Tu HM, Harney JW, et al. Severe hypothyroidism caused by type 3 iodothyronine deiodinase in infantile hemangiomas. N Engl J Med 2000;343(3):185–9.
6. Drolet BA, Esterly NB, Frieden IJ. Hemangiomas in children. N Engl J Med 1999;341(3):173–81.
7. Gonzalez-Crussi F, Reyes-Mugica M. Cellular hemangiomas ("hemangioendotheliomas") in infants. Light microscopic, immunohistochemical, and ultrastructural observations. Am J Surg Pathol 1991;15(8):769–78.
8. Yu Y, Flint AF, Mulliken JB, et al. Endothelial progenitor cells in infantile hemangioma. Blood 2004; 103(4):1373–5.
9. Boye E, Yu Y, Paranya G, et al. Clonality and altered behavior of endothelial cells from hemangiomas. J Clin Invest 2001;107(6):745–52.
10. Bielenberg DR, Bucana CD, Sanchez R, et al. Progressive growth of infantile cutaneous hemangiomas is directly correlated with hyperplasia and angiogenesis of adjacent epidermis and inversely correlated with expression of the endogenous angiogenesis inhibitor, IFN-beta. Int J Oncol 1999; 14(3):401–8.
11. Chang J, Most D, Bresnick S, et al. Proliferative hemangiomas: analysis of cytokine gene expression and angiogenesis. Plast Reconstr Surg 1999;103(1): 1–9 [discussion: 10].
12. Ritter MR, Dorrell MI, Edmonds J, et al. Insulin-like growth factor 2 and potential regulators of hemangioma growth and involution identified by large-scale expression analysis. Proc Natl Acad Sci U S A 2002;99(11):7455–60.
13. North PE, Waner M, Mizeracki A, et al. A unique microvascular phenotype shared by juvenile hemangiomas and human placenta. Arch Dermatol 2001; 137(5):559–70.
14. Berenguer B, Mulliken JB, Enjolras O, et al. Rapidly involuting congenital hemangioma: clinical and histopathologic features. Pediatr Dev Pathol 2003; 6(6):495–510.
15. North PE, Waner M, Mizeracki A, et al. GLUT1: a newly discovered immunohistochemical marker for juvenile hemangiomas. Hum Pathol 2000;31(1): 11–22.
16. Metry DW, Garzon MC, Drolet BA, et al. PHACE syndrome: current knowledge, future directions. Pediatr Dermatol 2009;26(4):381–98.
17. Burrows PE, Robertson RL, Mulliken JB, et al. Cerebral vasculopathy and neurologic sequelae in infants with cervicofacial hemangioma: report of eight patients. Radiology 1998;207(3):601–7.
18. Orlow SJ, Isakoff MS, Blei F. Increased risk of symptomatic hemangiomas of the airway in association with cutaneous hemangiomas in a "beard" distribution. J Pediatr 1997;131(4):643–6.
19. Brandling-Bennett HA, Metry DW, Baselga E, et al. Infantile hemangiomas with unusually prolonged growth phase: a case series. Arch Dermatol 2008; 144(12):1632–7.
20. Waner M, North PE, Scherer KA, et al. The nonrandom distribution of facial hemangiomas. Arch Dermatol 2003;139(7):869–75.
21. Hochman M, Mascareno A. Management of nasal hemangiomas. Arch Facial Plast Surg 2005;7(5): 295–300.
22. Waner M, Kastenbaum J, Scherer K. Hemangiomas of the nose: surgical management using a modified subunit approach. Arch Facial Plast Surg 2008; 10(5):329–34.
23. Rahbar R, Nicollas R, Roger G, et al. The biology and management of subglottic hemangioma: past, present, future. Laryngoscope 2004;114(11):1880–91.
24. Barnes PD, Burrows PE, Hoffer FA, et al. Hemangiomas and vascular malformations of the head and neck: MR characterization. AJNR Am J Neuroradiol 1994;15(1):193–5.

25. Leaute-Labreze C, Dumas de la Roque E, Hubiche T, et al. Propranolol for severe hemangiomas of infancy. N Engl J Med 2008;358(24):2649–51.
26. Denoyelle F, Leboulanger N, Enjolras O, et al. Role of propranolol in the therapeutic strategy of infantile laryngotracheal hemangioma. Int J Pediatr Otorhinolaryngol 2009;73(8):1168–72.
27. Buckmiller L, Dyamenahalli U, Richter GT. Propranolol for airway hemangiomas: case report of novel treatment. Laryngoscope 2009;119(10):2051–4.
28. Chamlin SL, Haggstrom AN, Drolet BA, et al. Multicenter prospective study of ulcerated hemangiomas. J Pediatr 2007;151(6):684–9, 689.e1.
29. Adams DM. The nonsurgical management of vascular lesions. Facial Plast Surg Clin North Am 2001;9(4):601–8.
30. Garzon MC, Lucky AW, Hawrot A, et al. Ultrapotent topical corticosteroid treatment of hemangiomas of infancy. J Am Acad Dermatol 2005;52(2):281–6.
31. Goyal R, Watts P, Lane CM, et al. Adrenal suppression and failure to thrive after steroid injections for periocular hemangioma. Ophthalmology 2004;111(2):389–95.
32. Chamot L, Zografos L, Micheli JL. Ocular and orbital complications after sclerosing injections in a case of a frontal cutaneous angioma. Ophthalmologica 1981;182(4):193–8.
33. Adams DM, Lucky AW. Cervicofacial vascular anomalies. I. Hemangiomas and other benign vascular tumors. Semin Pediatr Surg 2006;15(2):124–32.
34. Enjolras O, Breviere GM, Roger G, et al. Vincristine treatment for function- and life-threatening infantile hemangioma. Arch Pediatr 2004;11(2):99–107 [in French].
35. Chang E, Boyd A, Nelson CC, et al. Successful treatment of infantile hemangiomas with interferon-alpha-2b. J Pediatr Hematol Oncol 1997;19(3):237–44.
36. Barlow CF, Priebe CJ, Mulliken JB, et al. Spastic diplegia as a complication of interferon alfa-2a treatment of hemangiomas of infancy. J Pediatr 1998;132(3 Pt 1):527–30.
37. Barsky SH, Rosen S, Geer DE, et al. The nature and evolution of port wine stains: a computer-assisted study. J Invest Dermatol 1980;74(3):154–7.
38. Elluru RG, Azizkhan RG. Cervicofacial vascular malformations. II Vascular Malformations. Semin Pediatr Surg 2006;15(2):133–9.
39. Comi AM, Mehta P, Hatfield LA, et al. Sturge-Weber syndrome associated with other abnormalities: a medical record and literature review. Arch Neurol 2005;62(12):1924–7.
40. Anderson RR, Parrish JA. Selective photothermolysis: precise microsurgery by selective absorption of pulsed radiation. Science 1983;220(4596):524–7.
41. Burrows PE, Mason KP. Percutaneous treatment of low flow vascular malformations. J Vasc Interv Radiol 2004;15(5):431–45.
42. Ulrich H, Baumler W, Hohenleutner U, et al. Neodymium-YAG laser for hemangiomas and vascular malformations–long term results. J Dtsch Dermatol Ges 2005;3(6):436–40.
43. Marler JJ, Fishman SJ, Upton J, et al. Prenatal diagnosis of vascular anomalies. J Pediatr Surg 2002;37(3):318–26.
44. Alqahtani A, Nguyen LT, Flageole H, et al. 25 years' experience with lymphangiomas in children. J Pediatr Surg 1999;34(7):1164–8.
45. Deveikis JP. Percutaneous ethanol sclerotherapy for vascular malformations in the head and neck. Arch Facial Plast Surg 2005;7(5):322–5.
46. Mathur NN, Rana I, Bothra R, et al. Bleomycin sclerotherapy in congenital lymphatic and vascular malformations of head and neck. Int J Pediatr Otorhinolaryngol 2005;69(1):75–80.
47. Greinwald JH Jr, Burke DK, Sato Y, et al. Treatment of lymphangiomas in children: an update of Picibanil (OK-432) sclerotherapy. Otolaryngol Head Neck Surg 1999;121(4):381–7.
48. Dubois J, Garel L. Imaging and therapeutic approach of hemangiomas and vascular malformations in the pediatric age group. Pediatr Radiol 1999;29(12):879–93.

Rosacea
Pathophysiology and Management Principles

Nitin Chauhan, MD, FRCSC*,
David A.F. Ellis, MD, FRCSC, FACS

KEYWORDS

• Rosacea • Acne rosacea • Telangiectasias • Rhinophyma • Facial erythema

KEY POINTS

- Rosacea is a chronic cutaneous condition characterized by symptoms of facial flushing and a broad spectrum of clinical signs, including erythema, telangiectasias, edema, papules, pustules, ocular lesions, and rhinophyma.
- Medical management includes lifestyle modification; sunscreen products; medical-grade skin care; oral/topical antibiotics; and topical prescription medications, such as benzoyl peroxide and azelaic acid.
- Laser- and light-based therapies are effective for erythema reduction and also targeted treatment of telangiectasias and other prominent vasculature.
- Severe disease may result in rhinophyma, with irregular thickening of the nasal skin and nodular deformation, often necessitating surgical management.

DEFINITION OF ROSACEA

Rosacea is a chronic cutaneous condition characterized by symptoms of facial flushing and a broad spectrum of clinical signs. It is considered a syndrome encompassing various combinations of such cutaneous signs as[1]

- Flushing
- Erythema
- Telangiectasias
- Edema
- Papules
- Pustules
- Ocular lesions
- Rhinophyma

Typical patients usually present with some of these symptoms as opposed to the spectrum of possible manifestations. Its pathophysiology has been the subject of significant discussion because of its complexity and our relatively poor understanding of disease progression. Understanding the disease is of importance to facial plastic surgeons and clinicians in general because of its prevalence as well as significant lifestyle and treatment implications associated with the diagnosis.

Rosacea is defined by persistent erythema of the central portion of the face lasting for at least 3 months. Supporting criteria include flushing, papules, pustules, and telangiectasias on the convex facial surfaces. Secondary features may include burning and stinging, edema, plaques, skin dryness, ocular manifestations, and phymatous changes. The prevalence of these findings warrants disease subclassification, which, in turn, helps to rationalize the therapeutic options.[2]

Disclosures: None (NC); lecturer and consultant for Cutera (DAFE).
Department of Otolaryngology – Head and Neck Surgery, Division of Facial Plastic and Reconstructive Surgery, University of Toronto, 167 Sheppard Avenue West, Toronto, Ontario M2N1M9, Canada
* Corresponding author.
E-mail address: nitin.chauhan@utoronto.ca

Facial Plast Surg Clin N Am 21 (2013) 127–136
http://dx.doi.org/10.1016/j.fsc.2012.11.004

CLASSIFICATION OF ROSACEA

In 2002, an expert committee assembled by the National Rosacea Society explicitly defined and classified rosacea into 4 subtypes[3]:

1. Erythematotelangiectatic rosacea
2. Papulopustular rosacea
3. Phymatous rosacea
4. Ocular rosacea

General guidelines for diagnosis are based on the presence of primary features and the possible existence of secondary features (**Box 1**). Often, primary and secondary features occur together. The National Rosacea Society designated specific subtypes based on the most common patterns or groupings of clinical signs (**Table 1**). Certainly, patients may have characteristics of more than one rosacea subtype at the same time.

Subtype 1: Erythematotelangiectatic Rosacea

Erythematotelangiectatic rosacea is predominantly characterized by central facial flushing, often with burning or stinging. There is usually periocular sparing by the erythema. Red areas of the face are often rough with scaling, likely caused by chronic, low-grade dermatitis. Frequent triggers to flushing include emotional stress, hot drinks, alcohol, spicy foods, exercise, cold or hot weather, and hot baths and showers. This flushing is characteristically progressive, leading to gradual development of permanent telangiectatic red vessels on the affected areas, initially over cheeks primarily. In early stages, these vessels are red but can also become bluish as they persist and mature, especially around the nose and on the cheeks.

Box 1
Diagnostic guidelines for rosacea, including primary and secondary features

Presence of one or more of the following primary features

Flushing (transient erythema)

Nontransient erythema

Papules and pustules

Telangiectasia

May include one or more of the following secondary features

Burning or stinging discomfort

Plaque

Dry appearance and texture

Edema

Ocular manifestations

Peripheral location

Phymatous changes

Subtype 2: Papulopustular Rosacea

Papulopustular rosacea is often described as classic rosacea. Patients are typically middle-aged women predominantly presenting with an erythematous central face and small erythematous papules or pinpoint pustules (or both) in a central facial distribution. These patients often have telangiectasias; however, they may be obscured by persistent erythema, papules, or pustules.

Subtype 3: Phymatous Rosacea

Phymatous rosacea is characterized by skin thickening, irregular surface nodularities, and enlargement. The nose is affected most commonly, referred to as rhinophyma; however, this phymatous presentation can also affect the chin, forehead, cheeks, and ears. Significant telangiectasias are also often present over the affected regions. Four distinct histologic variants can occur with rhinophyma: glandular, fibrous, fibroangiomatous, and actinic.

Subtype 4: Ocular Rosacea

Ocular manifestations often precede the development of cutaneous signs but can also occur concurrently. These manifestations may include blepharitis, conjunctivitis, inflammation of the lids and meibomian glands, interpalpebral conjunctival hyperemia, and conjunctival telangiectasias. Patients may often experience eye stinging or burning sensation, excess dryness, irritation with light, or foreign body sensation. Meibomian gland dysfunction presenting as a chalazion or chronic staphylococcal infection as manifested by hordeolum are common signs of rosacea-related ocular disease.[4] Worrisome complications include decreased visual acuity caused by corneal complications (keratitis or corneal ulcers); to lessen the risk of vision loss, the involvement of an ophthalmologic specialist may be warranted in addition to treating the cutaneous disease.

EPIDEMIOLOGY OF ROSACEA

Rosacea is commonly misdiagnosed in many patients who experience facial erythema or even transient rashes of the face. It should be kept in mind that the diagnostic criteria are relatively strict. The epidemiologic data on rosacea remain fragmentary and the methodological quality

Table 1
Rosacea subtypes and associated clinical characteristics

Subtype	Characteristics
Erythematotelangiectatic	Flushing, persistent central facial erythema with or without telangiectasias
Papulopustular	Persistent central facial erythema with transient, central facial papules/ pustules
Phymatous	Thickened skin, irregular surface nodularities; may occur on the nose (rhinophyma), chin forehead, cheeks, or ears
Ocular	Eye foreign body sensation, burning/stinging, dryness, itching, ocular photosensitivity, telangiectasias of sclera, periorbital edema

debatable.[5] The prevalence statistics published in the United States and Europe are highly variable, ranging from less than 1% to greater than 20% of the adult population. Unfortunately, the methods used and populations studied are greatly variable between studies, consequently barring any meaningful comparisons. Individuals with rosacea are disproportionately of fair-skinned European and Celtic origin. Interestingly, the caseating granulomatous variant may more commonly occur in people of Asian or African origin. New studies examining the epidemiology are undoubtedly necessary; it would be prudent for researchers to use the diagnostic and severity criteria established in 2002 and 2004, respectively.

PATHOPHYSIOLOGY OF ROSACEA

Despite being one of the most common skin disorders, its pathogenesis remains unclear and controversial and has also been the subject of prolonged study. Several factors are known to be key components in its development, including[6]

- Vasculature
- Climatic exposures
- Dermal matrix degeneration and endothelial damage
- Chemicals and ingested agents
- Pilosebaceous unit abnormalities
- Microorganisms
- Reactive oxygen species (ROS)

The erythema and flushing associated with rosacea result from increased blood flow to the facial vasculature and increased blood vessel density near the skin surface. Patients with rosacea can have an exaggerated vasodilatation response to various triggers, such as hyperthermia.

There is evidence to suggest that harsh climatic exposures and extremes of temperature cause mechanical damage to cutaneous vasculature and dermal connective tissue.[7] This risk also includes exposure to solar irradiation, providing some explanation as to why facial convexities are primarily affected and why symptoms may flare in the spring.

Certain ingested agents, such as spicy foods, alcohol, and hot beverages, may trigger a flushed face in patients with rosacea (**Table 2**); however, a clear link demonstrating dietary factors playing a central role in pathogenesis does not exist. In addition to various foods, certain medications, such as amiodarone, topical steroids, nasal steroids, and high doses of vitamins B6 and B12, may result in exacerbations of symptoms for patients with rosacea.[8]

Demodex species (microscopic parasitic mites, **Fig. 1**) may play a role in the pathogenesis of

Table 2
Rosacea trigger factors for facial flushing and worsening of symptoms

Rosacea Trigger Factors	Patients Affected (%)
Sun exposure	81
Emotional stress	79
Hot weather	75
Wind	57
Strenuous exercise	56
Alcohol consumption	52
Cold weather	46
Spicy foods	45
Certain skin care products	41
Heated beverages	36
Certain cosmetics	27
Medications	15
Dairy products	8
Other factors	24

Data from Cohen AF, Tiemstra JD. Diagnosis and treatment of rosacea. J Am Board Fam Pract 2002;15(3):214–7.

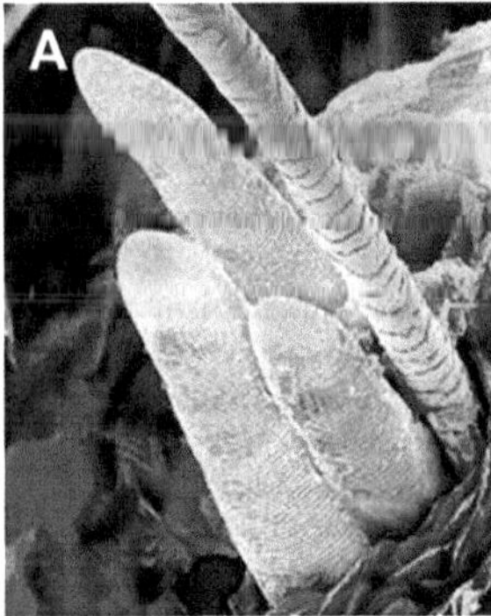

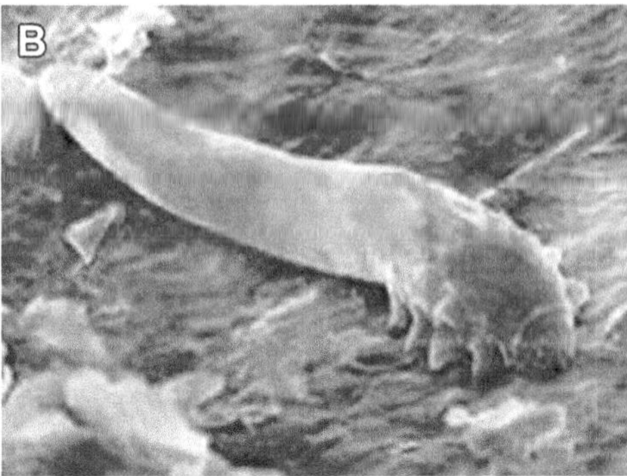

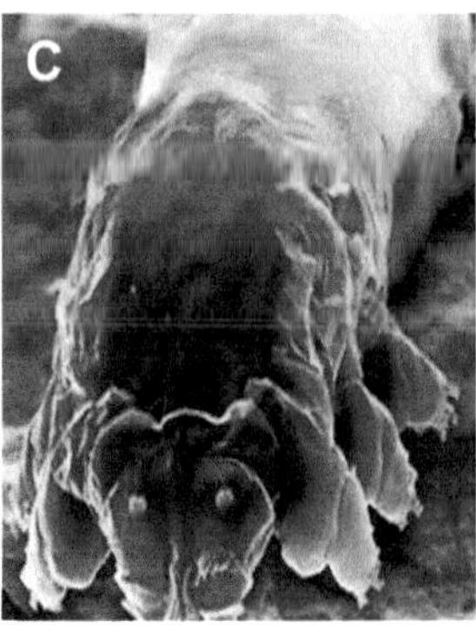

Fig. 1. *Demodex folliculorum* (*A*) living in hair follicle, (*B*) crawling on skin, and (*C*) frontal view of *Demodex* mite. (*Data from* Cohen AF, Tiemstra JD. Diagnosis and treatment of rosacea. J Am Board Fam Pract 2002;15(3):214–7.)

rosacea. Some studies suggest that *Demodex* preferentially resides in skin regions affected by rosacea, including the nose and cheeks.[9] Research also suggests that *Demodex* antigens result in an immune response of helper-inducer T-cell infiltrates occurs in patients with rosacea. The research is somewhat inconclusive; there is also a body of conflicting evidence suggesting a role for other microorganisms, such as *Helicobacter pylori*, *Staphylococcus epidermidis*, and *Chlamydia pneumoniae*.[10]

ROS are postulated to have a central role in the inflammatory response associated with rosacea. These species are comprised of free radicals, such as superoxide anions and hydroxyl radicals, in addition to other reactive molecules, such as molecular oxygen, singlet oxygen, and hydrogen peroxide; each of them can lead to oxidative tissue damage. Various mechanisms explain the role of ROS in skin inflammation, most notably deactivation of natural defenses caused by excessive oxidative stress by ROS, chemical and oxidative modification of proteins and lipids by ROS, and alteration of the lipid balance in patients with rosacea.[11]

Several researchers have demonstrated the role of neoangiogenesis, enlargement of blood vessel caliber, and vascular endothelial growth factor overexpression in the vascular endothelium of patients with rosacea.[12]

Histology

Rosacea histology is characterized by sebaceous hyperplasia, nonspecific perivascular and perifollicular lymphohistiocytic infiltrate with multinucleated cells, plasma cells, neutrophils, and eosinophils (**Fig. 2**). In patients with papulopustular lesions, there is granulomatous inflammation with occasional perifollicular abscesses. *Demodex folliculorum* may also reside in nearby hair follicles.

CLINICAL PRESENTATION OF ROSACEA

History

Rosacea is a common inflammatory facial dermatosis seen in adults that exhibits considerable variety in clinical presentation.[13] Patients commonly have a history of facial flushing or facial redness, which may have arisen in childhood or early adolescence, especially during physical exertion. The erythematous face of a 10-year-old who has been exercising strenuously during the summer months will often portend a delayed diagnosis of rosacea in that individual. Rosacea is often inherited through one of the parents. Patients may be able to identify triggering agents, such as hot beverages, environmental factors, emotional reactions, alcohol, and several other causes of rapid body temperature changes. Although these episodic exacerbations are transient, they can progressively lead to the appearance of permanently flushed skin, associated with vascular changes and the development of permanent telangiectasias. Rosacea has a major psychosocial impact on patients' quality of life.[14] Many patients are left with feelings of self-consciousness and isolation. According to the National Rosacea Society, 76% of patients had lowered self-confidence and self-esteem, 65% felt frustrated with the condition, and 41% reported that it had caused them to avoid social gatherings.

Physical Examination

The symptom spectrum of rosacea is broad, and patients typically do not develop every stage or aspect of the disease. Variable erythema and telangiectasias can be seen over the cheeks and forehead. Inflammatory papules and pustules are often present over the nose, forehead, and cheeks. It is not uncommon to also have neck and upper chest signs, including erythema and flushing in these regions. Prominence of

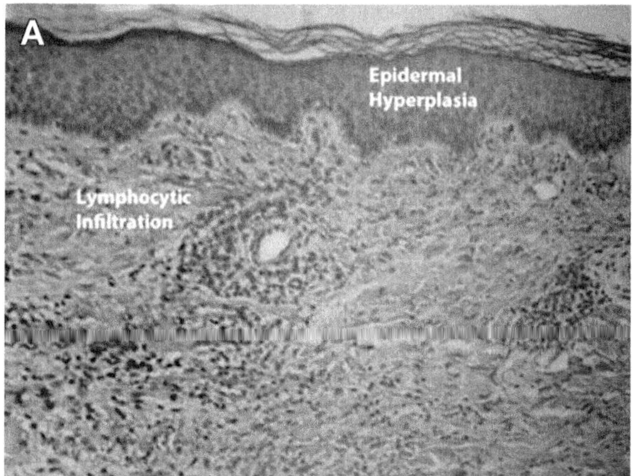

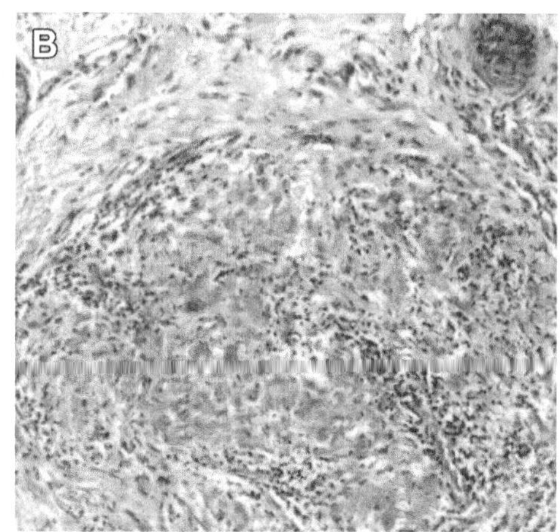

Fig. 2. Rosacea histology. (*A*) Epidermal hyperplasia with lymphocytic infiltration and (*B*) papulopustular lesion with granulomatous inflammation and perifollicular microabscesses. H and E stain, 40×.

sebaceous glands is common in severe disease, and this can lead to the development of thickened and disfigured nose.

Rhinophyma primarily affects Caucasian men in their fifth decade. Its main characteristic is a slowly progressive hyperplasia of the sebaceous glands and the adjacent tissue with irregular thickening of the nasal skin and nodular deformation. The associated problems are not only cosmetic because this can lead to functional impairments, such as nasal airway obstruction or even difficulty in eating.[15]

Patients with rosacea generally do not have increased oiliness of the skin but often complain of drying and peeling. Further, the absence of comedones is another helpful distinguishing feature, which separates patients with rosacea from patients with acne.

Ocular rosacea is most frequently diagnosed when it presents in the context of the cutaneous signs and symptoms of the condition. In approximately one-fifth of patients, ocular signs may be the presenting symptom occurring before cutaneous manifestations of rosacea. Patients may have minor irritation, excessive dryness, blurry vision, and in severe cases ocular surface disruption and inflammatory keratitis.[16] Blepharitis and conjunctivitis are the most common findings but others include lid margin and conjunctival telangiectasias, eyelid thickening, lid crusting and scaling, chalazia and hordeolum, corneal ulcers/scars, and neovascularization. Vision-threatening disease is very rare; however, keratitis can result in corneal ulceration and eventual perforation with inadequate treatment.[17]

Rosacea fulminans (pyoderma faciale) is an uncommon acute presentation of rosacea. Edema, nodules, and draining sinuses may occur. This severe manifestation typically affects women in their 20s, and severe scarring may result in untreated cases.[18]

DIFFERENTIAL DIAGNOSIS OF ROSACEA

The differential diagnosis is somewhat broad and varied. The erythematotelangiectatic subtype of rosacea can resemble seborrheic dermatitis, lupus erythematosus, and other photodermatoses. Seborrheic keratoses occur in as many as 26% of patients with rosacea, although this relationship is still somewhat unclear on a pathophysiologic level. Carcinoid syndrome, mitral valve incompetence, polycythemia vera, and exogenous niacin administration are often overlooked causes of erythema and telangiectasias.

Acneiform rosacea may be stimulated by acne, bromoderma and iododerma, perioral dermatitis, and pustular folliculitis. The classic presentation is usually described as rosacea, acneiform papules, and pustules on a background of telangiectasias.[19]

It is also important to rule out potential confounding variables, such as the long-term application of topical steroids, contact dermatitis, and photosensitivity for other reasons.

TREATMENT OF ROSACEA

Because of the complexity of the disease, rosacea management spans a broad spectrum of therapeutic modalities. Fluctuations in symptom severity, relapses, and the typically progressive nature of the disease necessitate a thorough understanding of the available treatment options available and their corresponding appropriate usage.

Lifestyle Modification

Before the initiation of medical therapy, a thorough history should be taken to evaluate for the presence of any identifiable triggering agents. Identification of these exacerbating agents, such as temperature extremes, wind, hot beverages, caffeine, exercise, spicy food, emotional upsets, irritating topical agents, and such, can facilitate their avoidance or modulation.[20]

The use of daily broad-spectrum sunscreen is recommended for all patients with rosacea, with an agent protective against both UV-A and UV-B light. Patients generally tolerate blocking agents quite well, such as titanium dioxide and zinc oxide. Preferably, the sunscreen should contain protective silicones, such as dimethicone or cyclomethicone.[21]

Skin Care Products

There are several over-the-counter skin-care products targeted at patients with rosacea, each with varying concentrations of active ingredients. There are some more therapeutic lines on the market, labeled as *medical-grade* skin-care products, which are typically distributed under the care of a treating physician.

The Obagi Rosaclear System (Obagi Medical Products, Inc, Long Beach, California) consists of a gentle cleanser designed to remove bacteria and other irritating residues, with its key ingredient *Aloe barbadensis* leaf juice. The prescription component of the system is metronidazole topical gel (0.75%), which is typically indicated for the treatment of inflammatory papules and pustules of rosacea. The third component is a "hydrating complexion corrector," designed to protect the skin barrier, provide some moisture, and reduce visible redness (active ingredients include glycerin, licorice, aloe, lavender, sea whip, and mica). Finally, the system includes a "Skin Balancing Sun Protection SPF 30" product that provides important protection against harmful UV-A/UV-B rays while helping to reduce the appearance of erythema (key ingredients include 15.5% zinc oxide and 2.0% titanium oxide).

The RevaleSkin (RevaleSkin Products, Inc, Richmond, Virginia) skin-care line is another medical-grade skin-care line marketed for its ability to improve the appearance of wrinkles, fine lines, and discoloration. The active ingredient within the products is CoffeeBerry (J&J Technologies) whole fruit extract, which is an agent derived from the fruit of the coffee plant, *Coffea arabica*. This extract is exceptionally rich in polyphenol antioxidants, such as chlorogenic acid, condensed proanthocyanidins, quinic acid, and ferulic acid. In general, topical antioxidants exert their effects by downregulating free radical–mediated pathways that damage skin.[22]

Medications

The goals of pharmacotherapy for rosacea are to reduce morbidity, diminish troublesome symptoms, achieve predictable disease control, and prevent complications.

Oral antibiotics

Oral antibiotics have been used commonly for first-line treatment since the 1950s because microorganisms were thought to be the underlying cause of disease. Treatment philosophy has evolved and though microbial infection is no longer thought to play a part in pathogenesis, oral and topical agents are often used alone or in combination because of their demonstrated efficacy.[23] Metronidazole gel 0.75% or 1.0% (MetroGel, Noritate, Flagyl) is an imidazole ring-based antibiotic active against various anaerobic bacteria and protozoa. It is helpful for mild disease and as an adjuvant to systemic therapy. Oral metronidazole has proven benefit in treating papules and pustules of acne rosacea. Erythromycin oral or 2% topical solution inhibits bacterial growth on a molecular level and has proven efficacy in treating ocular rosacea.[24] Topical clindamycin inhibits bacterial growth by arresting RNA-dependent protein synthesis. On topical application to skin, it is converted to its active component and has demonstrated efficacy against mild to moderate papulopustular rosacea.

Topical medications

In addition to antibiotics, topical retinoids are advocated by some authorities as being a useful adjunct to the management of recalcitrant disease.[25] Topical tretinoin may be useful for such cases; however, recurrence is common. Treatment inhibits comedone formation and makes keratinocytes in sebaceous follicles less cohesive and easier to remove. Long-term, low-dose therapy can have some benefit; however, many patients do experience skin irritation.

Topical medications commonly used to treat acne can have substantial benefit in patients with papules, pustules, and the phymatous and glandular types of rosacea. Benzoyl peroxide administration results in free-radical oxygen release, which oxidizes bacterial proteins in sebaceous follicles, decreasing the quantity of irritating free fatty acids and anaerobic bacteria.[26] Azelaic acid is available in 2 strengths (azelaic acid 15% gel [Finacea] and azelaic acid 20% cream [Azelex]) and is known to be effective against mild to moderate papulopustular rosacea.[27] In the authors' practice, they have had excellent results in treating patients with recalcitrant disease, severe flushing, and the presence of papules/pustules (**Fig. 3**). Its mechanism of action is related to its ability to reduce the production of reactive oxygen species by neutrophils.

Laser

Laser therapy has been proven to be an effective solution for patients with rosacea because of the positive therapeutic effects, such as dermal connective tissue remodeling and enhancing the robustness of the epidermal barrier.[28] A laser is a device that emits light (electromagnetic radiation) through a process of optical amplification based on the stimulated emission of photons (**Fig. 4**). Laser- and light-based technologies can be used to treat specific disease signs and symptoms, such as facial telangiectasias, persistent erythema, and midfacial flushing.

Facial erythema and flushing

Intense pulsed light (IPL) therapy is based on technology that produces high-intensity light during a very short period of time. The multichromatic light is broad spectrum, with its wavelength controlled by filters, and consequently has multiple targets, including melanin and hemoglobin. Variation of the filters alters the wavelength to target either oxyhemoglobin or melanin. Traditional IPL filters have a tendency to wear out, whereas the IPL system by Cutera (Cutera, San Francisco, California) delivers repetitive, consistent energy levels. IPL has demonstrated efficacy in its excellent ability to reduce persistent facial erythema. IPL treatments also have some demonstrated efficacy in reducing the severity of facial telangiectasias and troublesome flushing. In patients with erythematotelangiectatic rosacea and have also shown similar efficacy and safety as pulsed dye laser (PDL) treatments.[29]

Telangiectasias

Vascular lasers are the primary modality of treatment and these include the PDL (585 or 595 nm), the potassium-titanyl-phosphate laser (532 nm), and the diode-pumped frequency-doubled laser (532 nm). Lasers in these wavelength ranges selectively target oxyhemoglobin as their chromophore, resulting in significant vascular targeting and minimal collateral damage to surrounding tissue or scarring. Although these lasers can be effective in reducing erythema, they tend to work very well for treating facial telangiectasias.

The bluish vessels do not respond well with the shorter wave lengths, and the Nd:YAG 1064-nm laser is needed. Bluish vessels are characterized by slower blood flow, greater depth beneath the skin surface, and greater vessel diameter. The Nd:YAG 1064-nm laser penetrates 8 mm rather than the 2 mm reached by the PDLs, and a long pulse width or longer pulse duration is needed. A spot size of 5 mm with low fluence of approximately 100 to 150 J/cm^2 and a pulse duration of 30 ms would be the recommended initial settings. Because of the slow flow, the pulse duration is increased.

Deeper facial vessels typically require longer wavelengths, including the diode laser (810 nm), the long-pulsed alexandrite laser (755 nm), and the Nd:YAG laser (1064 nm). These lasers are far more effective at targeting facial telangiectasias and broken capillaries as opposed to reducing facial erythema and improving troublesome flushing.

Ablative lasers, such as the erbium:YAG, Yttrium Scandium Gallium Garnet, and carbon dioxide laser, have demonstrated efficacy in the treatment

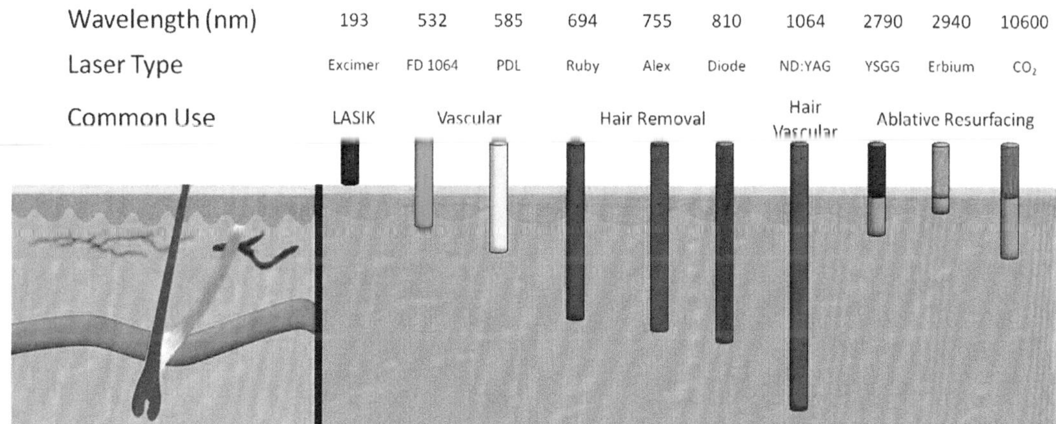

Fig. 3. Schematic depiction of various laser wavelengths, clinical applications, and tissue penetration depths.

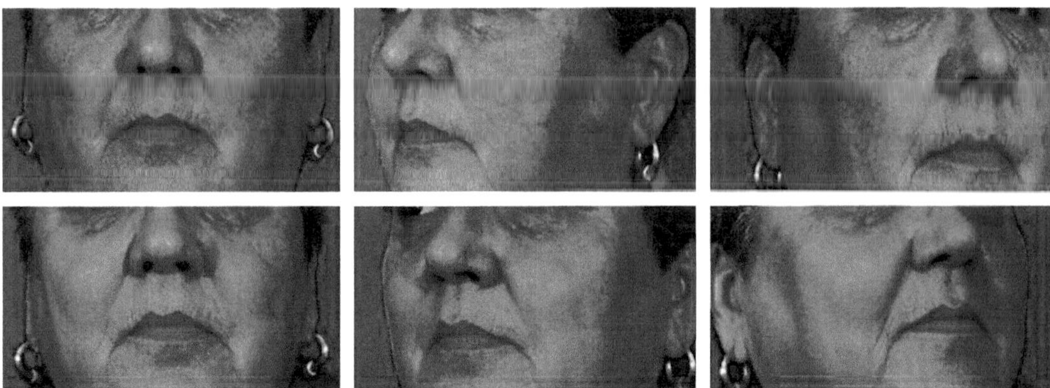

Fig. 4. Pretreatment and posttreatment views of a female patient with recalcitrant rosacea, troublesome flushing, persistent erythema, and intermittent pustules. Top row views show patient before Finacea treatment; bottom views demonstrate appearance 3 months after initiation of therapy.

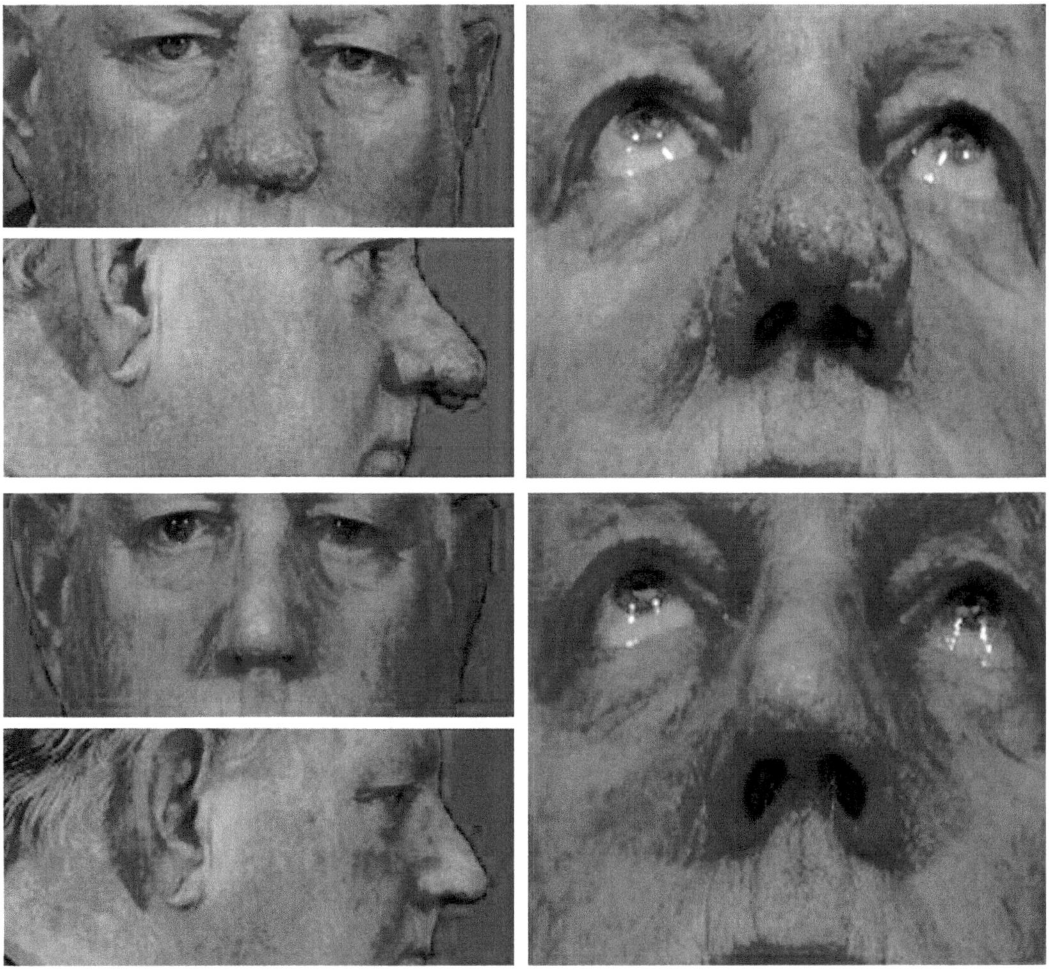

Fig. 5. Patient images demonstrating rhinophyma preoperatively (*top row: frontal, lateral, and basal*) and postoperatively (*bottom row: frontal, lateral, and basal*) after electrocautery surgical recontouring procedure.

of midfacial skin thickening and rhinophyma. However, these also have beneficial effects in collagen remodeling, leading to wrinkle improvement, to a greater degree than erythema reduction.

Surgical Care

Rhinophyma is a descriptive term for a large, bulbous, ruddy/erythematous appearance of the nose caused by granulomatous infiltration, commonly caused by untreated rosacea.[30] Mechanical dermabrasion, carbon dioxide laser resurfacing, and surgical shave techniques may produce cosmetic improvement of rhinophyma. In the authors' practice, they have had excellent results using electrocautery shave excision under conscious sedation. Patients are typically informed that they will likely require 2 sessions, approximately 6 months apart. The first session is typically geared toward debulking, whereas the second session is usually required for more finesse modifications aimed at achieving symmetry and a more normal nasal shape. Postoperative care includes a regimen of oral analgesia (acetaminophen with codeine), a very short course of Vaseline ointment (Unilever, London, United Kingdom) to the surface of the nose, vinegar soaks every 6 hours to clean and allow for reapplication of ointment, and patient counseling for reassurance that they will be socially acceptable within 3 weeks of the procedure (**Fig. 5**).

SUMMARY

Rosacea is a relatively common cutaneous disorder characterized by symptoms of facial flushing and a broad spectrum of clinical signs, including erythema, telangiectasias, skin coarseness, and an inflammatory papulopustular acneiform reaction. It is often misdiagnosed, and practitioners should be aware that there are relatively clear diagnostic criteria. The National Rosacea Society has defined and subclassified rosacea based on specific clinical signs and symptoms. The treatment is as varied as the clinical presentation spectrum. It is imperative that patient education constitute part of the treatment paradigm; patients should be advised to avoid known exacerbating factors, such as temperature extremes, wind, hot beverages, caffeine, vigorous physical activity, spicy foods, alcohol, emotional upset, irritating topical products, and medications that result in iatrogenic flushing. In addition to avoidance of triggers, treatment can be broadly divided into medical, surgical, and nonsurgical interventional (laser- and light-based therapy). Understanding of rosacea as a disease entity is imperative for facial plastic surgeons that treat a broad variety of cutaneous conditions as well as ensuring optimal outcomes in patients presenting for other reasons but with evidence of rosacea as a comorbid condition.

REFERENCES

1. Wilkin JK. Rosacea: pathophysiology and treatment. Arch Dermatol 1994;130:359–62.
2. Crawford GH, Pelle MT, James WD. Rosacea: I. Etiology, pathogenesis, and subtype classification. J Am Acad Dermatol 2004;51(3):327–41 [quiz: 342–4].
3. Wilkin JK, Dahl M, Detmar M, et al. Standard classification of rosacea: report of the National Rosacea Society Expert Committee on the classification and staging of rosacea. J Am Acad Dermatol 2002;56: 584–7.
4. Macsai MS, Mannis MJ, Huntley AC. Acne rosacea. In: Macsai MS, Mannis MJ, Huntley AC, editors. Eye and skin disease. Philadelphia: Lippincott-Raven; 1996. p. 335–41.
5. Chosidow O, Cribier B. Epidemiology of rosacea: updated data. Ann Dermatol Venereol 2011; 138(Suppl 2):S124–8 [in French].
6. Laquer V, Hoang V, Nguyen A, et al. Angiogenesis in cutaneous disease: part II. J Am Acad Dermatol 2009;61(6):945–58.
7. Gutierrez EL, Galarza C, Ramos W, et al. Influence of climatic factors on the medical attentions of dermatologic diseases in a hospital of Lima, Peru. An Bras Dermatol 2010;85(4):461–8.
8. Jansen T, Romiti R, Kreuter A, et al. Rosacea fulminans triggered by high-dose vitamins B6 and B12. J Eur Acad Dermatol Venereol 2001;15(5): 484–5.
9. Bonnar E, Eustace P, Powell FC. The Demodex mite population in rosacea. J Am Acad Dermatol 1993, 28(3):443–8.
10. Lazaridou E, Giannopoulou C, Fotiadou C, et al. The potential role of microorganisms in the development of rosacea. J Dtsch Dermatol Ges 2011;9(1): 21–5.
11. Jones DA. Rosacea, reactive oxygen species, and azelaic acid. J Clin Aesthet Dermatol 2009;2(1): 26–30.
12. Wilkin J. A role for vascular pathogenic mechanisms in rosacea: implications for patient care. Cutis 2008; 82(2):100–2.
13. Del Rosso JQ, Baum EW. Comprehensive medical management of rosacea: an interim study report and literature review. J Clin Aesthet Dermatol 2008; 1(1):20–5.
14. Aksoy B, Altaykan-Hapa A, Egemen D, et al. The impact of rosacea on quality of life: effects of demographic and clinical characteristics and various

treatment modalities. Br J Dermatol 2010;163(4):719–25.

15. Sadick H, Riedel F, Bran G. Rhinophyma in rosacea: what does surgery achieve? Hautarzt 2011;62(11):834–41.
16. Akpek EK, Merchant A, Pinar V, et al. Ocular rosacea: patient characteristics and follow up. Ophthalmology 1997;104(11):1863–7.
17. Browning DJ, Proia AD. Ocular rosacea. Surv Ophthalmol 1986;31(3):145–58.
18. Helm TN, Schechter J. Biopsy may help identify early pyoderma faciale (rosacea fulminans). Cutis 2006;77(4):225–7.
19. Diamantis S, Waldorf HA. Rosacea: clinical presentation and pathophysiology. J Drugs Dermatol 2006;5(1):8–12.
20. Greaves MW, Burova E. Flushing: causes, investigation and clinical consequences. J Eur Acad Dermatol Venereol 1997;8:91–100.
21. Powell FC. Clinical practice. Rosacea. N Engl J Med 2005;352(8):793–803.
22. Farris P. Idebenone, green tea, and Coffeeberry extract: new and innovative antioxidants. Dermatol Ther 2007;20(5):322–9.
23. Baldwin HE. Systemic therapy for rosacea. Skin Therapy Lett 2007;12(2):1–5, 9.
24. Hong E, Fischer G. Childhood ocular rosacea: considerations for diagnosis and treatment. Australas J Dermatol 2009;50(4):272–5.
25. Ceilley RI. Advances in the topical treatment of acne and rosacea. J Drugs Dermatol 2004;3(Suppl 5):S12–22.
26. Gooderham M. Rosacea and its topical management. Skin Therapy Lett 2009;14(2):1–3.
27. Del Rosso JQ, Bhatia N. Azelaic acid gel 15% in the management of papulopustular rosacea: a status report on available efficacy data and clinical application. Cutis 2011;88(2):67–72.
28. Lonne-Rahm S, Nordlind K, Edstrom DW, et al. Laser treatment of rosacea: a pathoetiological study. Arch Dermatol 2004;140(11):1345–9.
29. Neuhaus IM, Zane LT, Tope WD. Comparative efficacy of nonpurpuragenic pulsed dye laser and intense pulsed light for erythematotelangiectatic rosacea. Dermatol Surg 2009;35(6):920–8.
30. Cohen AF, Tiemstra JD. Diagnosis and treatment of rosacea. J Am Board Fam Pract 2002;15(3):214–7.

The Use of Negative-Pressure Therapy in the Closure of Complex Head and Neck Wounds

Graham Michael Strub, MD, PhD*, Kristen S. Moe, MD

KEYWORDS

• Negative pressure wound therapy • Vacuum-assisted closure • Complex head and neck wounds

KEY POINTS

Negative-pressure wound therapy

- Is a safe, efficacious, and cost-effective treatment strategy in the management of complex head and neck wounds.
- Reduces wound infections, shortens hospital stays, and simplifies wound reconstruction strategies.
- Should be included in the wound management strategies of otolaryngologists and facial plastic surgeons.

INTRODUCTION

The treatment of complex head and neck wounds has presented unique challenges throughout the evolution of modern wound care. In addition to the array of difficulties that large wounds present in general, such as tissue loss, poor vascularity, and chronic infection, wounds to the head and neck region are particularly challenging because of their highly visible location and relative paucity of available adjacent tissue for simple reconstruction. The traditional methods used to reconstruct large or chronic wounds in other regions of the body, namely, skin grafting, tissue expansion, and free flaps,[1–4] may be suboptimal in the head and neck. Specifically, skin grafts and free tissue transfers often result in poor color or thickness matching to adjacent structures, whereas tissue expansion is associated with significant morbidity during the lengthy expansion process.[5] In addition, the increasing complexity of surgical resections in head and neck cancer and the improvements in radiation treatment have resulted in an increased number and variety of challenging facial reconstructions. For these reasons, recent focus has turned to the use of vacuum-assisted closure, a technique that has been widely successful in the treatment of wounds in other regions of the body,[6–8] to address complex head and neck wounds.

The Advent of Suction Drainage

The evolution of negative-pressure therapy began early this century with the advent of suction drainage. In 1934, Chaffin[9] described the use of a suction drainage device that he developed to facilitate drainage in areas where gravity was inefficient,

The authors have no conflicts of interest in the publication of this work.
Department of Otolaryngology/Head and Neck Surgery, University of Washington, 1959 Northeast Pacific Street, Seattle, WA 98195, USA
* Corresponding author. University of Washington, Box 3566515, 1959 Northeast Pacific Street, Seattle, WA 98195-6515.
E-mail address: strub@uw.edu

Facial Plast Surg Clin N Am 21 (2013) 137–145
http://dx.doi.org/10.1016/j.fsc.2012.11.005

such as the abdomen, pelvis, and neck. Chaffin's device was simply a perforated suction catheter attached to a collection canister, which was in turn connected to a vacuum generated by a tank of running water. By inserting this catheter into a healing wound bed, he immediately noted improved wound healing and patient recovery. Silvis and colleagues[10] went on to describe the use of continuous negative suction following mandibular resection and radical neck dissections, demonstrating prevention of subcutaneous serum collections and increased collateral blood flow resulting in fewer postoperative infections and fewer instances of skin necrosis. Moloney[11] expanded on these observations by applying suction drainage devices after salivary gland resections and thyroidectomies. In 1959, Breslau and colleagues[12] introduced the first method of providing portable continuous suction. Initial studies of 50 cases using this technique reported a stronger and more rapidly forming scar, shorter hospital stays, and a very rare occurrence of necrosis, infection, or dehiscence.[13] In 1962, Von Leden and Kaplan[14] went on to describe the use of the portable HemoVac system (Snyder Manufacturing Corp). The HemoVac system was then used by McLean[15] in his landmark study comparing head and neck postoperative wounds with and without suction. This study demonstrated significant decreases in morbidity associated with suction drainage; patients developed fewer salivary fistulas, fewer soft tissue infections, and began oral feedings at earlier dates. Histologically, wounds in the suction-drainage group were less edematous, better approximated, and less frequently necrotic.

The underlying principles of closed suction that led to the improvements in overall wound healing were well articulated by McLean and colleagues,[15] namely, the removal of devitalized and necrotic tissue, reduction of secondary edema, minimization of dead spaces, close apposition of wound edges, and stimulation of intracellular histamine.[16] Thus, the use of suction drainage became the standard of care for the next 30 years, with few changes in its application. During this time, the observations by Winter[17] on moist wound healing principles led to the development of alginates, hydrogels, debriding agents, and antimicrobial agents, with modest effects on overall wound healing.

Development of Negative-Pressure Wound Therapy

It was not until the 1990s that Argenta and Morykwas[6,18] expanded on the principles of suction drainage by introducing negative-pressure wound therapy. This method uses an interface material, typically a hydrophobic collapsible foam, to distribute the force of a vacuum throughout the wound rather than simply placing a suction catheter drain within the closed wound bed. The term *negative pressure* is a misnomer because it is a relative pressure to the atmospheric pressure and not a true negative value; the importance of this pressure difference is underscored by the fact that wounds do not heal more efficiently at lower atmospheric pressures, such as at high elevations.[19] The device consists of a semiocclusive dressing with a connection for suction tubing, which is in turn connected to a portable vacuum source with a collection canister. The semiocclusive dressing is placed on top of the interface material that lies within the wound bed; when the vacuum is started, the dressing holds a seal, drawing the wound edges closer together while facilitating fluid removal through the drainage tube.

Mechanism of Action of Negative-Pressure Therapy

The precise mechanism of action whereby negative-pressure wound therapy facilitates improved wound healing has been the subject of many studies. Orgill and Bayer[19] reviewed the most recent peer-reviewed literature investigating negative-pressure therapy and categorized these mechanisms into 5 major physiologic categories: fluid removal, blood flow changes, microdeformation, macrodeformation, and maintenance of wound hemostasis. Fluid removal has been known to improve wound healing since the introduction of suction drainage and is now thought to act by improving nutrient transport, removing toxins, reducing bacterial load, and modulating local blood flow changes.[18,20] Blood flow changes during the application of negative pressure have been extensively studied.[21–25] During the application of negative pressure, blood flow decreases at the wound edge but then increases on its release. The intermittent application of negative pressure is thought to provide an overall increased blood flow to wound edges, whereas the transient hypoxia induced by the vacuum is thought to stimulate vasculogenesis and increase granulation tissue formation. The observations that cell proliferation and organization of cellular structural elements are related to cell shape[26,27] led Saxena and colleagues[28] to propose microdeformation as the mechanism by which dramatic granulation tissue forms in wounds under negative pressure despite minimal fluid removal. Their group demonstrated increased microdeformation, elongation of wound surface, increased neuropeptide levels, and more ordered blood vessel morphology in wounds treated with negative pressure compared with foam alone.[29–31]

Macrodeformation is the reduction in wound size when negative pressure is applied and is a function of both the compressibility of the interface material and the deformability of the surrounding skin. This reduction in wound size can allow the reconstructive surgeon to select a less complex reconstruction strategy, such as a local advancement flap in place of a free tissue transfer or primary closure in place of skin grafting. Finally, the application of the semiocclusive material decreases heat loss, minimizes evaporation, and reduces desiccation.[19] No clinical studies have been published on the efficacy of macrodeformation or hemostasis as they relate to negative-pressure therapy.

The most popular device for applying negative-pressure therapy has been the vacuum-assisted closure system (VAC; Kinetic Concepts, Inc, San Antonio, Texas). This device has been successfully used in the management of complex wounds in general surgery, orthopedic surgery, gynecologic surgery, and plastic and reconstructive surgery.[20] A meta-analysis of negative-pressure therapy trials versus standard wound-care therapy was recently published by Suissa and colleagues[32] and concluded that negative-pressure therapy leads to significant reduction in wound size and time to healing. Despite these studies, there exists a paucity of literature comparing standard wound-care therapy to vacuum-assisted therapy in the region of the head and the neck. This article reviews the literature on vacuum-assisted closure of head and neck wounds and discusses its potential benefits and pitfalls.

SURGICAL TECHNIQUE

The application of the VAC device is relatively straightforward. The dimensions of the wound are measured, and the interface material (polyvinyl alcohol and polyurethane in the case of the VAC system) is trimmed to the appropriate size. The skin surrounding the wound edges is cleaned, and excess hair is trimmed away. The wound is then packed with the interface material such that the shape of the material coincides with the contours of the wound. A semiocclusive dressing with an attached suction port is then applied over the interface material and adhered to the surrounding skin such that an adequate seal can be maintained with the application of the vacuum. A suction tube is then connected to the suction port and the portable vacuum device, and the vacuum is set to a specific pressure, typically 125 mm Hg. Most published studies have changed the interface material every 48 to 72 hours. The VAC device is then left in place until complete wound closure is achieved or until a sufficient granulation tissue bed has formed to allow for a reconstructive surgical procedure to facilitate closure. Moues and colleagues[33] reviewed the various manufacturers, materials, and settings that exist for negative-pressure wound therapy devices; however, to date no absolute consensus exists on optimal settings or interface compositions.

CLINICAL OUTCOMES WITH VAC THERAPY

Publication of studies examining negative-pressure therapy in the head and neck began in 2006. Schuster and colleagues[34] published the first report using the VAC system to successfully treat a large infected face wound.

VAC for Complicated Head and Neck Wounds with Comorbidities

That same year, the first retrospective study examining the outcomes of vacuum-assisted wound closure for head and neck wounds appeared by Andrews and colleagues.[35] This study examined the outcomes of 13 patients with complicated head and neck wounds, 9 of which had bony exposure caused by failed reconstructive pedicled flaps, ablative Mohs defects, or traumatic scalping injuries. Three patients with split-thickness skin grafts (STSGs), for which the VAC system was used as a bolster, were included as well as one patient with a large neck defect after resection of necrotizing fasciitis. The duration of VAC application ranged from 5 days for the STSG bolster to 6 weeks for soft tissue coverage for an exposed orbit caused by necrotizing fasciitis. Most of the selected patients (83.3%) had a variety of comorbidities, including cardiac disease, cancer, pulmonary disease, diabetes, and liver and kidney disease. All cases of exposed bone developed an intact granulation tissue bed and subsequently underwent successful STSG placement. All 3 cases whereby the VAC system was used as a bolster for an STSG demonstrated viable grafts with no crusting and healthy grafts at postoperative follow-up visits. Patients with large scalping defects also developed healthy granulation tissue beds and subsequently underwent successful delayed primary closure or local advancement flaps. There were no reported complications in this study.

VAC for Complicated Head and Neck Wounds Including Chemotherapy and Radiation

In 2009, Dhir and colleagues[36] published a cohort study in which 19 patients with a variety of complicated head and neck wounds, including those who had undergone extensive chemotherapy and radiation therapy, underwent VAC treatment. The wounds studied included failed pedicled flaps, necrotizing fasciitis, osteoradionecrosis, and wound dehiscence. Again, most patients (84.2%) had significant comorbidities, including hypertension, malnutrition, diabetes, peripheral vascular disease, and coronary artery disease. Of this cohort, 84% of patients healed completely after VAC therapy, whereas the remaining patients healed after subsequent adjunctive procedures, such as hyperbaric oxygen, dermal grafting, salivary diversion, or regional flap reconstruction.

VAC Therapy for Oromaxillofacial Surgery

Byrnside and colleagues[37] reported 3 cases in 2010 whereby the VAC system was applied in oromaxillofacial surgery. The first case was a successful treatment of an infected mandibular plate exposure, the second a necrotizing fasciitis of the orbit, and the third a large gunshot wound to the face. These cases were eventually managed with primary closure, full-thickness skin graft (FTSG), and gracilis free flap, respectively. All 3 cases healed well without complication.

VAC Therapy for Revision Free Flap Complications

In 2011, 2 case series were reported examining the utility of VAC devices in managing revision free flap complications. The first, published by Kakarala and colleagues,[38] demonstrated healthy granulation tissue bed formation on exposed muscle after cutaneous defects were created by retraction of fibrotic, irradiated skin flaps. Both cases were successfully treated with STSG. The second publication, by Poglio and colleagues,[39] details VAC treatment of an exposed fibula free flap and reconstruction plate 1 month after composite reconstruction caused by advanced mandibular osteoradionecrosis. Again, healthy granulation tissue was formed within the wound bed, and a subsequent pectoralis flap was healthy 9 months after surgery.

VAC Therapy for Traumatic Complex Forehead Wounds

Hsia and Moe[40] reported 3 cases in 2011 whereby VAC therapy was used in the management of complex forehead wounds caused by trauma. Each patient had a large (21–100 cm^2) soft tissue defect resulting from blunt force trauma. VAC therapy ranged from 27 to 95 days; each patient demonstrated healthy granulation tissue formation and underwent successful adjuvant surgical procedures, including scar revision and local advancement flaps, with excellent functional and cosmetic outcomes. This group has now used VAC therapy for 6 defects involving the forehead with similar results; **Figs. 1** and **2** demonstrate 2 of the authors' recent outcomes.

VAC for Therapy in Pediatric Resection of Large Lymphangiomas

Most recently, Katz and colleagues[41] used VAC therapy in a series of children following resection of large lymphangiomas. These lesions are typically difficult to completely resect because of their intertwinement with neurovascular structures and, therefore, have high recurrence rates. The investigators report an initial case of a 4-year-old girl who developed a severe postoperative infection after extensive lymphangioma resection that was successfully treated with VAC therapy. The infection resolved, but the lymphangioma did not recur despite a very difficult resection that likely left significant lymphangioma tissue behind. This finding led the investigators to examine VAC therapy not only as a means for facilitating wound closure postoperatively but also as a potential therapy to prevent recurrence of lymphangiomas in children. Thirteen children aged between 34 days and 20 years underwent lymphangioma resection from the head and neck, thorax, abdomen, or extremity; the resulting wound was treated with VAC therapy. All patients achieved adequate wound closure; after 289 days, no recurrences have been reported. The physiologic and histologic changes that occur in lymphangioma tissue under negative pressure have not been examined; however, one may hypothesize that negative-pressure application may facilitate lymphatic channel collapse and subsequent fibrosis. Further long-term studies will be required to determine the efficacy of VAC therapy in the prevention of lymphangioma recurrence.

COMPLICATIONS AND CONCERNS WITH VAC THERAPY

Despite the overall low morbidity and complication rate with VAC therapy, major complications, such as infection, damage to vital structures, toxic shock syndrome, and enteric fistula formation, have been reported.[6,42–44] These complications can be mostly avoided by the proper patient selection, proper wound preparation, adequate protection of underlying structures, and infrequent dressing changes.[36]

Pain and Skin Irritation

More commonly, pain and skin irritation have been reported with VAC therapy.[45] Skin irritation can be reduced by proper technique, including correct dimensions of the interface material, clean

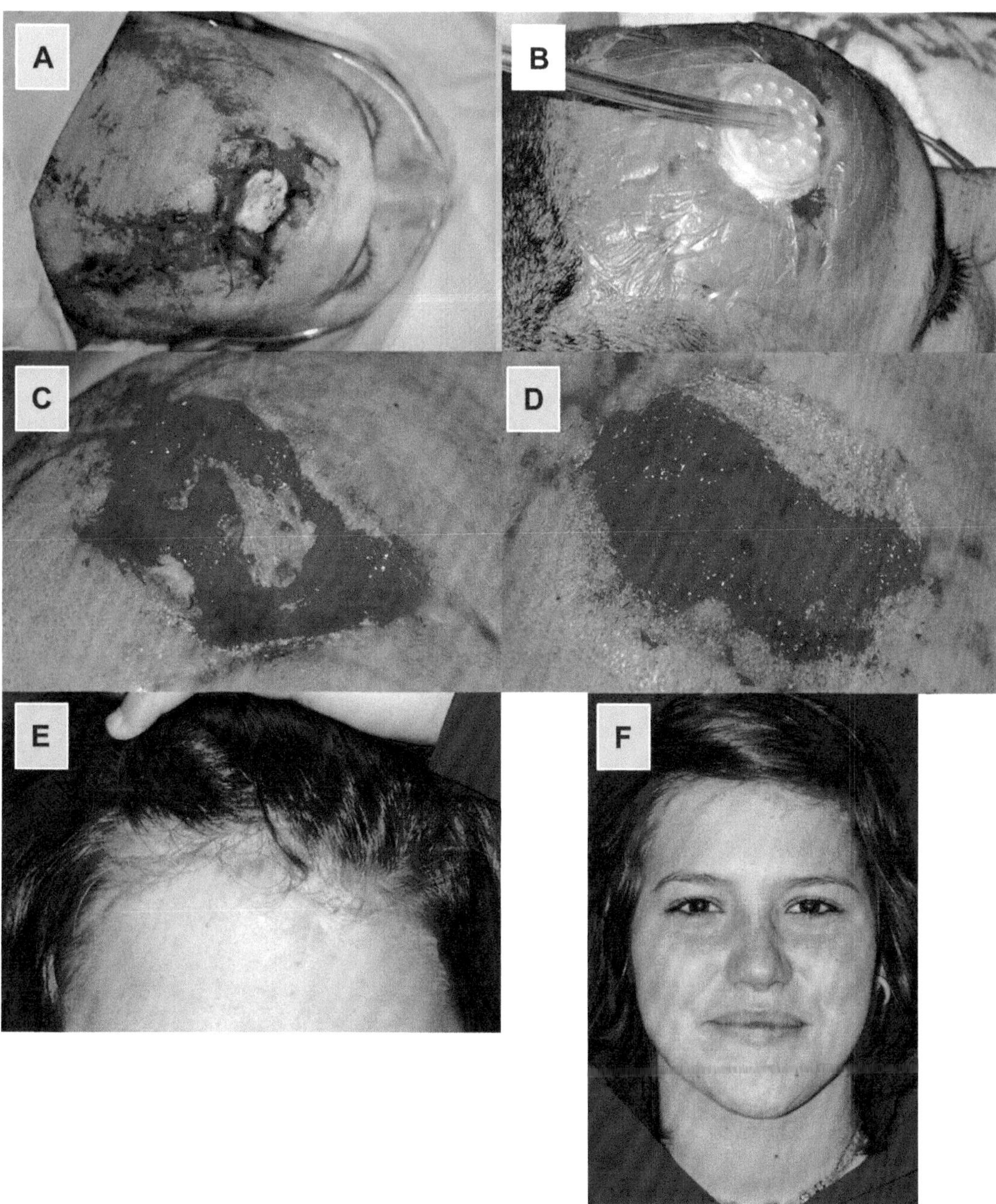

Fig. 1. Wound VAC therapy for blunt force trauma to the forehead. (*A*) Initial injury. (*B*) Wound VAC in place, 8 months after injury. (*C*) Wound bed after 8 weeks. (*D*) Wound bed after 11 weeks. (*E*, *F*) Final outcome, 1 year after injury.

skin, and selection of patients that can tolerate adhesive dressings. Pain can be reduced by beginning the VAC setting at a low suction (50 mm Hg) and gradually increasing to the desired level as well as using topical anesthetic solutions or hydrogen peroxide to the interface material. In addition, reduction of the number of interface changes reduces the pain associated with VAC therapy.[45]

Challenges Specific to Head and Neck

The implementation of a VAC system faces specific challenges in the head and neck region

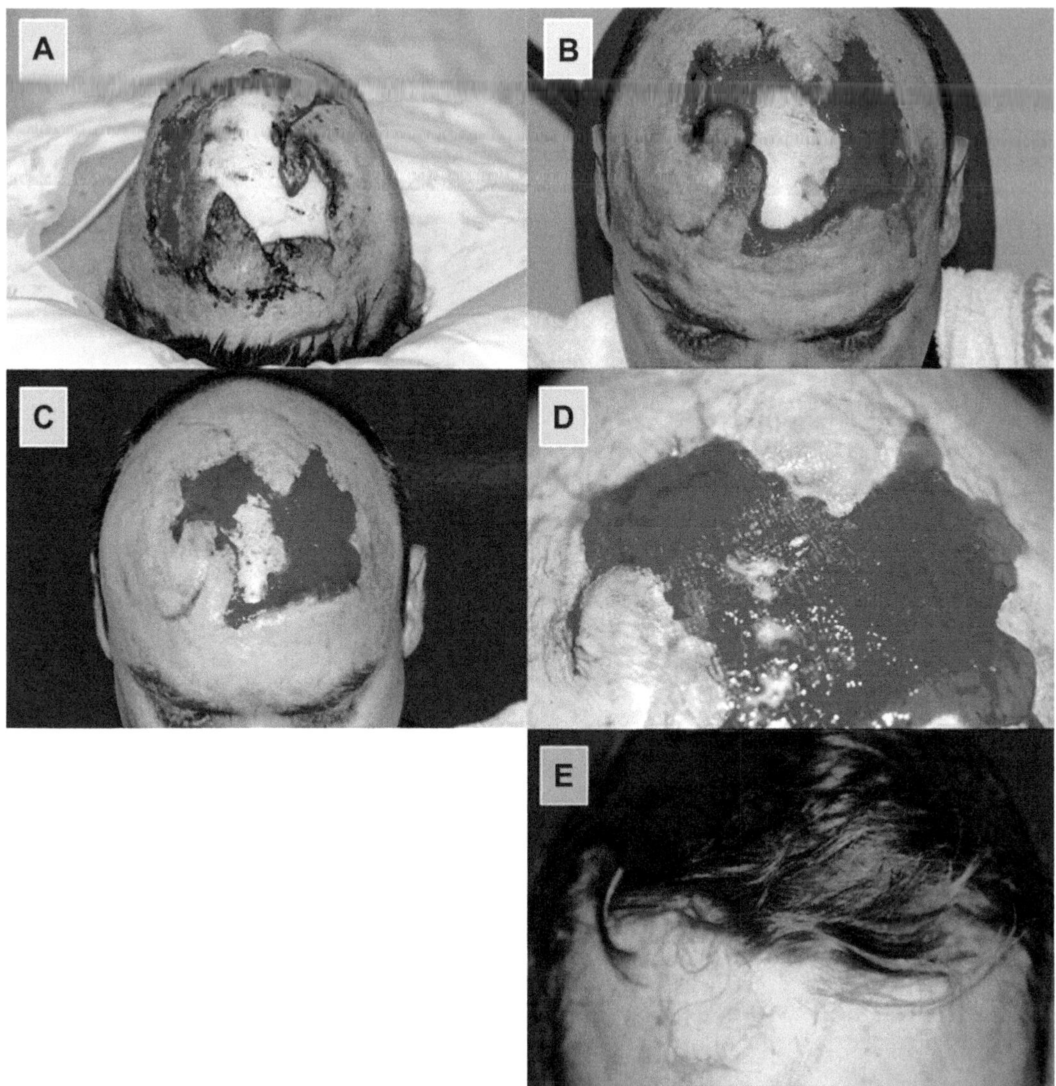

Fig. 2. Wound VAC therapy for blunt force trauma to the forehead. (*A*) Initial injury. (*B*) Wound bed, 2 weeks after wound VAC placement. (*C*) Wound bed after 4 weeks. (*D*) Wound bed after 8 weeks, note the new bone formation throughout wound bed. (*E*) Final outcome, 9 months after injury.

because of multiple facial contours, frequent movement, hair-bearing skin, and the presence of tracheotomy stomas. These challenges require attention to skin preparation, patient education, and may require complicated preparations of the semiocclusive dressing. As VAC therapy becomes more prevalent in the treatment of head and neck wounds, the design of precut adhesive dressings molded for particular head and neck regions would reduce the occurrence of air leaks and dressing revisions.

An additional concern in the head and neck region is the acceptance by patients as an outpatient wound-care modality. Although VAC placement on the torso or extremities can be easily hidden by clothing, VAC placement on the head and neck will be obvious and prominent. As manufacturers improve the cosmetic appearance of their dressings for facial wounds, the placement of these devices in an outpatient setting will likely grow.

Contraindications of VAC Therapy

There are few contraindications to the placement of a VAC device.[45] An absolute contraindication is the presence of residual malignancy in the wound bed because VAC placement may stimulate

Table 1
Clinical review of the literature: summary table of various reviews and comparisons using VAC therapy in head and neck wounds

Author, Year	Type of Study	Number of Patients	Wound Types	Outcomes	Complications
Schuster et al,[34] 2006	Case report	1	Infected facial wound	Healthy FTSG	None
Andrews et al,[35] 2006	Retrospective	13	Failed pedicle flaps, Mohs defects, scalping injuries, STSGs, NSTI	Healthy primary closure, STSG, local advancement flap	None
Dhir et al,[36] 2009	Cohort	19	Failed pedicle flaps, osteoradionecrosis, wound dehiscence, NSTI	Healthy primary closure, STSG, salivary diversion, regional flap	None
Byrnside et al,[37] 2010	Case series	3	Exposed infected mandible, NSTI, shotgun wound	Healthy primary closure, FTSG, free flap	Loss of first patient to follow-up
Kakarala et al,[38] 2011	Case report	1	Exposed free flap muscle	Healthy STSG	None
Poglio et al,[39] 2011	Case report	1	Exposed mandibular recon plate	Healthy STSG	None
Hsia and Moe,[40] 2011	Case series	3	Traumatic forehead wounds	Healthy primary closure, local advancement flap	None
Katz et al,[41] 2012	Retrospective	13	Postoperative lymphangioma resections	Healthy primary closure, secondary intention, no recurrence of lymphangiomas	3 machine malfunctions, 2 wound infections

Abbreviation: NSTI, Necrotizing soft tissue infection.

further tumor growth through the very mechanisms by which they promote wound healing. Relative contraindications include an ischemic wound (because these patients will experience further skin edge necrosis), fragile skin, and patients who cannot tolerate skin adhesives.

Costs of VAC Therapy

The cost of the VAC system can vary but is typically between $100 and $200 per day, including dressing supplies. Although this cost is significantly higher than standard wound care supplies for head and neck wound care, the overall decrease in hospitalization time, wound healing time, and wound-care time spent by health care workers may offset this difference.[46]

Table 1 presents a clinical review of the literature summarizing reviews and comparisons of VAC therapy in head and neck wounds.

SUMMARY

The use of vacuum-assisted closure devices is a safe, efficacious, and cost-effective technique in the management of head and neck wounds, leading to fewer wound infections, shorter hospital stays, less complex wound reconstructions, and overall improvements in wound healing. In the last 15 years, the use of negative-pressure therapy in managing complex wounds has become the standard practice in general surgery, orthopedic surgery, gynecologic surgery, and plastic and reconstructive surgery. Only recently have publications emerged demonstrating the efficacy of negative-pressure therapy on head and neck wound management; the preponderance of evidence to date supports its use. This method should be regularly considered for use by the otolaryngologist or facial plastic surgeon in managing complex head and neck wounds.

REFERENCES

1. Maillard GF, Clavel PR. Aesthetic units in skin grafting of the face. Ann Plast Surg 1991;26(4):347–52.
2. Kawashima T, Yamada A, Ueda K, et al. Tissue expansion in facial reconstruction. Plast Reconstr Surg 1994;94(7):944–50.
3. Kruse-Losler B, Presser D, Meyer U, et al. Reconstruction of large defects on the scalp and forehead as an interdisciplinary challenge: experience in the management of 39 cases. Eur J Surg Oncol 2006; 32(9):1006–14.
4. Beasley NJ, Gilbert RW, Gullane PJ, et al. Scalp and forehead reconstruction using free revascularized tissue transfer. Arch Facial Plast Surg 2004;6(1): 16–20.
5. Frodel JL Jr, Ahlstrom K. Reconstruction of complex scalp defects: the "banana peel" revisited. Arch Facial Plast Surg 2004;6(1):54–60.
6. Argenta LC, Morykwas MJ. Vacuum-assisted closure: a new method for wound control and treatment: clinical experience. Ann Plast Surg 1997; 38(6):563–76 [discussion: 577].
7. Baillot R, Cloutier D, Montalin L, et al. Impact of deep sternal wound infection management with vacuum-assisted closure therapy followed by sternal osteosynthesis: a 15-year review of 23,499 sternotomies. Eur J Cardiothorac Surg 2010;37(4):880–7.
8. Bollero D, Carnino R, Risso D, et al. Acute complex traumas of the lower limbs: a modern reconstructive approach with negative pressure therapy. Wound Repair Regen 2007;15(4):589–94.
9. Chaffin R. Drainage. Am J Surg 1934;40:100.
10. Silvis RS, Potter LE, Robinson DW, et al. The use of continuous suction negative pressure instead of pressure dressing. Ann Surg 1955;142(2):252–6.
11. Moloney GE. Apposition and drainage of large skin flaps by suction. Aust N Z J Surg 1957;26(3):173–9.
12. Breslau RC, Pories WJ, Schwartz SI. A portable technique for the maintenance of constant sterile postoperative wound suction. Surgery 1959;46:711–7.
13. de AS, Barbosa JF, Faccio CH. Continuous suction after neck dissection. J Int Coll Surg 1960;33:737–40.
14. Von Leden H, Kaplan J. Closed wound suction in head and neck surgery. Arch Otolaryngol 1962;75: 103–7.
15. McLean WC. The role of closed wound negative pressure suction in radical surgical procedures of the head and neck. Laryngoscope 1964;74:70–94.
16. Kahlson G, Nilsson K, Rosengren E, et al. Wound healing as on rate of histamine formation. Lancet 1960;2(7144):230–4.
17. Winter GD. Formation of the scab and the rate of epithelization of superficial wounds in the skin of the young domestic pig. Nature 1962;193:293–4.
18. Morykwas MJ, Argenta LC, Shelton-Brown EI, et al. Vacuum-assisted closure: a new method for wound control and treatment: animal studies and basic foundation. Ann Plast Surg 1997;38(6):553–62.
19. Orgill DP, Bayer LR. Update on negative-pressure wound therapy. Plast Reconstr Surg 2010; 127(Suppl 1):105S–15S.
20. Argenta LC, Morykwas MJ, Marks MW, et al. Vacuum-assisted closure: state of clinic art. Plast Reconstr Surg 2006;117(Suppl 7):127S–42S.
21. Borgquist O, Ingemansson R, Malmsjo M. Wound edge microvascular blood flow during negative-pressure wound therapy: examining the effects of pressures from -10 to -175 mmHg. Plast Reconstr Surg 2010;125(2):502–9.
22. Malmsjo M, Ingemansson R, Martin R, et al. Wound edge microvascular blood flow: effects of negative pressure wound therapy using gauze or polyurethane foam. Ann Plast Surg 2009;63(6):676–81.
23. Wackenfors A, Gustafsson R, Sjogren J, et al. Blood flow responses in the peristernal thoracic wall during vacuum-assisted closure therapy. Ann Thorac Surg 2005;79(5):1724–30 [discussion: 1730–1].
24. Petzina R, Ugander M, Gustafsson L, et al. Topical negative pressure therapy of a sternotomy wound increases sternal fluid content but does not affect internal thoracic artery blood flow: assessment using magnetic resonance imaging. J Thorac Cardiovasc Surg 2008;135(5):1007–13.
25. Kairinos N, Voogd AM, Botha PH, et al. Negative-pressure wound therapy II: negative-pressure wound therapy and increased perfusion. Just an illusion? Plast Reconstr Surg 2009;123(2):601–12.
26. Huang S, Ingber DE. The structural and mechanical complexity of cell-growth control. Nat Cell Biol 1999; 1(5):E131–8.
27. Folkman J, Moscona A. Role of cell shape in growth control. Nature 1978;273(5661):345–9.
28. Saxena V, Hwang CW, Huang S, et al. Vacuum-assisted closure: microdeformations of wounds and cell proliferation. Plast Reconstr Surg 2004;114(5): 1086–96 [discussion: 1097–8].
29. Scherer SS, Pietramaggiori G, Mathews JC, et al. The mechanism of action of the vacuum-assisted closure device. Plast Reconstr Surg 2008;122(3):786–97.
30. Younan G, Ogawa R, Ramirez M, et al. Analysis of nerve and neuropeptide patterns in vacuum-assisted closure-treated diabetic murine wounds. Plast Reconstr Surg 2010;126(1):87–96.
31. Erba P, Ogawa R, Ackermann M, et al. Angiogenesis in wounds treated by microdeformational wound therapy. Ann Surg 2011;253(2):402–9.
32. Suissa D, Danino A, Nikolis A. Negative-pressure therapy versus standard wound care: a meta-analysis of randomized trials. Plast Reconstr Surg 2010;128(5):498e–503e.
33. Moues CM, Heule F, Hovius SE. A review of topical negative pressure therapy in wound healing: sufficient evidence? Am J Surg 2011;201(4):544–56.

34. Schuster R, Moradzadeh A, Waxman K. The use of vacuum-assisted closure therapy for the treatment of a large infected facial wound. Am Surg 2006; 72(2):129–31.
35. Andrews BT, Smith RB, Goldstein DP, et al. Management of complicated head and neck wounds with vacuum-assisted closure system. Head Neck 2006;28(11):974–81.
36. Dhir K, Reino AJ, Lipana J. Vacuum-assisted closure therapy in the management of head and neck wounds. Laryngoscope 2009;119(1):54–61.
37. Byrnside V, Glasgow M, Gurunluoglu R. The vacuum-assisted closure in treating craniofacial wounds. J Oral Maxillofac Surg 2010;68(4):935–42.
38. Kakarala K, Richmon JD, Lin DT, et al. Vacuum-assisted closure in revision free flap reconstruction. Arch Otolaryngol Head Neck Surg 2011;137(6): 622–4.
39. Poglio G, Grivetto F, Nicolotti M, et al. Management of an exposed mandibular plate after fibula free flap with vacuum-assisted closure system. J Craniofac Surg 2011;22(3):905–8.
40. Hsia JC, Moe KS. Vacuum-assisted closure therapy for reconstruction of soft-tissue forehead defects. Arch Facial Plast Surg 2011;13(4):278–82.
41. Katz MS, Finck CM, Schwartz MZ, et al. Vacuum-assisted closure in the treatment of extensive lymphangiomas in children. J Pediatr Surg 2012;47(2):367–70.
42. Fleischmann W, Lang E, Russ M. Treatment of infection by vacuum sealing. Unfallchirurg 1997;100(4): 301–4 [in German].
43. Clare MP, Fitzgibbons TC, McMullen ST, et al. Experience with the vacuum assisted closure negative pressure technique in the treatment of non-healing diabetic and dysvascular wounds. Foot Ankle Int 2002;23(10):896–901.
44. Armstrong DG, Lavery LA, Abu-Rumman P, et al. Outcomes of subatmospheric pressure dressing therapy on wounds of the diabetic foot. Ostomy Wound Manage 2002;48(4):64–8.
45. Venturi ML, Attinger CE, Mesbahi AN, et al. Mechanisms and clinical applications of the vacuum-assisted closure (VAC) device: a review. Am J Clin Dermatol 2005;6(3):185–94.
46. Braakenburg A, Obdeijn MC, Feitz R, et al. The clinical efficacy and cost effectiveness of the vacuum-assisted closure technique in the management of acute and chronic wounds: a randomized controlled trial. Plast Reconstr Surg 2006;118(2):390–7 [discussion: 398–400].

Periorbital Rejuvenation
Reticular Vein Treatment

Nitin Chauhan, MD, FRCSC*,
David A.F. Ellis, MD, FRCSC, FACS

KEYWORDS

- Periorbital rejuvenation • Reticular veins • Laser • Periorbital veins

KEY POINTS

- The periorbital region is anatomically complex, and age-related changes often prompt patients and practitioners to find solutions to combat the visible signs of aging.
- Unsightly periorbital reticular veins, and those extending to the temples, represent a relatively frequent complaint of patients.
- Various treatments such as sclerotherapy and phlebectomy have been promoted with varying degrees of success, but also may have potential for undesirable complications.
- The authors' experience with laser-based treatment of these veins has been excellent; this article presents the treatment paradigm and explores patient outcomes.

BACKGROUND

The periorbital region plays an essential role in communication, emotional expression, health, and aging. Clearly defined goals of facial, specifically periorbital, aesthetics are the basis of successful results in therapeutic rejuvenation of the upper face. A common complaint of patients relates to the prominence or appearance of unsightly periorbital reticular veins, which may become increasingly prominent throughout life. A reticular vein is a dilated bluish intradermal vein, typically between 1 to 3 mm in diameter, and often tortuous in its course.

Age-related changes, including decreased skin thickness, subcutaneous fat depletion, soft-tissue and muscle atrophy, and venous dilatation all contribute to the increased prominence of veins in the periorbital region, leading many patients to seek intervention for this unsightly feature. Increasing use of neurotoxin injectables for periocular rejuvenation has led to heightened clinical awareness of these vessels, from a technical perspective to minimize bruising as well as from an aesthetic viewpoint when they are particularly prominent. In addition, clinicians have noted increasing prominence of veins in the lateral orbital or temporal region subsequent to therapeutic maneuvers that occlude vessels, such as ligation of the sentinel vein during endoscopic brow lifting.[1]

There exist numerous therapeutic options for the treatment of unwanted veins. In general terms, lasers for the treatment of facial telangiectasias and prominent veins have had good success. The authors have had excellent results using a 1064-nm Nd:YAG laser (Cutera, Brisbane, CA), with good clinical outcomes and an excellent level of patient comfort. In the past the treatment of smaller facial vessels (≤1 mm) was generally effective using laser technology. Effective treatment of larger facial reticular veins has remained somewhat elusive.

Sclerotherapy is a commonly suggested and performed treatment modality, with reasonable

Disclosures: (N.C.) Nothing to disclose. (D.A.F.E) Dr Ellis is a lecturer and trainer for Allergan and Cutera.
Department of Otolaryngology – Head and Neck Surgery, Division of Facial Plastic and Reconstructive Surgery, University of Toronto, 190 Elizabeth St., Rm 3S438, RFE Building, Toronto, Ontario M5G2N2, Canada
* Corresponding author.
E-mail address: dr.nitinchauhan@gmail.com

Facial Plast Surg Clin N Am 21 (2013) 147–155
http://dx.doi.org/10.1016/j.fsc.2012.11.006
1064-7406/13/$ – see front matter

results in expert hands. However, this procedure does confer some associated risk. Many facial plastic, oculoplastic, and dermatologic surgeons tend to avoid the use of this agent in the periorbital region, secondary to concern regarding diffusion of solution to unintended areas of venous circulation, with possible ophthalmologic and other complications.[2]

Ambulatory phlebectomy is another alternative; however, some view this option as less desirable on the face, for a variety of aesthetic and technical reasons.

Very little literature exists documenting the use of the 1064-nm Nd:YAG laser in the periorbital region, an area with no standardized treatment and an often fragmented therapeutic algorithm on the part of clinicians. The authors' treatment algorithm has yielded great success with the use of the Cutera long-pulsed, contact-cooled, variable spot-sized Nd:YAG laser.

METHODS

Twelve patients were voluntarily enrolled after informed consent was obtained.

Informed consent involved discussions regarding the unlikely possibility of discomfort during treatment, skin-pigmentation anomalies, possible burns, and the possibility for repeat treatments to achieve adequate elimination of the unsightly veins.

Treatment sites ranged from infraorbital vessels to lateral orbital and temple reticular veins, and in some cases extended to superior temporal forehead regions.

Treatment parameters varied according to the size of the veins being treated. Posttreatment cooling was used. The treatment goal was to achieve blanching of vessels without causing a skin burn. Patients required 1 to 2 passes during the treatment. To prevent excessive heat accumulation, the vessels were treated via multiple shots in nonadjacent order. The entire vessels were treated but without overlap. The periorbital treatments involve carefully aiming the laser beam away from the orbit. All patients were required to wear protective eyewear before treatment.

The laser used was the Cutera 1064-nm Nd:YAG. Precisely controlled variables used to achieve predictable and effective results included spot size, fluence, and pulse duration (**Table 1**).

Some patients developed an immediate posttreatment urticarial or erythematous response, which resolved in 1 to 2 hours. Each patient received one treatment and was examined 1 month after the treatment. Photographs were taken both pretreatment and posttreatment.

Table 1
Treatment parameters for the Cutera 1064-nm Nd:YAG, for treatment of periorbital and temple reticular veins

Spot size	5–7 mm (2–3 mm depth)
Fluence	100–120 J/cm^2
Pulse duration	20–25 ms

Results were judged by 2 experienced physicians both visually on patients and by comparison of pre- and posttreatment 35-mm color slides and photographs. Determination was made on follow-up visit as to whether another treatment session would be required to further improve the appearance of these veins to the patient's satisfaction.

RESULTS

The treatments were tolerated well by patients, with occasional pain being well managed using the direct-contact copper-plate cooling mechanism of the laser. The total treatment duration was typically less than 15 minutes per patient, although those patients with very extensive superficial veins requiring a large number of impulses often required slightly longer treatments.

The end point of treatment was determined by appropriate vessel response (gray coloration of the vessel, or visible vessel collapse). In addition, areas of skin that had an erythematous appearance after spot treatment were avoided to prevent thermal injury.

Twelve patients were initially enrolled in the study (**Table 2**). There were 10 female and 2 male patients. The average age was 42.3 years, with a large age range of 13 to 68 years.

Table 3 details the clinical and therapeutic characteristics of the treated patient population. Twelve patients were treated in total, with 6 having treatment of periorbital veins only, 2 having treatment of temple veins only, and 4 having treatment of both periorbital and temple veins.

The average age of the patients was 32.8 years for those undergoing eye-vein treatments, 58.0 years

Table 2
Patient demographics of periorbital vein treatment population

Gender	Male	2
	Female	10
Age (y)	Mean	42.3
	Range	13–68

Table 3
Clinical and therapeutic characteristics of periorbital vein treatment population

Patient	Age (y)	Orbital	Side	Temple	Side	Fluence (J/cm²)	Pulse Duration (ms)	No. of Treatments	Longevity
DW	49	×	L			120	20	2	12/12
SD	68	×	L+R	×	L+R	110	20	3	8/12
LR	42	×	L+R	×	L+R	110	20	1	12/12
RS	29	×	R			125	20	1	27/12
VG	52	×	L+R			120	25	2	12/12
LD	28	×	L+R	×	L+R	110–115	20–30	1	3/12
BP	36	×	L			120	25	1	2/12
HS	62			×	L+R	110–120	25	2	6/12
MS	54			×	L+R	110	30	1	2/12
BM	18	×	R			110	20	1	12/12
JM	13	×	L+R			110	20	1	1/12
SH	56	×	L+R	×	L+R	110–125	25	2	1/12

for those undergoing temple-vein treatments only, and 48.5 years for the remaining patients undergoing treatment of both regions.

Complications discussed with patients before treatment included pain, bruising, burning, skin irritation, pruritus, and swelling.

The only complication reported by patients was a short course (<48 hours) of irritation and slight swelling. No patient complained of significant posttreatment discomfort, bruising, or persistent erythema, and no catastrophic complications such as blindness occurred.

Fig. 1 demonstrates a pretreatment and immediate posttreatment view of a patient undergoing laser treatment of veins in the left temporal region. Immediate vessel collapse, regional erythema, and vessel collapse can all be ascertained in the posttreatment photograph.

Fig. 2 shows pre- and posttreatment images of infraorbital vein treatments. Each patient required only one treatment session to achieve satisfactory correction. The patient shown in **Fig. 3** was concerned about the appearance of left-sided infraorbital and temple veins. Initially the infraorbital veins were treated in a single session with good resolution (see **Fig. 3**B), and a subsequent session was used to treat her temple veins, again with excellent results (see **Fig. 3**C). **Fig. 4** depicts another patient with extensive prominent veins in her right and left temporal regions, with significant, though not complete resolution bilaterally after one treatment to either side.

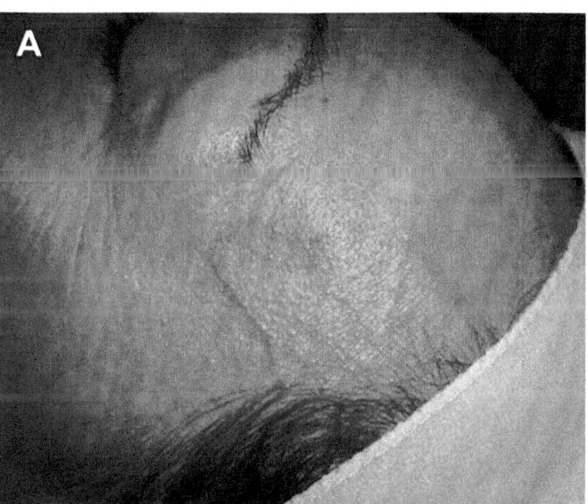

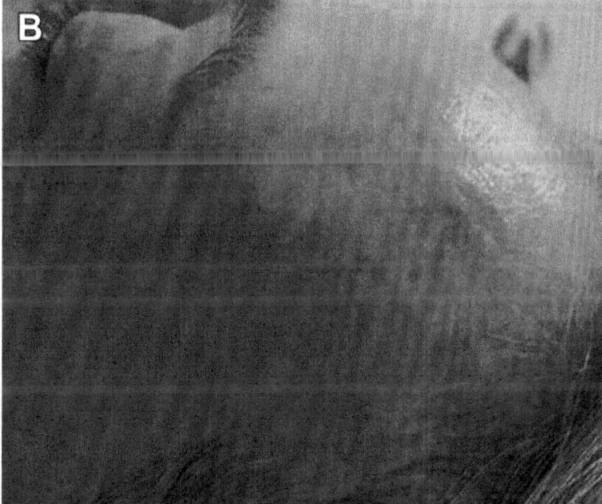

Fig. 1. Pretreatment (*A*) and immediate posttreatment (*B*) images depicting laser treatment of left temporal vein.

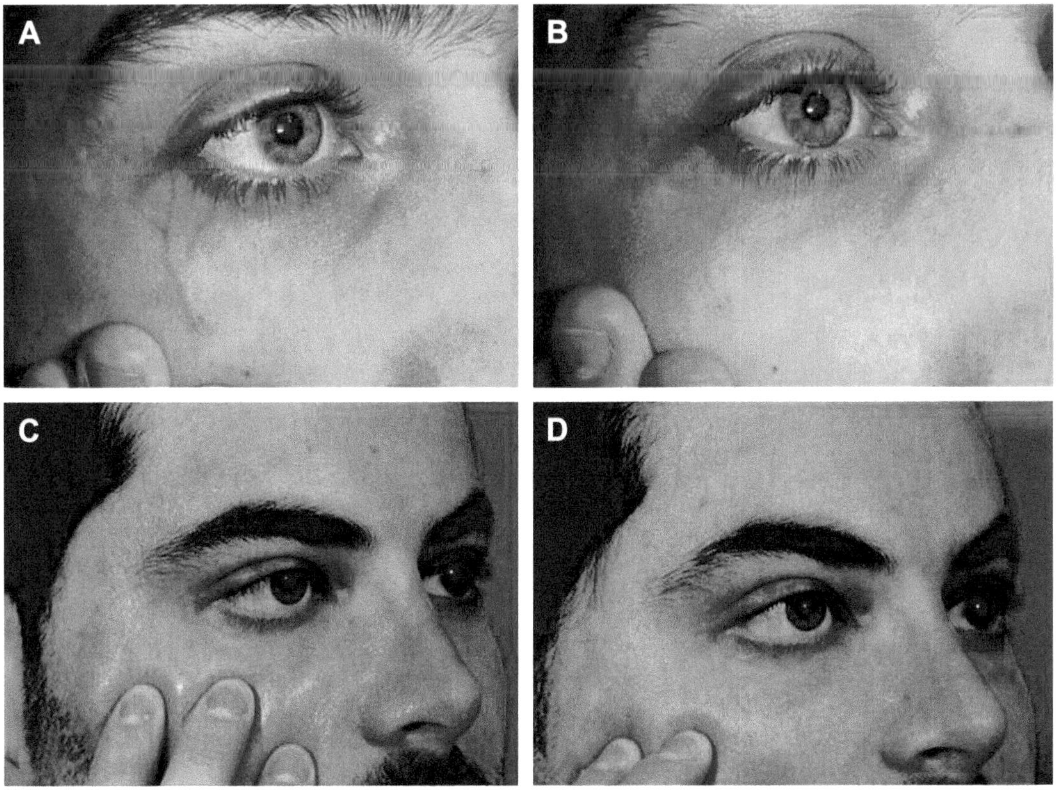

Fig. 2. (*A, B*) Patient 1. Pretreatment appearance (*A*) and posttreatment resolution of right periorbital vein (*B*). (*C, D*) Patient 2. Pretreatment appearance (*C*) and posttreatment resolution of right infraorbital vein (*D*).

DISCUSSION

Anatomic Discussion of Periorbital Region

A thorough understanding of the venous drainage and anatomic variation of the periorbital region is paramount for the clinician treating the vasculature in this area.

The superficial temporal vein originates on the side and vertex of the skull, in a plexus that communicates with the frontal vein and supraorbital vein, with the contralateral superficial temporal vein, and the posterior auricular and occipital vein. Owing to this rich anastomotic network, as well as a certain degree of normal variability in drainage patterns, it is important to consider these anatomic relationships when performing therapeutic maneuvers targeted at diminishing the appearance of prominent veins in the

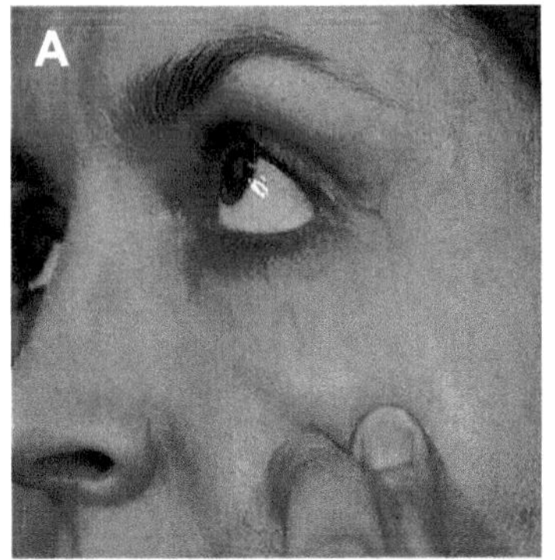
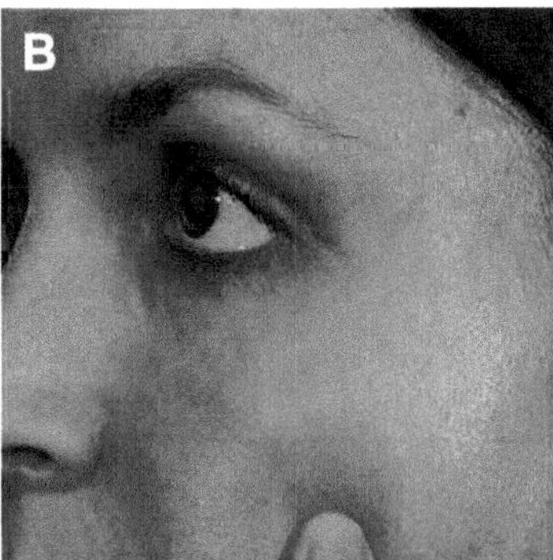
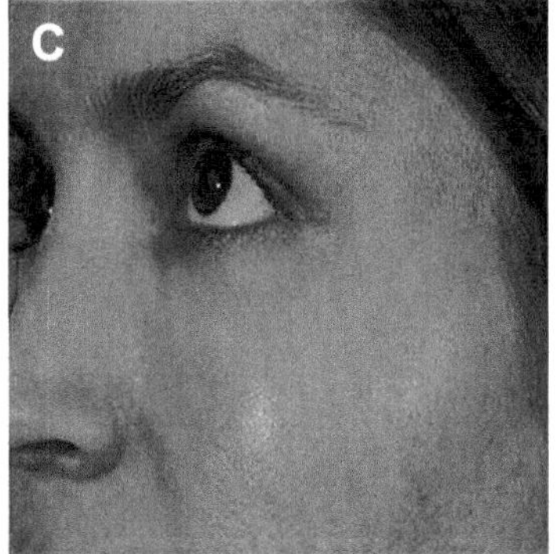

Fig. 3. A patient with left infraorbital and temple veins. Pretreatment (*A*), resolution of infraorbital veins after single treatment (*B*), and resolution of temple veins after single treatment to the area (*C*).

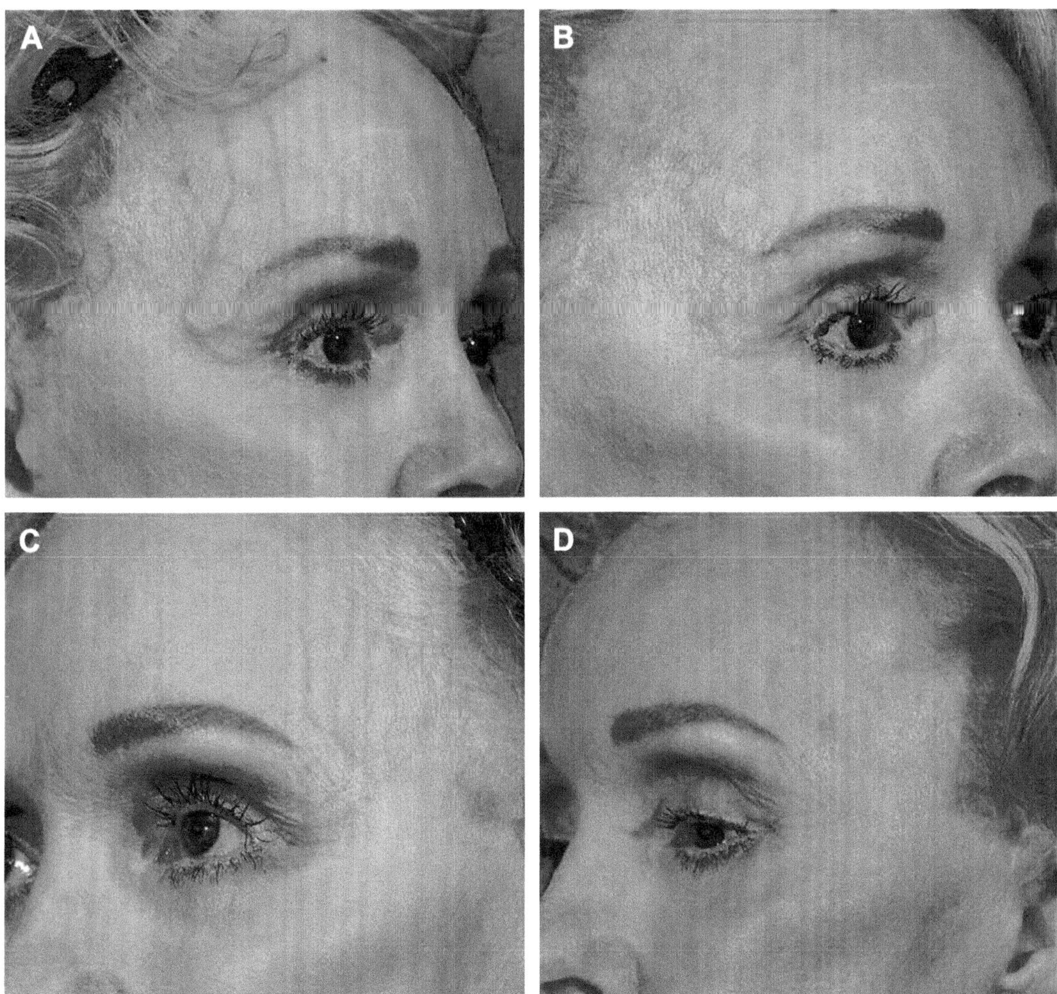

Fig. 4. This patient had extensive prominent veins in her right (*A*) and left (*B*) periorbital and temporal regions. One month posttreatment, her right (*C*) and left (*D*) temporal regions show significant improvement.

region. Frontal and parietal branches arise from this plexus, uniting above the zygomatic arch to form the trunk of the vein, which is joined by the middle temporal vein emerging from the temporalis muscle. This vein drains the temple as well as lateral scalp regions (**Fig. 5**).

The frontal vein (supratrochlear vein) also arises from the aforementioned venous plexus, which communicates with the frontal branches of the superficial temporal vein. These veins typically converge to form a single trunk, running in an inferior direction parasagittally, parallel with the frontal vein on the opposite side. Typically these 2 veins are joined at the nasal root by a transverse branch, called the nasal arch, receiving some small veins from the dorsum of the nose. These veins diverge at the root of the nose, and each joins its ipsilateral supraorbital vein at the medial orbit to form the angular vein (**Fig. 6**).

The supraorbital vein begins on the forehead where it communicates with the frontal branch of the superficial temporal vein. Its level of depth is superficial to the frontalis muscle, and it joins the frontal vein to form the angular vein, at the medial angle of the orbit. This vein is important as well, as it sends through the supraorbital notch into the orbit a branch that communicates with the ophthalmic vein (**Fig. 7**). The anatomic regions drained by the supraorbital vein include the forehead, eyebrow, and upper eyelid.

The central retinal vein runs through the optic nerve, draining blood from the capillaries of the retina into the larger veins outside the eye. Normal anatomic variations do exist; in some individuals the vein drains into the superior ophthalmic vein, whereas in others it drains directly into the cavernous sinus. Central retinal vein occlusion is one of the major causes of severe vision

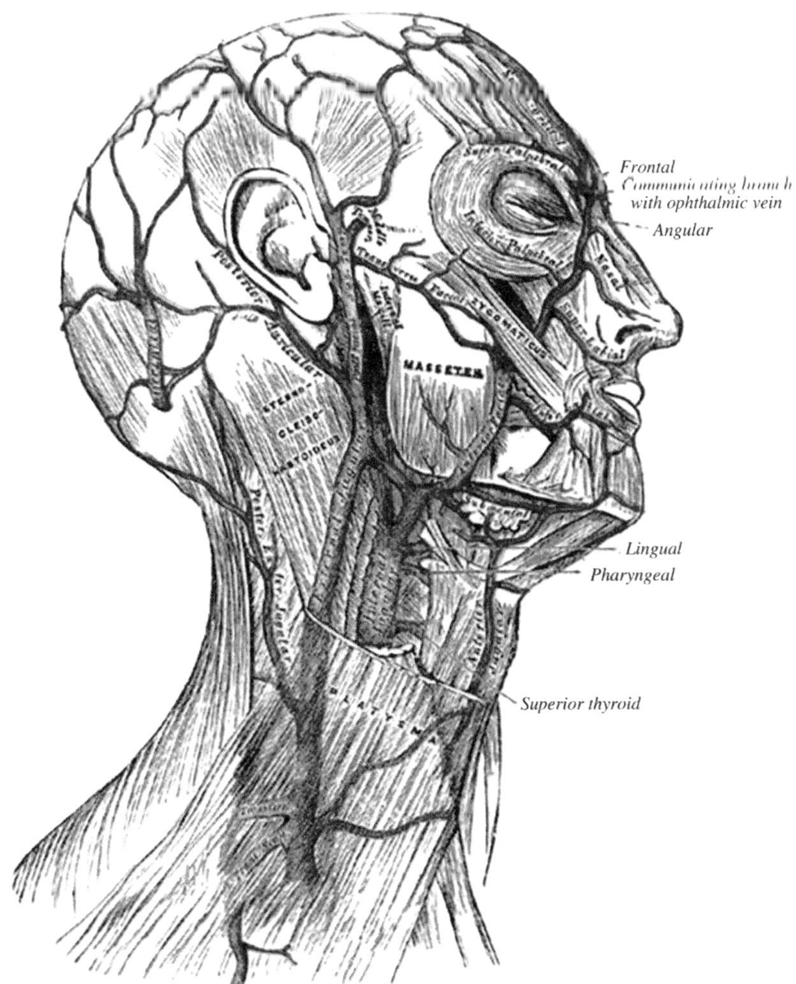

Fig. 5. Scalp, face, and neck venous drainage pathways. (*From* Gray H. Anatomy of the Human Body. Philadelphia: Lea & Febiger, 1918.)

impairment and blindness.[3] Thrombosis of the central retinal vein results in venous stasis, leading to disc swelling, diffuse nerve-fiber layer, and preretinal hemorrhage (**Fig. 8**).[4]

Clinical Implications

Lasers in general have been proved to be a safe therapeutic modality with which to treat vascular lesions, including benign, unsightly periorbital reticular veins. There have been problems in the past using continuous-wave argon lasers, and early pulsed-dye lasers in the 585- to 600-nm range were mostly limited to port-wine stains because of issues with posttreatment purpura.[5] In the 1990s there was substantial progress and a variety of laser systems, including the 532-nm diode, KTP, double-frequency Nd:YAG, and newer pulsed-dye lasers, were used successfully for treating small facial vessels, but often had disappointing results for the treatment of larger vessels.[6]

Sclerotherapy is a commonly suggested and performed treatment modality, with reasonable results in expert hands. However, this procedure does confer some associated risk. Many facial plastic, oculoplastic, and dermatologic surgeons tend to avoid the use of this agent in the periorbital region, secondary to concern regarding diffusion of solution to unintended areas of venous circulation, with possible complications.[2] Some investigators have cited the safety and efficacy of sodium tetradecyl sulfate (STS) sclerotherapy for periocular vessels of 1- to 2-mm diameter, citing an excellent response rate and low side-effect profile.[7] Caution must be exercised, as it is possible that intravenous periorbital injection could reach the orbit within close proximity of the central retinal

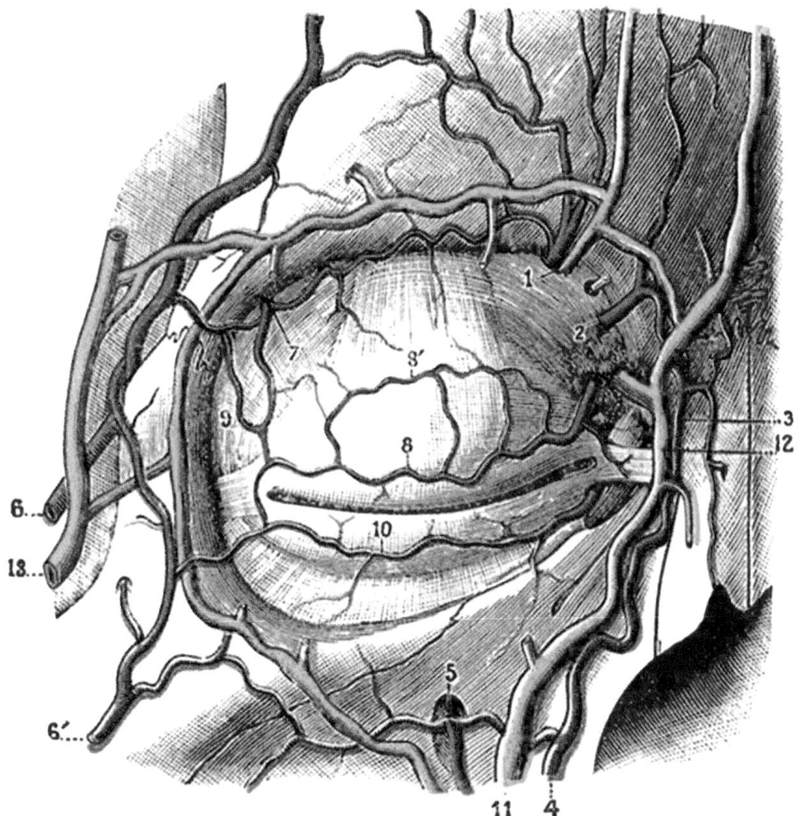

Fig. 6. Right periorbital venous drainage pathways, front view. 1, supraorbital artery and vein; 2, nasal artery; 3, angular artery, the terminal branch of 4, the facial artery; 5, suborbital artery; 6, anterior branch of the superficial temporal artery; 6′, malar branch of the transverse artery of the face; 7, lacrimal artery; 8, superior palpebral artery with 8′, its external arch; 9, anastomoses of the superior palpebral with the superficial temporal and lacrimal; 10, inferior palpebral artery; 11, facial vein; 12, angular vein; 13, branch of the superficial temporal vein. (*From* Gray H. Anatomy of the Human Body. Philadelphia: Lea & Febiger, 1918.)

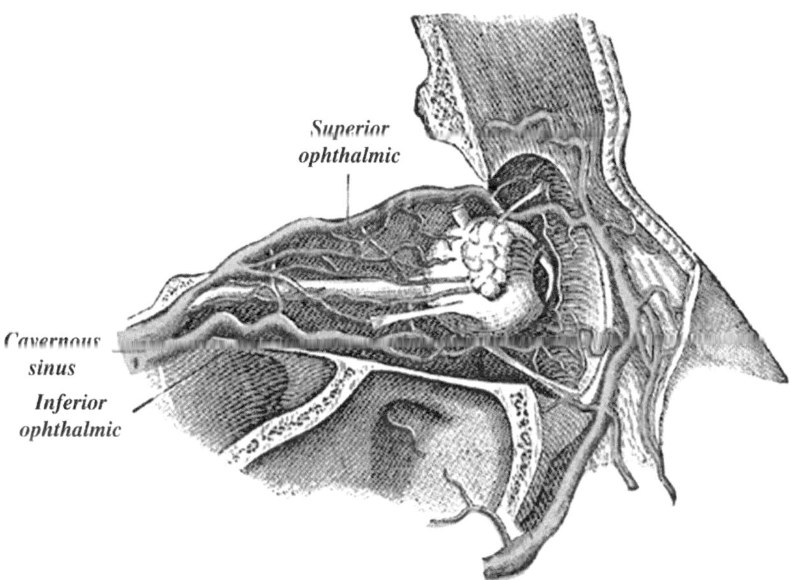

Fig. 7. Parasagittal depiction of venous drainage through the orbit. Connections may exist between both the supraorbital vein and angular vein, with the ophthalmic vein, and ultimately the cavernous sinus. (*From* Gray H. Anatomy of the Human Body. Philadelphia: Lea & Febiger, 1918.)

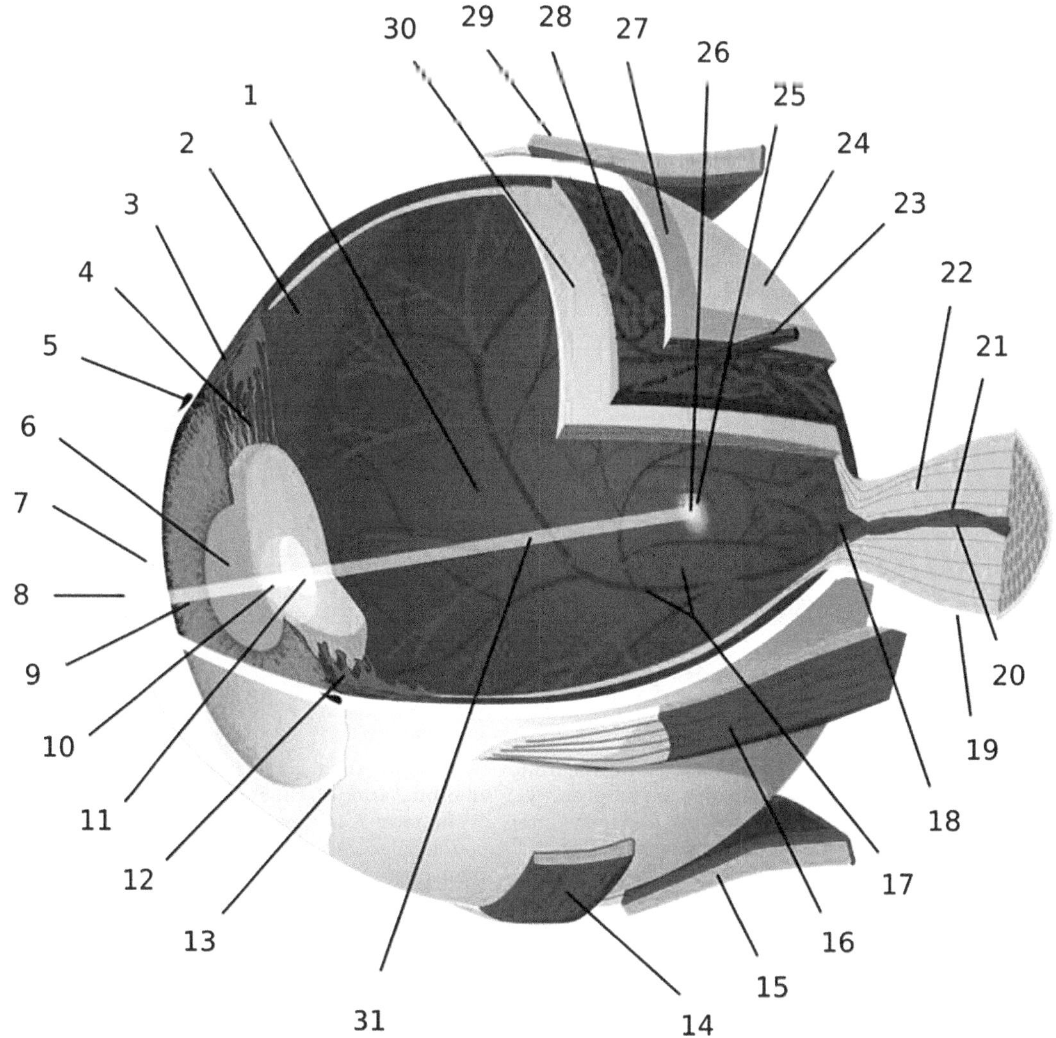

Fig. 8. Diagram of the eye, and associated important ocular structures. 1, posterior chamber; 2, ora serrata; 3, ciliary muscle; 4, ciliary zonules; 5, canal of Schlemm; 6, pupil; 7, anterior chamber; 8, cornea; 9, iris; 10, lens cortex; 11, lens nucleus; 12, ciliary process; 13, conjunctiva; 14, inferior oblique muscle; 15, inferior rectus muscle; 16, medial rectus muscle; 17, retinal arteries and veins; 18, optic disc; 19, dura mater; 20, central retinal artery; 21, central retinal vein; 22, optical nerve; 23, vorticose vein; 24, bulbar sheath; 25, macula; 26, fovea; 27, sclera; 28, choroid; 29, superior rectus muscle; 30, retina.

vein, the choroidal vortex veins, or even the cavernous sinus via valveless anastomoses.[8] Blindness has been reported following STS injection into a venous malformation partially located within the orbit.[9]

Ambulatory phlebectomy is another alternative; however, this option is less desirable on the face, for a variety of aesthetic and technical reasons. Some investigators propose this as the favorable alternative to sclerotherapy; however, it does require a fair amount of technical expertise and there are definite equipment requirements as well.[10] In addition, this technique requires several serial puncture sites of the targeted length of the vein, and is associated with the risk of hematoma and ecchymoses formation, possible requirement of repeat procedures in cases of difficult dissection, and possible scarring of the puncture sites.

This area of treatment represents a fascinating adjunct to the practice of facial plastic surgery. Many patients present with issues regarding the appearance of these periorbital veins, and the treatments proposed often vary dramatically in their success rates, complication profiles, and therapeutic efficacy. Thorough analysis of the literature highlights the diverging opinions of clinicians regarding ideal treatments, and very few data exist documenting the use of the 1064-nm Nd:YAG laser in the periorbital region. The authors' treatment algorithm has yielded great success with the use of the Cutera long-pulsed, contact-cooled, variable sport-sized Nd:YAG laser. The patient population typically experienced dramatic resolution in vessel prominence after only one treatment session, although they were counseled regarding the possibility of repeat treatments. Discomfort during the procedure was minimal and the side-effect profile negligible, rendering this technique an ideal approach to managing such patients. Furthermore, the evolution in therapeutic options arising from emerging technologies represents the critical interplay between scientific progress and clinical efficacy.

REFERENCES

1. Winslow CP, Burke A, Bartels S, et al. Bipolar scissors in facial plastic surgery. Arch Facial Plast Surg 2000;2(3):209–12.
2. Fante RG, Goldman MP. Removal of periocular veins by sclerotherapy. Ophthalmology 2001;108:433–4.
3. The Central Vein Occlusion Study Group. Natural history and clinical management of central retinal vein occlusion. Arch Ophthalmol 1997;115:486–91.
4. Alasil T, Lee N, Keane P, et al. Central retinal vein occlusion: a case report and review of the literature. Cases J 2009;2:7170.
5. Dixon JA, Huether S, Rotering R. Hypertrophic scarring in argon laser treatment of port-sine stains. Plast Reconstr Surg 1984;73:771–80.
6. Landthaler M, Hohenleutner U, El Raheem TA. Therapy of vascular lesions in the head and neck area by means of argon, Nd:YAG, CO_2 and flashlamp-pumped pulsed dye laser. Adv Otorhinolaryngol 1995;49:81–6.
7. Green D. Removal of periocular veins by sclerotherapy. Ophthalmology 2001;108:442–8.
8. Hadjikoutis S, Carroll C, Plant GT. Raised intracranial pressure presenting with spontaneous periorbital bruising: two case reports. J Neurol Neurosurg Psychiatry 2004;75(8):1192–3.
9. Siniluoto IM, Svendsen PA, Wilkholm GM, et al. Percutaneous sclerotherapy of venous malformations of the head and neck using sodium tetradecyl sulphate sotradecol. Scand J Plast Reconstr Surg Hand Surg 1997;31:145–50.
10. Weiss RA, Ramelet AA. Removal of blue periocular lower eyelid veins by ambulatory phlebectomy. Dermatol Surg 2002;28(1):43–5.

Index

Note: Page numbers of article titles are in **boldface** type.

Facial Plast Surg Clin N Am 21 (2013) 157–170
http://dx.doi.org/10.1016/S1064-7406(13)00011-4
1064-7406/13/$ – see front matter

C

D

G

H

M

O

P

Q

T

U

V

W

Printed and bound by CPI Group (UK) Ltd, Croydon, CR0 4YY

03/10/2024

01040347-0015

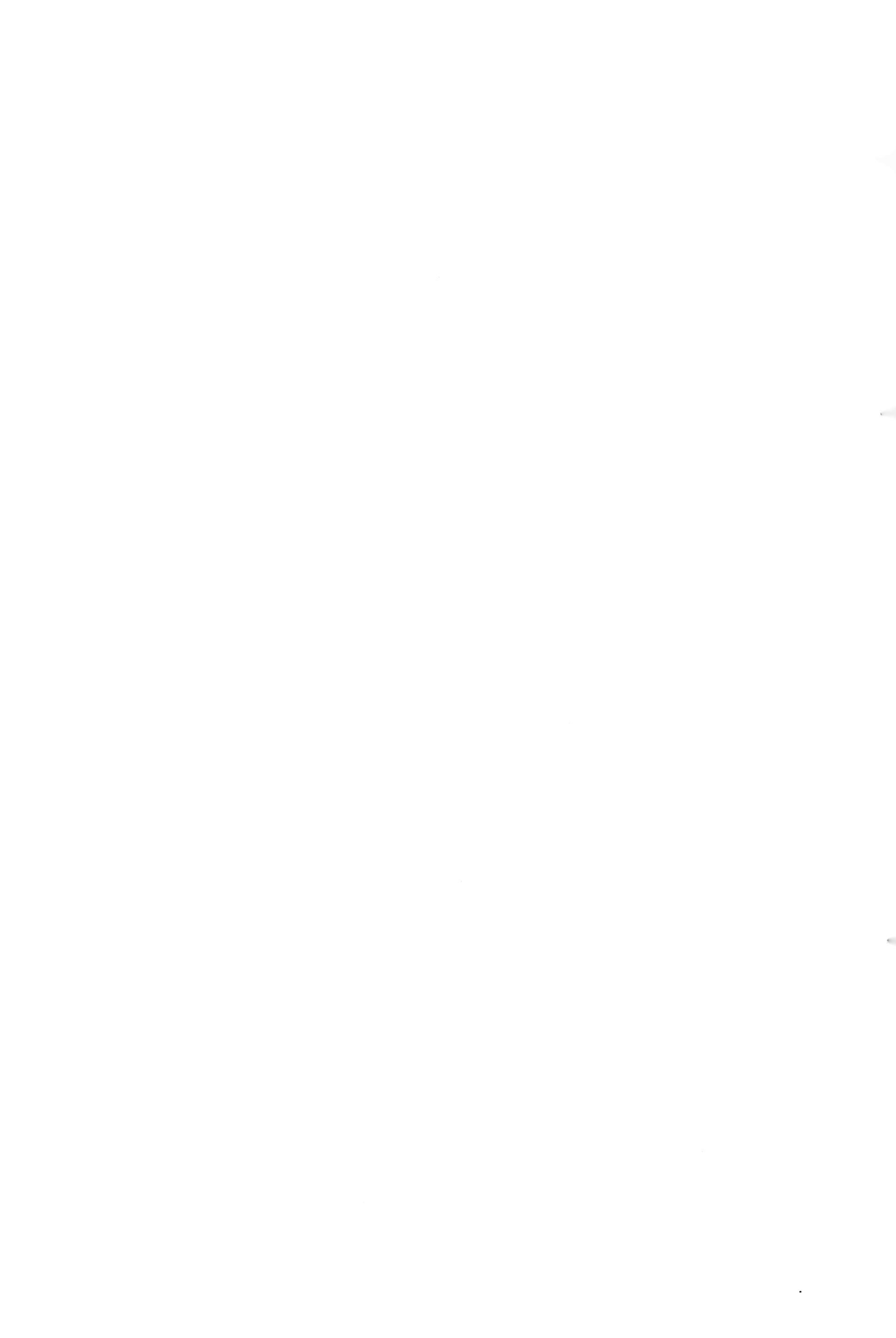